Biomaterials in plastic surgery

Related titles:

Coatings for biomedical applications
(ISBN 978-1-84569-568-2)
The biomaterials sector is rapidly expanding due to the increase in healthcare spending worldwide. Coatings and surface modification of biomaterials provides a means to improve the wear of joints, change the biological interaction between implant and host and combine the properties of various materials to improve device performance. The considerable interest in coatings for biomedical applications has resulted in a great deal of research in industry and academia. This book provides a comprehensive review of coatings and surface modification for biomedical applications, including background, theory, materials and applications.

Durability and reliability of medical polymers
(ISBN 978-1-84569-929-1)
Given the rapid development and use of polymers within medicine, the durability and reliability of polymer biomaterials and devices is an area of critical importance to the biomedical industry. This book reviews types of polymer biomaterials before going on to discuss examples of failure. Other chapters discuss degradation mechanisms, wear and ageing processes that affect the use and reliability of medical polymers.

Biocompatibility and performance of medical devices
(ISBN 978-0-85709-070-6)
Implant and device manufacturers are increasingly being faced with the challenge of proving that their implants or devices are safe/biocompatible and perform as expected. This book will describe and explain the factors that influence the biocompatibility of materials and medical devices, the methods to predict or screen biocompatibility, how to build a biological safety evaluation plan for medical devices, strategies and tactics in biocompatibility and biological performance evaluation of medical devices. It will also provide insights on recent changes in regulations and standards, standards interpretation and worldwide health authorities' expectations with regard to the biocompatibility and performance of new products.

Details of these books and a complete list of titles from Woodhead Publishing can be obtained by:

- visiting our web site at www.woodheadpublishing.com
- contacting Customer Services (e-mail: sales@woodheadpublishing.com; fax: +44 (0) 1223 832819; tel.: +44 (0) 1223 499140 ext. 130; address: Woodhead Publishing Limited, 80, High Street, Sawston, Cambridge CB22 3HJ, UK)
- in North America, contacting our US office (e-mail: usmarketing@woodheadpublishing.com; tel.: (215) 928 9112; address: Woodhead Publishing, 1518 Walnut Street, Suite 1100, Philadelphia, PA 19102-3406, USA

If you would like e-versions of our content, please visit our online platform: www.woodheadpublishingonline.com. Please recommend it to your librarian so that everyone in your institution can benefit from the wealth of content on the site.

Woodhead Publishing Series in Biomaterials: Number 42

Biomaterials in plastic surgery

Breast implants

Edited by
W. Peters, H. Brandon, K. L. Jerina, C. Wolf
and V. L. Young

WP
WOODHEAD
PUBLISHING

Oxford Cambridge Philadelphia New Delhi

Published by Woodhead Publishing Limited,
80 High Street, Sawston, Cambridge CB22 3HJ, UK
www.woodheadpublishing.com
www.woodheadpublishingonline.com

Woodhead Publishing, 1518 Walnut Street, Suite 1100, Philadelphia, PA 19102-3406, USA

Woodhead Publishing India Private Limited, G-2, Vardaan House, 7/28 Ansari Road, Daryaganj, New Delhi – 110002, India
www.woodheadpublishingindia.com

First published 2012, Woodhead Publishing Limited

British Library Cataloguing in Publication Data
A catalogue record for this book is available from the British Library.

Library of Congress Control Number: 2012938390

ISBN 978-1-84569-799-0 (print)
ISBN 978-0-85709-641-8 (online)
ISSN 2049-9485 Woodhead Publishing Series in Biomaterials (print)
ISSN 2049-9493 Woodhead Publishing Series in Biomaterials (online)

The publisher's policy is to use permanent paper from mills that operate a sustainable forestry policy, and which has been manufactured from pulp which is processed using acid-free and elemental chlorine-free practices. Furthermore, the publisher ensures that the text paper and cover board used have met acceptable environmental accreditation standards.

Typeset by Toppan Best-set Premedia Limited

Contents

Contributor contact details *ix*
Woodhead Publishing Series in Biomaterials *xi*
Introduction *xv*

1 The history of biomaterials used for breast augmentation 1
W. PETERS, University of Toronto, Canada

1.1 Introduction 1
1.2 Injectable materials 1
1.3 Sponges 10
1.4 Breast implants 16
1.5 Other forms of texturing 23
1.6 Inflatable implants 27
1.7 Trilucent (*LipoMatrix*) implants – 1995 to 2000 33
1.8 Acknowledgements 35
1.9 References 35

2 The development of breast implants 40
G. P. MAXWELL and A. GABRIEL, Loma Linda University Medical Center, USA

2.1 Introduction 40
2.2 Breast implant evolution 41
2.3 Alternative types of implant and safety aspects 44
2.4 Future trends 47
2.5 References 48

3 The chemistry and physical properties of biomedical silicones 52
M. A. BROOK, McMaster University, Canada

3.1 Introduction 52
3.2 Properties of silicones 56

3.3 The main forms of silicones/siloxanes 58
3.4 Silicones in breast implants 62
3.5 References 66

4 Cohesive gel breast implants 68
P. Hedén, Akademikliniken, Sweden

4.1 Introduction 68
4.2 Available form stable breast implants 70
4.3 Selection of the appropriate form stable breast implant 77
4.4 Preoperative planning 84
4.5 Incisions and surgical technique 86
4.6 Problems and complications 93
4.7 References 95

5 Polyurethane foam covered breast implants 96
D. Fleming, The Cosmetic Surgery Institute of Australia, Australia

5.1 Introduction 96
5.2 Capsular contracture and the role of polyurethane foam in its prevention 98
5.3 Comparison of polyurethane foam covered implants with smooth and textured surfaced implants 105
5.4 Safety when using polyurethane foam breast implants 110
5.5 Use in secondary procedures 112
5.6 Disadvantages of polyurethane foam breast implants 114
5.7 Conclusions 116
5.8 References 118

6 The safety of breast implants: epidemiologic studies 121
L. Lipworth and J. K. McLaughlin, International Epidemiology Institute, USA and Vanderbilt University Medical Center, USA

6.1 Introduction 121
6.2 Connective tissue disease 122
6.3 Offspring effects 127
6.4 Neurological disease 129
6.5 Implant rupture 129
6.6 Local complications 134
6.7 Incidence of cancer 136
6.8 Occurrence of suicide 141
6.9 Conclusion 143

6.10 Acknowledgments 144
6.11 References 144

7 Retrieval and analysis of breast implants emphasizing strength, durability, and failure mechanisms 154
H. J. Brandon, K. L. Jerina and C. J. Wolf, Washington University, USA and V. L. Young, BodyAesthetic Plastic Surgery and Skin Care Center, USA

7.1 Introduction 154
7.2 Silicone gel explants with longest implantation times 155
7.3 Shell properties of silicone gel implants as a function of implantation time 160
7.4 Lot-matched control study 175
7.5 Effect of implantation time on shell properties of saline implants 179
7.6 Breast implant rupture 186
7.7 Rupture rates and reoperation rates 210
7.8 References 214

Index *219*

Contributor contact details

(* = main contact)

Editors

Professor Walter Peters*
Division of Plastic Surgery
University of Toronto, Canada
Suite 802, 600 Sherbourne Street
Toronto
Ontario M4X 1W4
Canada

Email: walter.peters@utoronto.ca

Professor Harold J. Brandon and Professor Kenneth L. Jerina
Department of Mechanical Engineering and Materials Science
Washington University
Jolley Hall, Room 305
Campus Box 1185
One Brookings Drive
St Louis
MO 63130
USA

Email: hjb@wustl.edu; jerinak@seas.wustl.edu

Clarence J. Wolf (retired)
Department of Chemical Engineering
Washington University
Seattle
USA

Email: seawolf1931@aol.com

Leroy Young
Director of BodyAesthetic Research Center
969 Mason Road Ste. 170
Saint Louis
MO 63141
USA

Email: leroyyoungmd@bodyaesthetic.com

Introduction and Chapter 1

Professor Walter Peters
Division of Plastic Surgery
University of Toronto, Canada
Suite 802, 600 Sherbourne Street
Toronto
Ontario M4X 1W4
Canada

Email: walter.peters@utoronto.ca

Chapter 2

Dr G. Patrick Maxwell and Dr Allen Gabriel*
Department of Plastic Surgery
Loma Linda University Medical Center
Loma Linda
CA 92354
USA

Email: gabrielallen@yahoo.com

Chapter 3

Professor Michael A. Brook
Chemistry and Chemical Biology
McMaster University
1280 Main St. W.
Hamilton
Ontario L8S 4M1
Canada

Email: mabrook@mcmaster.ca

Chapter 4

Per Hedén
Associate Professor in Plastic Surgery
Akademikliniken
Storängsvägen 10
115 42 Stockholm
Stockholm
Sweden

Email: per.heden@ak.se

Chapter 5

Daniel Fleming
The Cosmetic Surgery Institute of Australia
PO Box 213
Fortitude Valley
Queensland 4006
Australia

Email: daniel@breastimplantsaustralia.com

Chapter 6

Dr Loren Lipworth* and Dr Joseph K. McLaughlin
International Epidemiology Institute
1455 Research Boulevard
Suite 550
Rockville
MD 20850
USA

Email: loren@iei.ws

Chapter 7

Professor Harold J. Brandon* and Professor Kenneth L. Jerina
Department of Mechanical Engineering and Materials Science
Washington University
Jolley Hall, Room 305
Campus Box 1185
One Brookings Drive
St Louis
MO 63130
USA

Email: hjb@wustl.edu; jerinak@seas.wustl.edu

Clarence J. Wolf (retired)
Department of Chemical Engineering
Washington University
St Louis
Seattle
USA

Email: seawolf1931@aol.com

Leroy Young
Director of BodyAesthetic Research Center
969 Mason Road Ste. 170
St Louis
MO 6314
USA

Email: leroyyoungmd@bodyaesthetic.com

Woodhead Publishing Series in Biomaterials

1 **Sterilisation of tissues using ionising radiations**
Edited by J. F. Kennedy, G. O. Phillips and P. A. Williams

2 **Surfaces and interfaces for biomaterials**
Edited by P. Vadgama

3 **Molecular interfacial phenomena of polymers and biopolymers**
Edited by C. Chen

4 **Biomaterials, artificial organs and tissue engineering**
Edited by L. Hench and J. Jones

5 **Medical modelling**
R. Bibb

6 **Artificial cells, cell engineering and therapy**
Edited by S. Prakash

7 **Biomedical polymers**
Edited by M. Jenkins

8 **Tissue engineering using ceramics and polymers**
Edited by A. R. Boccaccini and J. Gough

9 **Bioceramics and their clinical applications**
Edited by T. Kokubo

10 **Dental biomaterials**
Edited by R. V. Curtis and T. F. Watson

11 **Joint replacement technology**
Edited by P. A. Revell

12 **Natural-based polymers for biomedical applications**
Edited by R. L. Reiss et al

13 **Degradation rate of bioresorbable materials**
Edited by F. J. Buchanan

14 **Orthopaedic bone cements**
Edited by S. Deb

15 **Shape memory alloys for biomedical applications**
Edited by T. Yoneyama and S. Miyazaki

16 **Cellular response to biomaterials**
Edited by L. Di Silvio

17 **Biomaterials for treating skin loss**
Edited by D. P. Orgill and C. Blanco

18 **Biomaterials and tissue engineering in urology**
Edited by J. Denstedt and A. Atala

19 **Materials science for dentistry**
B. W. Darvell

20 **Bone repair biomaterials**
Edited by J. A. Planell et al

21 **Biomedical composites**
Edited by L. Ambrosio

22 **Drug-device combination products**
Edited by A. Lewis

23 **Biomaterials and regenerative medicine in ophthalmology**
Edited by T. V. Chirila

24 **Regenerative medicine and biomaterials for the repair of connective tissues**
Edited by C. Archer and J. Ralphs

25 **Metals for biomedical devices**
Edited by M. Ninomi

26 **Biointegration of medical implant materials: science and design**
Edited by C. P. Sharma

27 **Biomaterials and devices for the circulatory system**
Edited by T. Gourlay and R. Black

28 **Surface modification of biomaterials: methods analysis and applications**
Edited by R. Williams

29 **Biomaterials for artificial organs**
Edited by M. Lysaght and T. Webster

30 **Injectable biomaterials: science and applications**
Edited by B. Vernon

31 **Biomedical hydrogels: biochemistry, manufacture and medical applications**
Edited by S. Rimmer

32 **Preprosthetic and maxillofacial surgery: biomaterials, bone grafting and tissue engineering**
Edited by J. Ferri and E. Hunziker

33 **Bioactive materials in medicine: design and applications**
Edited by X. Zhao, J. M. Courtney and H. Qian

34 **Advanced wound repair therapies**
Edited by D. Farrar

35 **Electrospinning for tissue regeneration**
Edited by L. Bosworth and S. Downes

36 **Bioactive glasses: materials, properties and applications**
Edited by H. O. Ylänen

37 **Coatings for biomedical applications**
Edited by M. Driver

38 **Progenitor and stem cell technologies and therapies**
Edited by A. Atala

39 **Biomaterials for spinal surgery**
Edited by L. Ambrosio and E. Tanner

40 **Minimized cardiopulmonary bypass techniques and technologies**
Edited by T. Gourlay and S. Gunaydin

41 **Wear of orthopaedic implants and artificial joints**
Edited by S. Affatato

42 **Biomaterials in plastic surgery: breast implants**
Edited by W. Peters, H. Brandon, K. L. Jerina, C. Wolf and V. L. Young

43 **MEMS for biomedical applications**
Edited by S. Bhansali and A. Vasudev

44 **Durability and reliability of medical polymers**
Edited by M. Jenkins and A. Stamboulis

45 **Biosensors for medical applications**
Edited by S. Higson

46 **Sterilisation of biomaterials**
Edited by S. Lerouge and A. Simmons

47 **The hip resurfacing handbook: a practical guide to the use and management of modern hip resurfacings**
Edited by K. De Smet, P. Campbell and C. Van Der Straeten

48 **Developments in tissue engineered and regenerative medicine products**
J. Basu and John W. Ludlow

49 **Nanomedicine: technologies and applications**
Edited by M. Webster

50 **Biocompatibility and performance of medical devices**
Edited by J.-P. Boutrand

51 **Medical robotics**
Edited by P. Gomes

52 **Implantable sensor systems for medical applications**
Edited by A. Inmann and D. Hodgins

53 **Non-metallic biomaterials for tooth repair and replacement**
Edited by Pekka Vallittu

54 **Joining and assembly of medical materials and devices**
Edited by Y. Norman Zhou and M..D. Breyen

55 **Diamond based materials for biomedical applications**
Edited by Roger Narayan

56 **Nanomaterials in tissue engineering: characherization, fabrication and applications**
Edited by A. K. Gaharwar, S. Sant, M. J. Hancock and S. A. Hacking

57 **Biomimetic biomaterials: structure and applications**
Edited by Andrew Ruys

58 **Standardisation in cell and tissue engineering: methods and protocols**
Edited by Vehid Salih

59 **Inhaler devices: fundamentals, design and drug delivery**
Edited by Polina Prokopovich

60 **Bio-tribocorrosion in biomaterials and medical implants**
Edited by Yu Yan

61 **Microfluidics for biomedical applications**
Edited by XiuJun James Li and Yu Zhou

62 **Decontamination in hospitals and healthcare**
Edited by J. T. Walker

63 **Biomedical imaging: applications and advances**
Edited by Peter Morris

Introduction

W. PETERS, University of Toronto, Canada

This book reviews the history of breast augmentation surgery from injection materials used in the early 1900s up to the current state-of-the-art silicone gel breast implants. The various types of implants are described along with their advantages, disadvantages, and potential outcomes. Recent epidemiological studies are very thoroughly reviewed to underline the safety of silicone gel implants. Breast augmentation surgery is once again one of the most popular types of aesthetic plastic surgery performed in many countries in the world. This book helps to explain the reasons for the current popularity of this operation.

The history of breast augmentation occupies the past 110 years. Fewer surgical procedures have a history as fascinating as breast augmentation. In the early 1900s, initial efforts at augmentation involved injection of substances such as paraffin or oil into the breast tissue. From 1915 to the 1920s, materials such as ivory, glass balls, rubber, or glazier's putty were implanted into breasts. In fact, this list of materials was limited only by man's imagination. During the mid-1940s, liquid silicone was used, initially in Japan. Over time, the horrendous complications of paraffin injections would be repeated again with silicone injections. In some patients, the complications were even worse, because the material used was industrial grade silicone, and contaminants were often injected to restrict silicone migration. In the early 1950s, a number of different types of preformed implants were introduced. All of them were ultimately associated with serious complications and usually poor results.

In 1963, the introduction of silicone gel breast implants revolutionized the field of breast augmentation. Over the next 30 years, over two million women received these implants worldwide. There were three main generations of silicone gel implants, and a number of lesser variations. Over ten companies manufactured silicone gel implants in the United States. Many changed their names and ownership over the years. Others entered and left the market at intervals. The implant business was competitive. In the search of better aesthetics, companies introduced numerous changes, usually without much actual testing. Ultimately, more than 240 styles and 8300 models of silicone gel breast implants were manufactured in the United States alone.

On January 6, 1992, Dr David Kessler, the then Commissioner of the United States Food and Drug Administration (FDA), announced a moratorium on the use of silicone gel filled breast implants. This moratorium was also adopted in Canada and in many other countries. This ban was introduced not because these implants had been found to be dangerous, but because they 'had not been proven to be safe'! Dr Kessler heightened patients' fears by announcing at a press conference that 'we know more about the tires on our cars than we know about these breast implants!'

Silicone gel breast implants had been used for 30 years, but now, Kessler decided that it was the responsibility of manufacturers to show that the medical devices were actually safe. Fallout from the ban was swift and devastating. By 1992, about two million women had received silicone gel implants worldwide. Dr Kessler subsequently tried to reassure them that there was no evidence of danger. However, to them, it was not logical that the FDA would take this drastic action unless there was substantial risk. Letters poured into the FDA from patients experiencing problems with their implants. The impact of the media fueled the growing fire of unrest. This was followed by general pandemonium among patients, their families, and their plastic surgeons. Breast implant manufacturers were sued. Many plastic surgeons were also sued, particularly in the United States, as the blame was extended to them down the line from the manufacturers. Litigation lawyers seized the opportunity to expand their business.

An alarming plethora of symptoms and findings were progressively blamed on silicone gel breast implants and many women demanded immediate removal of their implants and many patients joined implant support groups. Others sought professional psychological support. In the United States, professional support groups were also organized for plastic surgeons. Explantation surgery soon became an integral part of a plastic surgeon's practice. Women who underwent explantation often became even more distraught. They had undergone breast augmentation to improve the size and shape of their breasts, but now, after implant removal, their breast tissue was stretched, loose, and generally 'worse than ever'.

Many patients requested capsulectomy along with their explantation. Lawyers, patients, and 'consultants' argued that retained capsules could serve as a reservoir for future silicone problems. This often resulted in further irregularities in breast shape and contour. Many of the women undergoing explantation elected to forego insertion of further implants. Others decided to replace their silicone gel implants with saline implants, which compounded their problems even further. Now, for the first time, their breasts, which had become thinned out by their original implants, developed horrendous ripples and folds on the breast surface. Ironically, many of these patients ultimately had those saline implants replaced with another set of silicone gel implants, once they became available again. Ultimately, implant manufacturers agreed to a $4.2B class action lawsuit, primarily on the grounds of product failure.

Many interesting findings emerged after patients had their implants removed. Some patients experienced an initial, almost euphoric improvement in their symptoms, during the first few months after explantation. However, their symptoms subsequently recurred over the following 6 to 12 months. Apart from local complications of capsular contracture, most other symptoms proved to be unrelated to their breast implants.

Over the past 20 years, a huge number of very large-scale epidemiological studies have been performed on patients who had received silicone gel breast implants. In fact, the safety of silicone gel breast implants has been studied more extensively than any other medical device in the world literature. The Institute of Medicine (IOM) study of 1999 extensively examined the safety concerns of breast implants. This study analyzed the relationship of breast implants to connective tissue disease (CTD), rheumatic disease, neurological disease, pregnancy, lactation, offspring, and various forms of cancer. No association was found between silicone gel implants and any of these conditions.

Chapter 6 of this book summarizes the current epidemiologic evidence regarding the safety of gel filled implants. This very thorough chapter by Lipworth and McLaughlin emphasizes the additional data, which has been published after the IOM report. The authors conclude that silicone gel breast implants are not associated with an increased occurrence of CTD, including systemic lupus erythematosus (SLE), rheumatoid arthritis, Sjögren's syndrome and fibromyalgia. They have also shown no association of gel implants with any type of 'atypical CTD', neurological disease, or any form of cancer, including any form of lymphoma. Similarly, the offspring of women with breast implants are not at increased risk for esophageal disorder or any other diseases.

During the past decade, extensive studies from Denmark and other countries have suggested that implant rupture is likely a relatively harmless event in most patients. It does not seem to produce significant clinical symptoms or activate the immune system. These studies have indicated that explantation surgery is not necessary in asymptomatic women with disrupted implants. Many patients and surgeons have now adopted a policy of simply following these patients along at regular intervals, with clinical and mammographic examinations.

Modern silicone gel implants are different from their predecessors. Today's implants are manufactured under much more stringent guidelines, to be more refined and durable. After the 1992 moratorium, the fourth generation silicone gel implants were developed. They had stronger and more durable elastomeric shells and a thicker and more cohesive gel with greater choices of implant height, width, and projection. This allowed 'tailoring' of the implant to each patient. Anatomic or 'teardrop' implants were reintroduced. This shape had previously been used on most gel implants from 1964 to 1973. They were discontinued in the mid-1970s. Various forms of texturing have been developed in an attempt to reduce capsular contracture and to maintain implant position. Subsequently, the fifth generation was developed. Its enhanced cohesive nature provides a 'form stable' device, which maintains its shape in all positions. These implants were formulated with different compartments of gel cohesiveness within the implant. Silicone gel breast implants are now undergoing a major reacceptance among women seeking breast enhancement surgery.

1
The history of biomaterials used for breast augmentation

W. PETERS, University of Toronto, Canada

Abstract: There is probably no other surgical procedure that has a history as fascinating and as terrifying as breast augmentation. This chapter traces the evolution of the biomaterials that have been used for breast augmentation from 1899 to the present time. There have been three main eras of biomaterials: injectable materials, sponges, and breast implants. Within each era, there have been a number of categories of materials. The current study reviews the biomaterials that have been used in each of these eras, and provides the current status of each.

Key words: silicone gel, breast implants, augmentation, moratorium, history.

1.1 Introduction

There is probably no other surgical procedure that has a history as fascinating and as terrifying as breast augmentation. This chapter will review the evolution of biomaterials that have been used for breast augmentation from 1899 to the present time. There have been three main eras of biomaterials:

- Injectable materials 1899–2010
- Sponges 1951–1963
- Breast implants 1963–2010

This chapter reviews the biomaterials used in each of these eras, and provides the current status of each.

1.2 Injectable materials

There have been four main groups of injectable materials for breast augmentation:

- Paraffin 1899–1914
- Other materials 1915–1943
- Liquid silicone 1944–1991
- Polyacrylamide hydrogel (PAH) 1988–2009

1.2.1 Paraffin, 1899–1914

Paraffin is a group of hydrocarbons, which is saturated with carbon to hydrogen bonds, making them relatively inert. The basic repeating unit in the polymers is: $-(CH_2)n-$. Paraffin exists as a hard form (wax) and a soft form (vaseline). Waxes are long-chain hydrocarbons, with $n > 20$. The softer form of paraffin, vaseline, is composed of shorter molecules. It looks and feels like the product that goes by that trade name today. Both the soft and hard forms of paraffin have a low melting point. Prior to injection, they were heated inside a chamber surrounded by warm water (Fig. 1.1), to form a semi-liquid material, which allowed easier injection (Kolle, 1911).

The first published report of paraffin injections into a patient dates back to a report by Gersuny of Vienna, in 1903. This patient was a young man, who had undergone a bilateral orchiectomy for tuberculous disease. Gersuny injected paraffin into his scrotum in 1899, so that the patient could pass the physical examination necessary to join the army. Paraffin injections were subsequently used extensively from 1899 until 1914, primarily for breast augmentation.

The early results of paraffin injections were often quite acceptable. The complications usually did not show up until 5–10 years later. Kolle's 1911 textbook, *Plastic and Cosmetic Surgery*, contained a whole section on the complications of paraffin injections. These complications included: pulmonary embolism, migration, ulceration, fistulae, infection, necrosis, and death. These complications would frequently lead to breast amputation. Figure 1.2 shows the clinical status of a woman in our practice, who had received paraffin injections in the Far East 40 years earlier. She had undergone multiple debridements and bilateral mastectomies over the years to treat multiple ulcers and fistulae. She continued to suffer from ulcers, and fistulae.

In his 1926 textbook, H. Lyons Hunt called paraffin injections an 'inexcusable practice' and blamed 'beauty doctors and other such imposters' for its continued use (Matton, 1985). However, in the Far East, the practice was continued into the 1950s and 1960s. Deaths continued to be sporadically reported after paraffin injections. In Europe and the United States, a number of patients injected themselves with paraffin, as a self-inflicted injury to escape the military service or deportation. Other patients injected themselves, to enlarge their penis or breasts. The disastrous experience with paraffin was to live on for a century, in the collective memory of the plastic surgery profession.

1.2.2 Other injectable materials, 1915–1943

After the paraffin saga, there was a period of about 30 years, when a huge plethora of materials was used for breast augmentation. The list of these

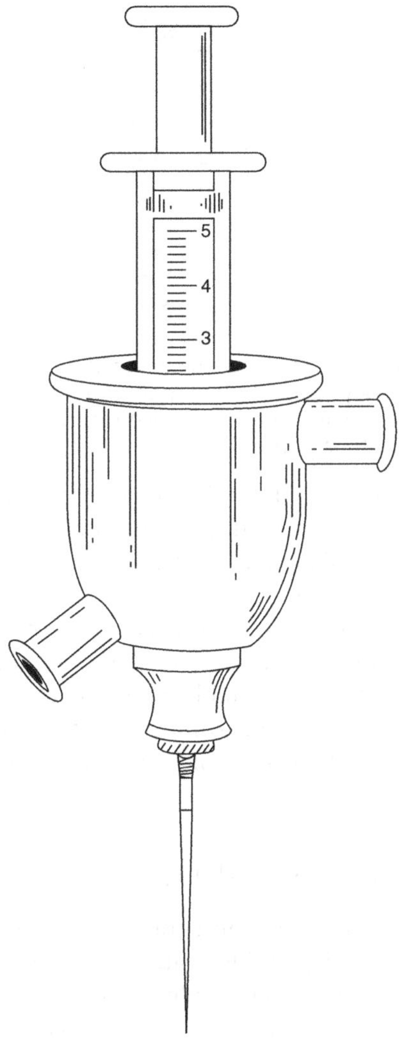

1.1 Warming chamber for liquefaction of paraffin prior to injection.

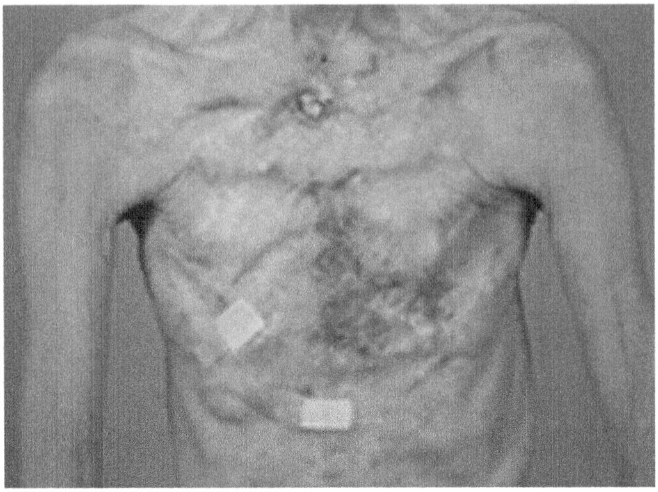

1.2 Clinical status of a woman who had received paraffin injections in the Far East 40 years previously. She has had many operations over the years, including bilateral mastectomies, to treat ulcers and fistulae. She continues to suffer from these problems.

materials was limited only by the extent of man's imagination. Injectable materials included: vegetable oils, mineral oil, lanolin, beeswax, shellac, epoxy resin, goat's milk, soybean oil and peanut oil (Bondurant *et al.*, 1999). During this same time interval, many solid materials were also implanted to augment women's breasts. These materials included: ivory balls, glass balls, silk fabric, epoxy resin, ground rubber, ox cartilage, sponges, sacs, rubber, Teflon, and glazier's putty. Like the injectable materials, the outcome with each of these materials was similar, with chronic inflammation, severe tissue reactions, and infections. Ultimately, none of these materials proved to be useful for breast augmentation.

1.2.3 Liquid silicone injections, 1944–1991

Surely the terrifying history of paraffin injections should have taught both physicians and patients to be wary of injectable materials for breast augmentation. However, in the 1940s and 1950s, many physicians and lay clinics turned to liquid silicone injections for breast augmentation (Duffy, 1998; Milojevic, 1982). Silicones are extensively cross-linked polymers of dimethyl siloxane. Their basic repeating unit is:

$$-O-\left[-\underset{CH_3}{\overset{CH_3}{\mathrm{Si}}}-\right]_n-O-$$

In 1943, the Dow Corning Corporation and Corning Glass formed a joint venture in the United States, to develop silicone products to be used for military purposes during World War II (Peters, 2009). Ultimately, these silicones were used for waterproofing equipment, to prepare high temperature grease and oil products for aircraft, to insulate electrical transformers, and to prepare high-temperature resistant rubbers. When the war came to an end, Dow Corning redirected their efforts to the formulation of medical grade silicone. Medical grade refers to material that is pure in quality, sterile, and of constant viscosity.

Near the end of World War II, prostitutes in Japan began to use industrial grade liquid silicone injections. United States servicemen preferred women with larger breasts than those of Asian women. Barrels of industrial grade silicone began to mysteriously disappear from Japanese docks, destined for injection into the breasts of these enterprising ladies, to cater to their potential clients. These injections were done with industrial grade liquid silicone, which was never intended to be injected into the body. Medical grade silicone was not available until 1960.

Many of the complications of paraffin were repeated, a half-century later, with silicone injections. Some of them were even worse, because of impurities and additives in the silicone preparations. In many of the preparations, contaminants were purposely added to the liquid silicone (Vinnick, 1978), to cause a sclerosis reaction, in an attempt to restrict migration to other sites. Common sclerosing agents included croton oil, cobra venom, olive oil and peanut oil. The adverse effects of injected liquid silicone were very similar to those of paraffin. These included: migration to other parts of the body, inflammation, discoloration, granulomas, ulceration, fistulae, and infection.

In 1960, Dow Corning developed its first commercial medical grade silicone, which was known as 'Dow Corning 360'. It was marketed under the name of Dermagen. Its intended purpose was for waterproofing skin and burn mattresses for burn victims, for treating racehorse injuries, and to manufacture fertilizers. Although this material was not approved or intended for injection in patients, it was used very extensively for this purpose, by certain physicians and by lay clinics. When it was used in breasts, huge volumes were often used. Large volumes of the silicone liquid were obtained under the false pretense that it was being used for burn mattresses, to treat racehorse injuries, and to make fertilizer products. All of these uses had been approved. Unscrupulous physicians in Las Vegas withdrew as much as a pint of the substance from 5-gallon drums stored in their offices (Christensen *et al.*, 2005; Romm, 1992). This was injected into breasts under great pressure, using equipment resembling a caulking gun. In the entertainment business, these silicone injections were referred to as 'Cleopatra's Needle'. It has been estimated that in Las Vegas in the 1960s, two physicians alone used silicone to inject the breasts of over 10 000 women over a 10-year period. No records were kept on any of these patients.

By 1965, many complications began to surface from liquid silicone injections (Matton, 1985; Mastrucerio and Pesqueira, 1996; Milojevic, 1982). Some injections had been done by plastic surgeons. Others were done by laypersons, who were minimally qualified to undertake this type of procedure. Because of the problems from uncontrolled silicone injections the United States Food and Drug Administration (FDA) designated silicone injections as a 'new drug' in 1966 (Coleman, 2001). This ruling stipulated that silicone must undergo certain laboratory investigations before it could be approved for use. To date, these studies have never been done.

In 1966, the FDA authorized nine plastic surgeons and a dermatologist to investigate the cosmetic use of Dow Corning's highly purified medical grade liquid silicone (Dow Corning 360) for certain problems in patients. The study was limited to only these particular physicians, treating certain facial deformities that were not treatable by other methods. In 1978, the FDA expanded this study to 27 physicians. However, other plastic surgeons, who were not part of the official study, were also able to obtain this silicone material (Wilkie, 1977). In 1975, because of the horrendous complications from silicone injections into breasts in Las Vegas, the state of Nevada declared that it was a felony to inject silicone or to transport liquid silicone across the state line.

By 1990, over 20 000 patients had received silicone breast injections and over 100 000 had received facial injections using liquid silicone of known or unknown origin. In August 1991, the FDA issued guidelines clearly forbidding the marketing or sale of injectable liquid silicone for aesthetic injection purposes, until appropriate studies had been completed. To date, these long-term clinical investigations have never been done. In 1991, silicone injections were labeled as 'adulterated' by the FDA, to indicate that they had not received FDA approval for marketing or scientific study. In 1992, the FDA issued press releases mandating that 'Physicians will no longer be allowed to use injectable silicone for cosmetic treatment unless the product is approved by the FDA for marketing or investigational studies'. The FDA has never approved the use of injections of liquid silicone for patients, except in their approved investigational study. In 1991–2, it officially banned the use of all silicone injection products by all physicians.

In spite of all of the warnings and cautions, liquid silicone injections were easily obtainable by any woman who wanted them. They were frequently injected in lay clinics in numerous regions of the United States. They were particularly popular in Mexico and even in San Francisco. Injectable silicone has also always been freely available from Asia.

In 1994, the FDA approved a form of silicone oil for the treatment of a particularly devastating AIDS-related disorder – complicated retinal detachment secondary to cytomegalovirus retinitis. The purpose of the oil was to provide 'prolonged retinal tamponade' so that the retina could reattach. In 1997, the FDA approved a commercial formulation of this silicone oil, Silikon 1000 (Alcon, Fort Worth, TX), for the treatment of this disorder. In March 2001, the FDA cleared another commercial formulation, Adatosil 5000 (Bausch & Lomb, Tampa, FL), for treatment of this form of detached retina. For the past several years, a number of practitioners in the U.S. have purchased these liquid silicone preparations, on the grounds that they were being used for the treatment of retinal detachment. However, they have actually been injecting the silicone to treat wrinkles and other cosmetic concerns (Coleman, 2001). In the case of retinal detachment, the silicone is meant to be removed after reattachment of the retina. This removal is not possible when this material is injected into soft tissues.

The FDA has never approved liquid silicone for general cosmetic injection purposes. However, the FDA has no jurisdiction over the practice of medicine. Therefore, physicians frequently use devices that are FDA-cleared for one indication, but they use it in a totally different application or off-label use. This off-label use is beyond the authority of the FDA. The FDA Modernization Act of 1997 permits FDA-cleared devices to be used off-label, for any condition within the doctor–patient relationship. Currently, FDA-approved clinical trials are reported to be in progress for a liquid silicone product specifically for treatment of HIV-associated facial lipoatrophy and for use with certain other indications (Coleman, 2001). Little is known about the study except that it involves the use of a microdroplet serial puncture technique, as described by Orentreich in 2000.

Like paraffin, the early results following silicone injections are often satisfactory.

Subsequently, the reactions of silicone injections into breasts vary considerably. Not all patients appear to be equally susceptible to the deleterious effects of silicone. Some patients appear not to be susceptible. In general, the average time from injection of silicone to the development of complications is about 9 years (Vinnick, 1978; Wilkie, 1977). There are two main types of clinical presentations: (a) multiple painful breast lumps, and (b) skin inflammation and impending breakdown. These findings may not occur until 10–15 years after injection. As the silicone invades the dermis and epidermis, the breast may show skin circulatory difficulties, ranging from telangiectasia to necrosis. Granulomas and fistulas can subsequently develop. Migration of the silicone is common.

Smaller granulomas can be treated by localized resection. However, once fistulae have developed, treatment may involve large area resection or even bilateral mastectomy. Many cases of major complications are related to the use of industrial silicone. However, there are also well-documented cases

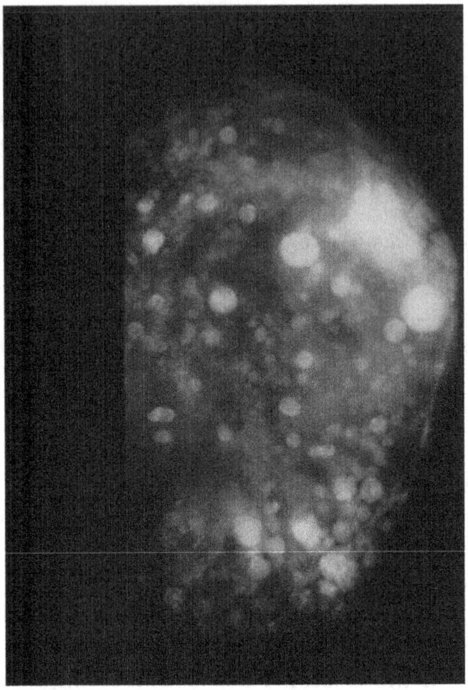

1.3 Mammography following silicone injections often demonstrates multiple cystic masses ranging from 0.2 to 2.0 cm in diameter, often with calcification. This appearance can interfere with the interpretation of mammograms.

of major complications, resulting in bilateral mastectomy, following the use of medical grade silicone (Achauer, 1982).

Mammography of breasts injected with silicone usually demonstrates a pattern of multiple cystic masses ranging from 0.2 to 2.0 cm in diameter, often with calcification (Fig. 1.3). This appearance can interfere with the interpretation of mammograms.

Injectable liquid silicone has many qualities that could make it a suitable material for long-term soft-tissue augmentation. At the same time, there are still many unanswered questions pertaining to potential complications that need to be addressed before it can be considered for this purpose. A well conducted, controlled, long-term study is needed to answer these questions.

1.2.4 Polyacrylamide hydrogel

Polyacrylamide hydrogel (PAH) is an extensively cross-linked polymeric soft tissue filler substance, that has been used in the Ukraine, Russia, and

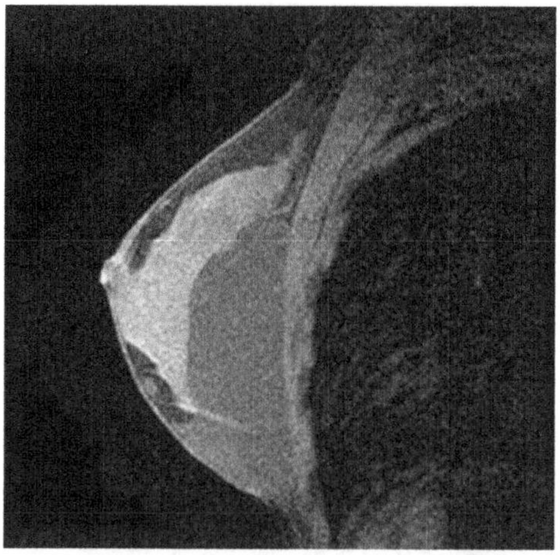

1.4 MRI T1 weighted image of the breast of a patient who had PAH breast injections. There is low signal intensity material (PAH), mostly superficial to the pectoral muscles, in the subglandular plane.

China for the past 15–20 years (Christensen *et al.*, 2003; Christensen and Breiting, 2006). It was originally introduced to aesthetic surgery under the name of Royamid in the Ukraine in the late 1980s. It has subsequently been marketed under many different names. PAH consists of 2.5% PAH and 97.5% water. The repeating unit for the polymers is $[–CH_2–CH(CONH_2)–]_n$. Water is bonded between cross-linked polymers, by hydrogen bonding. Theoretically, 1.0 ml of 2.5% PAH can bind up to 1.25 ml of normal saline. Preparations of PAH have been shown to be stable, non-toxic, non-allergenic, non-absorbable, and non-biodegradable.

Initially, PAH appeared to be an ideal soft tissue filler material. However, several reports have now demonstrated that numerous complications can occur after PAH injections. These can develop from several months to several years after injection. They include the following: migration, breast lumps, pain, infection, firmness and disfigurement (Cheng *et al.*, 2002; Cheng *et al.*, 2006; Qiao *et al.*, 2005).

The author recently treated a 29-year-old patient, who presented with multiple tender and painful lumps in the lower half of her breasts. She had received PAH injections in Iran 1 year previously. Figure 1.4 shows an MRI T1 weighted image of this patient's left breast. There is low signal intensity material, mostly superficial to the pectoral muscles, in the subglandular plane. This material was present in a large pocket, and was easily removed through bilateral inframammary incisions. It had the consistency of 'Cream of Wheat' (Fig. 1.5). The pockets were then thoroughly irrigated with Bacitracin/saline solution. She had an uneventful recovery. Two years later, she

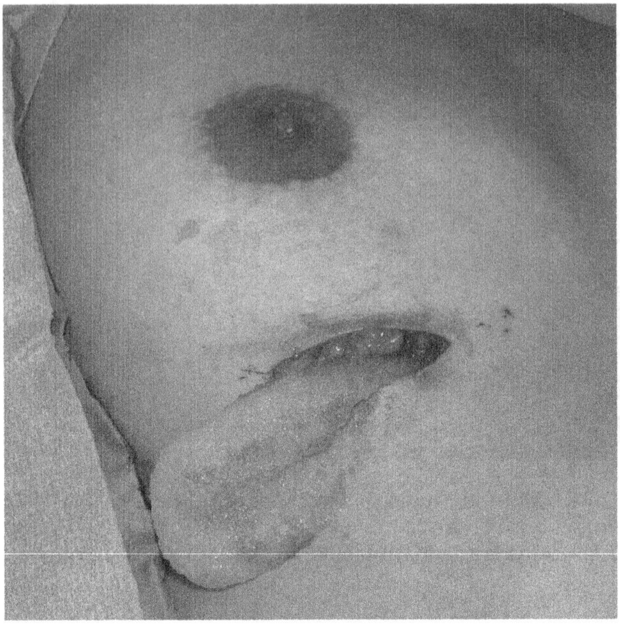

1.5 The PAH was removed through bilateral inframammary incisions. It was easily expressed out of the pockets. It had the consistency of 'Cream of Wheat'.

underwent a subglandular breast augmentation with 300 cc Mentor Moderate Plus Gel implants with an excellent result. Other patients have a poorer outcome after PAH injections. The author has recently seen a patient from Russia, who had received PAH injections into multiple sites, 6 years previously. She presented with major recurrent infections and multiple recurrent sinuses on her buttocks and legs (Fig. 1.6).

The Chinese State Food and Drug Administration (SFDA) recently banned the production, sale, and use of PAH (Peters, 2009). They received 183 reports of adverse effects from the use of PAH from 2002 to November 2005. Of those, 161 involved breast injection patients who suffered infections and disfigurement. The SFDA stipulated that all existing supplies of PAH were to be recalled and destroyed under SFDA supervision. Failure to comply with this mandate would result in criminal prosecution. History has repeated itself in each era of breast augmentation by injections.

1.3 Sponges

From 1951 to 1963, a number of different sponges were used for breast augmentation. The first of these was Ivalon, a polyvinyl alcohol sponge. Grindlay and Clagett originally evaluated this material in dogs in 1951.

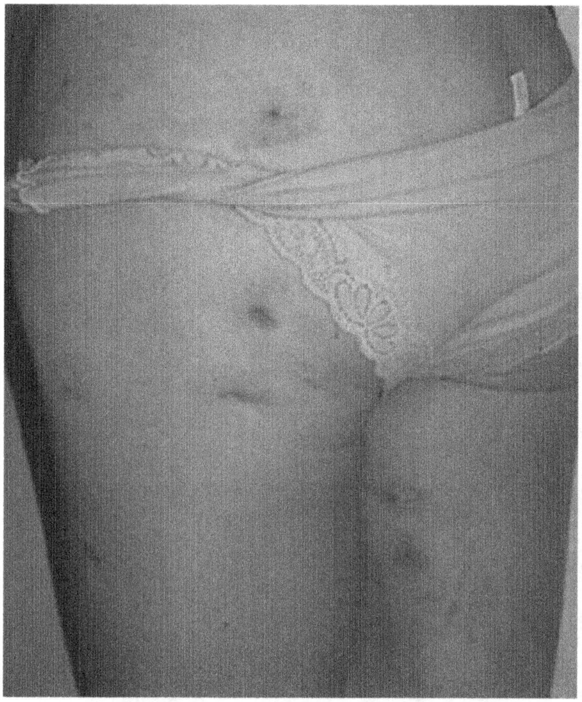

1.6 Clinical status of a 45-year-old Russian woman, who received PAH injections into multiple sites, 6 years earlier. She now presents with multiple recurrent sinuses and infections.

Pangman and Wallace began inserting it into women's breasts in 1951. Pangman subsequently formed the Poly-Plastic Company to manufacture these Ivalon implants. They were distributed by the Beverly Hills Surgical Supply Company, in Beverly Hills, California.

In 1955, Pangman and Wallace reported on the results of their first 400 Ivalon breast sponges. Because the Ivalon sponges became infiltrated with vascularized tissue, Pangman referred to the implant as a 'living sponge'. Although the initial results with Ivalon were encouraging, after 6–12 months, they underwent 'shrinkage and compression' and became 'very hard'. This was likely due to capsular contracture, a process that was not well understood at that time. It produced 'shrinkage' because it resulted in collapse of the sponge material. To address this problem, Pangman tried many different modifications. These included wrapping the inner core of the sponge in polyethylene, wrapping the entire sponge in polyethylene, and developing a double-layered sponge. However, none of these changes prevented capsular contracture and firmness (Liu and Truong, 1996). Figure 1.7 shows the original presentation case containing a Pangman Ivalon double-layered

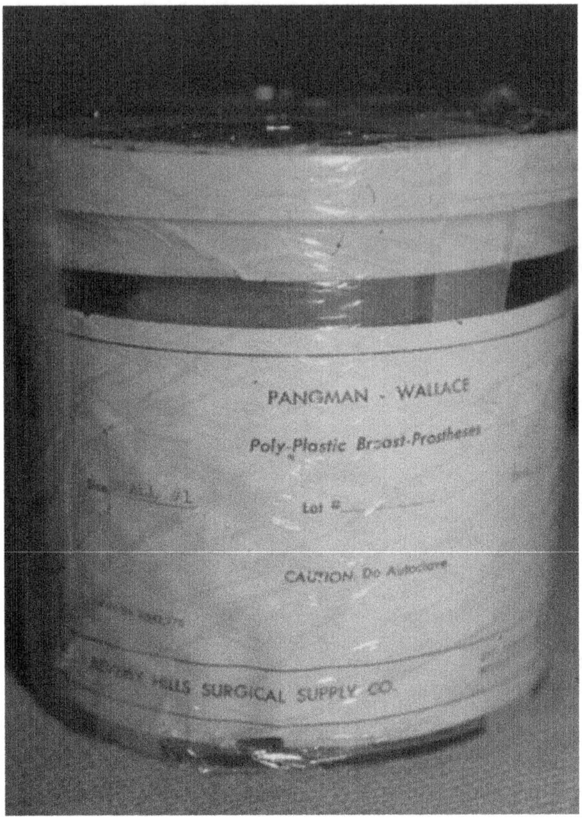

1.7 Original presentation case containing a Pangman Ivalon double-layered implant (circa 1955), manufactured by the Poly-Plastic Company and distributed by Beverley Hills Surgical Supply Company. The implant shown in Fig. 1.8 has been sitting in this case for 55 years.

implant (circa 1955), manufactured by the Poly-Plastic Company and distributed by Beverley Hills Surgical Supply Company. The implant shown in Fig. 1.8 has been sitting in this case for the past 55 years. Over time, the outer layer has become fragmented.

Figure 1.9 shows a 46-year-old woman, who presented to the author in 1979, with Class IV contractures, 19 years after she had received Pangman double-layered Ivalon implants. This appearance was rather classical, almost a trademark, for patients who received these early implants. The breasts looked like firm baseballs due to excessive capsular contracture. When these implants were removed, they were surrounded by a thick (4–5 mm) capsule (Peters and Smith, 1981). Scanning electron microscopy showed that this fibrous capsule had infiltrated into only the outer 2 mm of the

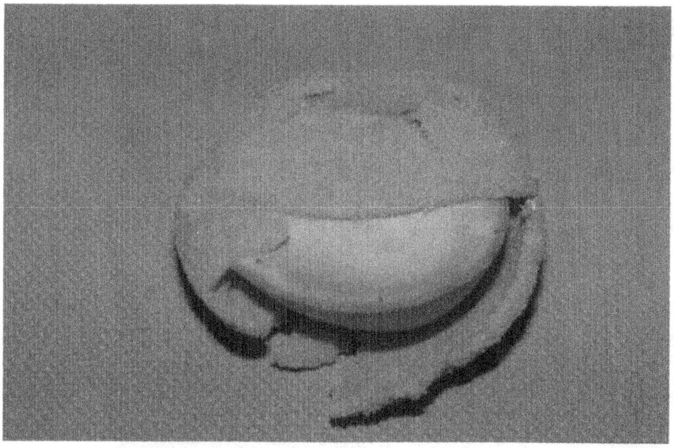

1.8 Double-layered Ivalon implant (circa 1955), from the presentation case shown in Fig. 1.7. The outer layer has become fragmented over the 55 years.

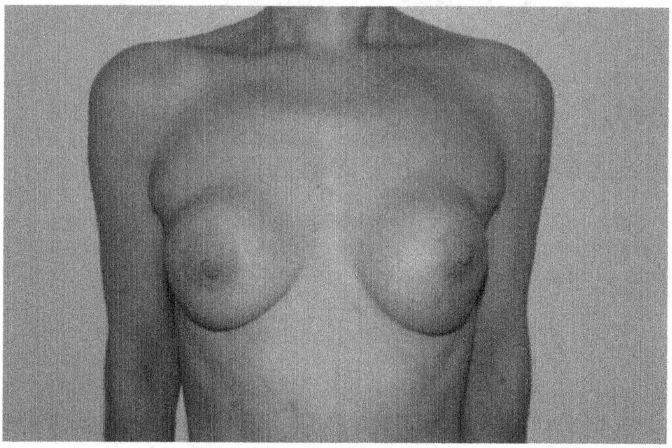

1.9 Breast appearance 19 years after augmentation with double layered Ivalon implant (circa 1958). There is major capsular contracture (Class IV), with marked distortion of the breasts.

surface of the sponge (Fig. 1.10). Previously, it was surmised that fibrous tissue infiltrated well into the Ivalon. Once the capsule was incised through, the compression properties of the implants were similar to virginal Ivalon sponge. The firmness of this woman's breasts was due to contracture of the fibrous capsules, not to any change in the implants themselves. Previously, it was also believed that the firmness was also due to calcification of the implant. However, analyses of Ivalon sponges explanted from the patient in Figure 1.9 failed to demonstrate calcification. In 1961, a survey performed

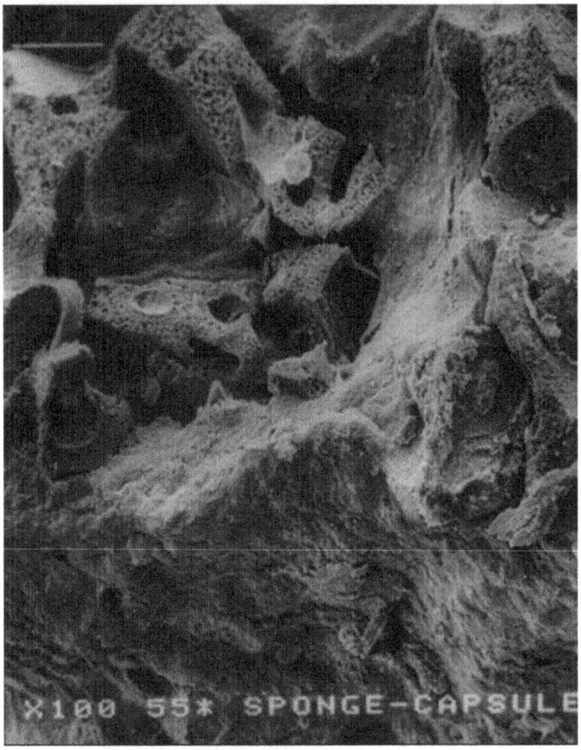

1.10 Scanning electron microscopy image of the capsule from the Ivalon implants in Fig. 1.9 showing that fibrous tissue had infiltrated only the outer 2 mm of the sponge (original magnification × 270).

by Harris estimated that approximately 16 600 Ivalon implants had been inserted by 184 of the 294 plastic surgeons in practice at that time.

From 1952 to 1962 other sponges were also used for breast augmentation. In 1952, Naso reported on the use of a polyethylene sponge. Other surgeons used Etheron, a form of polyether sponge (Conway and Dietz, 1962; Pickrell, 1962; Regnault, 1967). In 1967, Paule Regnault, who practiced in Montreal, reported on the insertion of 174 Etheron sponge prostheses for breast augmentation. In addition to developing major capsular contracture, these implants were also associated with infection and erosion. Another implant that was used at this time was the Polystan sponge (Edgerton and McClary, 1958). This was composed of fabric tapes, which were cut by machine and then wound by hand into a ball. In 1963, Edwards introduced an implant with an inner sponge of Silastic surrounded by a thin layer of Teflon. The Teflon shell was designed to prevent fibrous ingrowth, and to restrict 'post-operative shrinking' from capsular contracture. However,

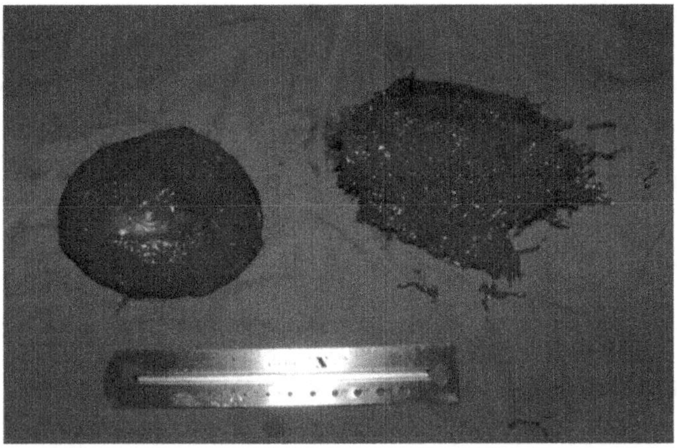

1.11 Polyethylene implants, which were inserted in Turkey in 1963.

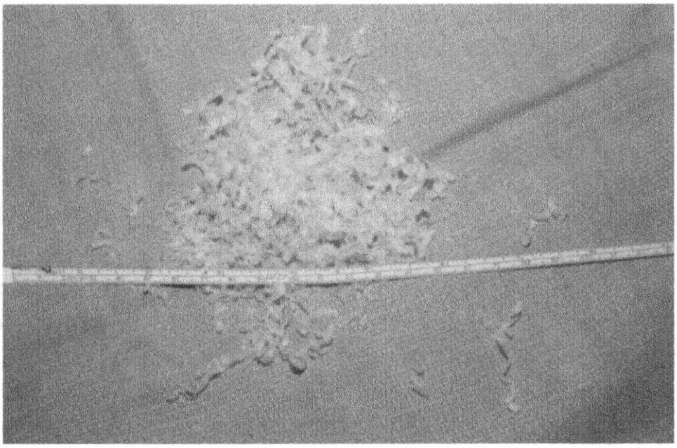

1.12 Inside the casing of the implants in Fig. 1.11 there were numerous strips of polyethylene, each about 2 mm wide.

breasts implanted with these sponges also became very firm and lost significant volume after 6–12 months.

In 1977, Smahel *et al.* reported on another type of implant that was used from 1958 to 1962. It consisted of shredded polyethylene strips enclosed in a casing. Figure 1.11 shows two such implants that were removed from a patient by the author in 1984. These had been inserted in Turkey in 1963, as a 17th birthday present from the recipient's parents! Once the casing was incised through, there were numerous shredded strips of polyethylene, each about 2 mm in width (Fig. 1.12). (Many of the breast implants shown in this study are from the author's personal collection of implants.)

All of the foam implants from this era had a similar outcome. Within a year of implantation, they tended to develop major capsular contracture. This resulted in breast firmness, and loss of breast volume, from compression of the implants. Because of this high complication rate, the popularity of breast augmentation surgery progressively declined until 1963, when the silicone gel implant was introduced.

1.4 Breast implants

The evolution of breast implants has been a colorful one, extending over the past 60 years. It has been a stormy course, with many exciting advances and many bitter disappointments (Peters, 2002).

1.4.1 Silicone gel implants

Cronin and Gerow introduced the silicone gel breast implant in 1963 as a new 'natural feel' implant. Since then, many different types and models of implants have been developed. From 1963 to 1992, there was no such thing as a 'standard' silicone gel breast implant. Implants consisted of a rubber-like silicone elastomer envelope (shell), which varied in thickness from 0.075 to 0.75 mm, enclosing a known volume of silicone gel, ranging from 80 cc to 800 cc (Bondurant *et al.*, 1999). The elastomer was composed of extensively cross-linked high molecular weight components, together with 16.4% to 26.9% amorphous fumed silica filler, which was used as a reinforcing agent. The gel was composed of a mixture of low-molecular weight (6000–38 000) silicone oil and high-molecular weight (up to 404 000) components. The chemical composition and average molecular weight of the gel differed from manufacturer to manufacturer and from time to time. Solvent extraction of the envelope and the gel has revealed 30 different linear and cyclic components.

From 1963 to 1992, silicone gel implants were extremely heterogeneous. About ten different companies manufactured many different types of silicone gel breast implants. They obtained raw materials for the gels and shells from a similar number of other companies, who entered and left the market at intervals. Many of the suppliers and manufactures changed their names and ownership over the years. Most of the companies no longer exist. Companies often introduced designs conceived by individual surgeons, usually without testing. The breast implant business was competitive and companies introduced changes such as softer gels, barrier low-bleed shells, greater or lesser shell thickness, surface texturing, different sizes, contours, shapes and multiple lumens in search of better marketing and better aesthetics. These changes were introduced at different times and usually affected some but not all of the company's products. Ultimately, over 240 styles and 8300 models of silicone gel breast implants were manufactured in the United States alone (Middleton, 1993). No formal process of FDA pre-market testing was in effect until 1988.

Implant vintage

There have been five main generations of silicone gel breast implants and a number of lesser variations (Peters, 2002; Report of the Independent Review Group, Cambridge, U.K., 1998; Cunningham and McCue, 2009). First-generation implants were made from about 1963 to 1972. During that time, Dow Corning had an almost exclusive monopoly on their manufacture. The implants were composed of a thick (firm) gel and a thick elastomeric wall (Fig. 1.13). From 1963 to 1968, the shells were 0.75 mm thick. They were prepared by a molding-technique, to produce a seamed shell, which was subsequently filled with gel. From 1969 onwards, all shells were seamless (the Silastic 0 implant). They were produced by 'dip-coating' a mandrel into a dispersion fluid. The shell was then removed, gel was injected into it, and the injection site was sealed with adhesive silicone. First-generation implants had woven Dacron® (DuPont, USA) patches on their posterior surface to anchor them to the chest wall, in an attempt to restrict ptosis. First-generation implants have proved to be much stronger than second-generation implants (Peters, 2000; Peters and Lugowski, 2002). This is likely due to the increased thickness of their elastomer shell. Most women with first-generation implants developed very firm breasts within a year of their surgery. This was likely due to capsular contracture, a process that was not well understood at the time. It was surmised that this firmness was due

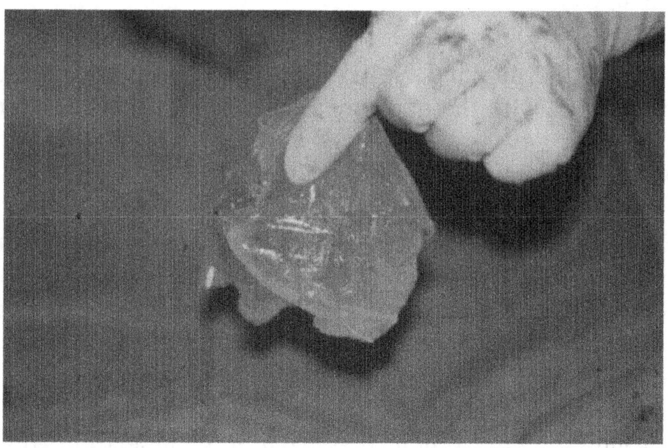

1.13 First generation silicone gel implant (1966) with a thick gel and a thick wall, with a Dacron patch.

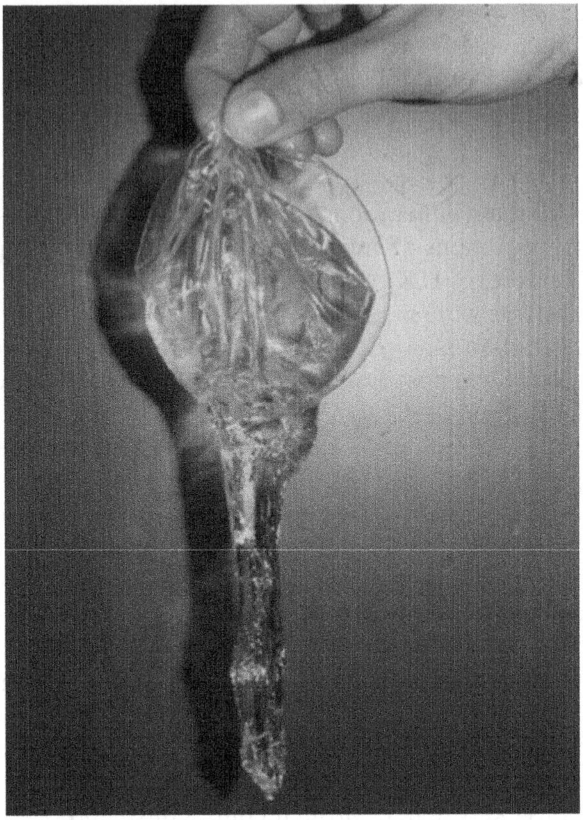

1.14 Second generation gel implant (1975) with a thin wall and a thin gel; the gel is quite liquid and could easily migrate if the implant shell is disrupted.

to the firmness of the implants. Softer (second-generation) implants were therefore developed, with the naive idea that their softness could result in softer breasts.

Second-generation implants were introduced in the U.S. from 1972 to 1975. They were used until the mid-1980s. They had a thin, watery, 'responsive' gel (Fig. 1.14), which was less viscous than first-generation implants, and a thin (0.13 mm to 0.20 mm) and softer wall. The thickness or firmness of the gel was related to the relative amount of highly cross-linked material in the gel. The thick or firm gel contained about 50% highly cross-linked silicone and about 50% low molecular weight chains. By contrast, the thin gel contained only about 20% highly cross-linked silicone and 80% low molecular weight chains. When these patients underwent revisionary surgery, some of these implants were found to be disrupted. This set the stage for the development of the third-generation implant. Ultimately,

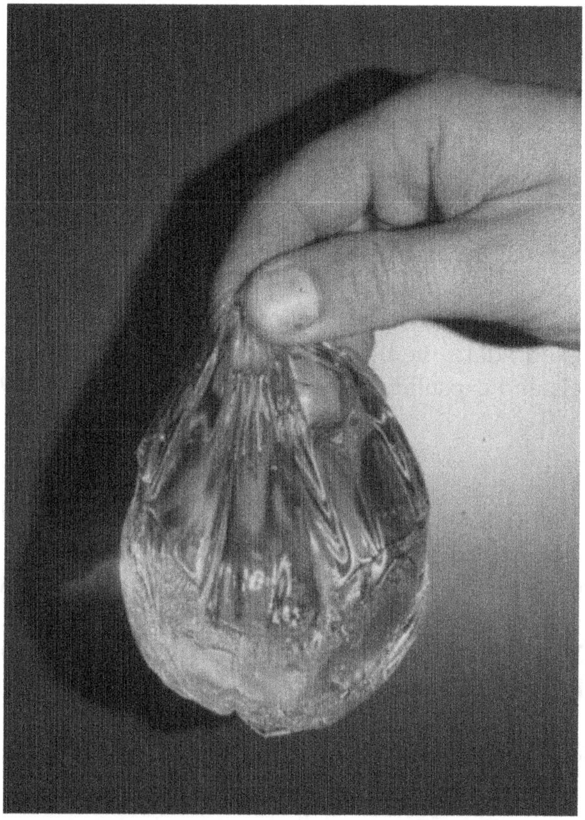

1.15 Third generation (1989) gel implant with a thick wall and a thick (cohesive) gel.

several studies showed that second-generation implants were much less durable than first- or third-generation implants (Peters *et al.*, 1996a; Peters, 2000; Peters and Lugowski, 2002; Robinson, 1995).

The third-generation implant had a stronger and thicker (0.30 to 0.50 mm) (High Performance (HP)) shell and a much more cohesive gel than a second-generation implant (Fig. 1.15). Third-generation implants also had a 'barrier layer' to reduce the diffusion of low molecular weight (4000 to 24 000) silicone oil, which was thought to contribute to capsular contracture. McGhan (*Intrashiel*) implants were introduced in the U.S. in 1979. The corresponding Dow Corning (*Silastic II*) implants were introduced in the U.S. in 1981. Surgitek (*SCL*) implants were introduced in the U.S. in 1986. Both Surgitek and McGhan implants had a diphenyl barrier layer incorporated within the shell, to restrict silicone bleed. Dow Corning (*Silastic II*) implants had a 0.010 mm barrier coat of fluorosilicone on the interior surface of the shell. The actual thickness of the shells of third-generation implants (like second-generation implants) was quite variable. The manufacturer listed the shell thickness of the McGhan *Intrashiel* shells to be 0.35 mm. However, subsequent analysis showed a range of shell thickness from 0.13 to 0.35 mm (Bondurant *et al.*, 1999).

Third-generation implants proved to be much more durable than second-generation implants (Peters, 2000; Peters and Lugowski, 2002). However, the effectiveness of the barrier layer to restrict silicone bleed remains unproven. Peters and coworkers have shown that Surgitek third-generation implants lost the effectiveness of their barrier layer after only 2–3 years (Peters *et al.*, 1996b). To date, there is no proof of any relationship between tissue silicone levels and capsular contracture (Bondurant *et al.*, 1999).

Multi-lumen implants

Double-lumen implants have two shells. The inner lumen is gel-filled and the outer is saline-filled. The outer lumen was intended to form an additional layer against silicone oil diffusion or gel leakage. However, this feature proved to be ineffective. In fact, no data can be found to support such a function (Yu *et al.*, 1996). In the late 1980s, double-lumen implants, mostly made by McGhan Corporation, constituted about 15% of all implants that were used. Subsequently, a reverse double-lumen implant was developed, with silicone gel in the outer lumen and saline in the inner lumen (the Becker implant). Other companies made a triple-lumen implant.

1.4.2 Polyurethane coated – 1968 to 1988

The first textured breast implant was developed and patented in 1968 by Ashley and Pangman. It was known as the Ashley Natural Y implant (Ashley, 1970). It was a high profile, clear-shell silicone gel-filled implant with a 1.5–2.0 mm layer of polyurethane (PU) on the surface (Ashley, 1972). These implants had an inverted Y-shaped baffle or internal divider, which was designed to control the shape of the implant. Early models had a flat posterior surface, which helped to control the orientation of the implant. These implants were manufactured by Pangman's Poly-Plastic Company, which had previously manufactured his Ivalon implants.

In 1971, Heyer-Schulte acquired the rights for the Ashley Natural Y implants from Poly-Plastics (Middleton, 1993) and manufactured about 2000 of these PU implants over the next few years. One such PU implant is shown in Fig. 1.16. This implant has been stored in its presentation case for the past 38 years. It is likely the only virginal Heyer-Schulte PU implant in existence from this era. In 1974, Heyer-Schulte was acquired by American Hospital Supply, which did not manufacture further PU implants.

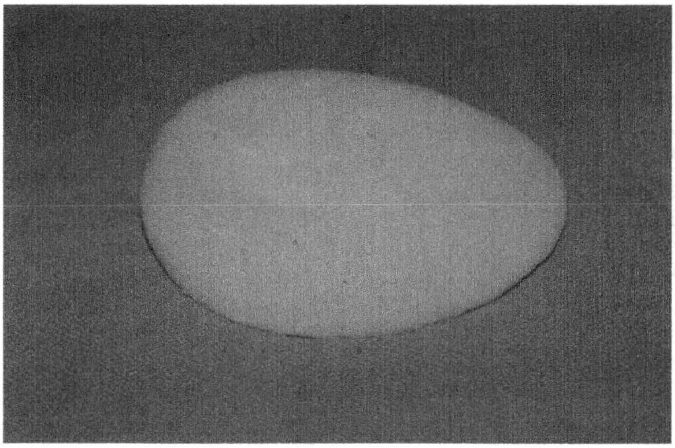

1.16 Polyurethane (PU) coated silicone gel-filled implant (Heyer-Schulte, 1972). This implant has been in its original presentation case for the past 38 years.

PU-coated implants became very popular during the 1980s, because their coating appeared to markedly reduce capsular contracture (Capossi and Pennisi, 1981; Pennisi, 1990; Capozzi, 1991; Vasquez, 2000). PU capsular contracture rates of 1–2% were common after breast augmentation and 2–3% after mastectomy reconstruction. From 1987 to 1991, about 19% of all implants inserted in the U.S. were PU-coated. The most likely explanation for their reduced rate of capsular contracture is that tissue grows into the interstices of the PU, prolonging chronic inflammation, disorienting collagen molecules, and weakening their contractile forces (Barone *et al.*, 1992; Raso and Greene, 1997). In addition, particles of PU, which are shed from the implant surface, become incorporated into the capsule, further breaking up the linearity of the collagen. Figure 1.17 shows the linear appearance of the collagen in a contracted capsule around a gel implant. By contrast, Fig. 1.18 shows fragments of shed PU, which have become incorporated into the capsule. This has broken up the linearity of the collagen, contributing to a reduction in capsular contracture.

Subsequently, many companies manufactured their own versions of PU implants. Cox-Uphoff International manufactured PU implants from 1979 until 1981. The Aesthetech Corporation manufactured the Optimam model from 1982 to 1991. Surgitek's Meme implant was made from 1982 to 1985. The PU foam used in these models had 80–100 open pores per linear inch, with a pore size of 200–500 μm in diameter. About 1.35 g of PU foam covered the average implant. All PU implant brands were acquired by Cooper Laboratories in 1987 and then by Surgitek in 1988. Surgitek continued to manufacture the Meme, Replicon (Fig. 1.19), and Optimam

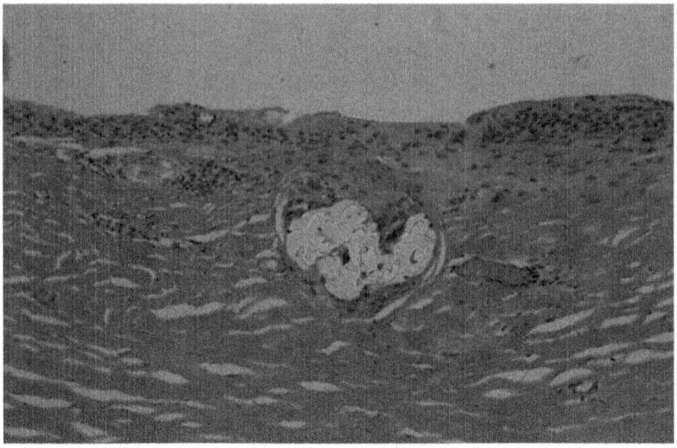

1.17 Contracted capsule from a silicone gel implant shows linear orientation of collagen in a contracted silicone gel implant (hematoxylin and eosin stain, ×100).

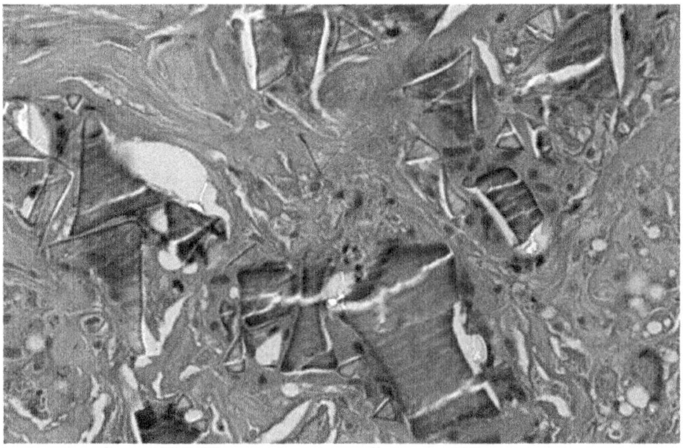

1.18 Capsule from a PU implant shows fragments of shed PU incorporated into the capsule. This has broken up the linearity of the collagen, contributing to a reduction in capsular contracture (World Health Organization Stain, original magnification × 250).

implants until domestic sales were suspended in 1991. The elastomer shell thickness for the Meme was 0.075 mm, for the Replicon, 0.23 mm, and for the Meme MP, 0.23 mm. These thin walls probably accounted for the high rupture rates of the Meme implants.

In the human breast, the layer of foam coating on a PU implant has been shown to disintegrate physically and chemically over time (Benoit, 1993). The half-life for biodegradation is about 23 months (Spear *et al.*, 2000). It

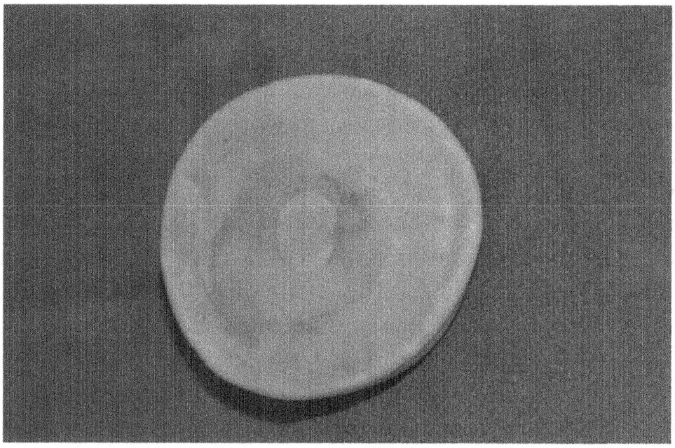

1.19 Replicon PU-coated gel implant, with circular white ring on posterior surface, explanted after 11 years. The PU has a half-life of about 23 months. Only a small amount of the PU remains on the implant surface.

should be emphasized that most of the published studies of the low rates of contracture were made over only the first 1–3 years. It is uncertain if long-term contracture results (after disintegration of the PU coating) are better than with regular smooth implants. PU foam undergoes partial chemical degradation under physiologic conditions, releasing compounds that could be carcinogenic to animals. One such compound is 2,4-toluenediamine (2,4-TDA), which was shown to be toxic to a particular strain of rat (Hester *et al.*, 1997). This finding led to the withdrawal of PU implants from the domestic market in 1991. Subsequent reports have indicated that the very small amounts of 2,4-TDA that would be released from PU implants would not provide a significant health risk.

1.5 Other forms of texturing

The success of PU implants in reducing the incidence of capsular contracture stimulated several companies to develop other forms of texturing for breast implants. In 1987, McGhan developed their Biocell surface (Spear *et al.*, 2000). This is an aggressive open-pore textured surface, similar to the PU surface. It is created using a lost salt technique. The elastomeric shell is placed on a bed of finely graded salt. Light pressure is then applied to produce depressions on the shell surface. Biocell texturing has 3.1 pores/mm^2. The pore size is 300–600 μm and an average height of 500–800 μm (Bondurant *et al.*, 1999). In 1988, Mentor developed their Siltex surface, which is a shallower and less-aggressive irregular surface.

It is created as a negative contact imprint of a textured foam. It has surface irregularities measuring 60–275 μm wide and 65–150 μm high.

Dow Corning developed their Micro Structured Implant (MSI) in 1989. This was perhaps the most scientifically developed form of surface texturing. It had an extremely regular surface of projecting, minute, silicone rubber papillae created with laser technology. It had regular pillars 250 μm in diameter, 750 μm high and 500 μm apart. This texturing was much more coarsely spaced than other implant surfaces, and was easily detectable on mammography (Middleton, 1998). These implants had a tendency to collect a thick layer of fluid between the implant and the capsule surface (Ahn *et al.*, 1995), possibly because of the added friction from the height of the pillars. The MSI Silastic implant was withdrawn from the market in 1992. The Biocell and Siltex textured surfaces continue to be used on silicone gel-filled and saline-filled implants today.

1.5.1 Effect of texturing on capsular contracture

A preventative relationship between surface texturing and capsular contracture has not been totally proven. Randomized control trials, comparing textured with smooth implants, have shown conflicting results. Earlier studies with silicone gel implants reported an advantage with textured implants. In 1993, Pollock published a study comparing 98 consecutive patients with Mentor, low-bleed, double-lumen gel implants to 99 consecutive patients with Siltex gel implants. The capsular contracture rate was lower in the Siltex group. However, there were numerous deficiencies in this study. There was no double blinding. There was observer bias. The results were recorded as number of patients with capsules, whereas it is generally held that contracture occurs as an independent breast-based phenomenon (Burkhardt, 1984), (rather than patient-based). Baker class 2 results were grouped together with class 3 and 4. Attrition was not evaluated.

In 1993, Coleman and coworkers reported on a 1-year study involving 53 patients with subglandular implants. Half received Mentor smooth implants and half had Mentor Siltex implants. The Siltex implants had a significantly reduced rate of capsular contracture. In 1997, Hakelius and Ohlsen reported on a 5-year study involving 50 patients with subglandular implants. Half had McGhan Intrashiel style 40 smooth gel implants and half had third-generation McGhan Biocell implants. The patients with Biocell implants had a reduced rate of capsular contracture. In 2000, Collis *et al.* published a 10-year review on 53 patients. Half had received Mentor smooth silicone gel implants and half had Siltex gel implants. The patients with Siltex implants had a significantly reduced rate of Baker 3 and 4 capsules. However, most of these studies suffered from similar shortcomings. There was a lack of double blinding. There was major attrition bias and there was significant observer bias (Wong *et al.*, 2006).

By contrast, other studies have failed to show a reduction in capsular contracture with textured gel implants. In 1995, Handell *et al.* analyzed 1655 breast implants in 752 patients, which were inserted over a 15-year period. They found no significant differences in the capsular contracture rates among smooth and textured implants. In 1996, Asplund and coworkers reported on 61 women who underwent submuscular augmentation with Dow Corning Silastic II High Performance gel implants or Dow Corning textured implants (Microstructured Silastic Implants (MSI)). There was no significant difference between the capsular contracture rates in the two groups.

More recently, two independent studies have reviewed a number of previously published data for randomized controlled trials, comparing textured with smooth implants. In 2006, Wong *et al.* reported on pooled data from six randomized controlled studies with a total of 235 patients (470 breasts). Textured implants were associated with less capsular contracture at 1, 3, and 7 years. However, the authors, themselves, listed many limitations with this study. The patient cohorts were diverse and may not have been comparable. There was significant attrition bias. Surgical techniques and incision approaches were not standardized. Long-term results were sparse, and by their nature, prone to bias. Wong *et al.* stated 'the quality of data significantly deteriorated after the 1-year follow-up mark'.

In 2006, Barnsley and coworkers conducted a meta-analysis on seven previous studies of textured implants. Only three of these studies had shown lower rates of capsular contracture with the use of textured implants. However, when all seven studies were pooled, there was a significant protective effect for surface texturing on the development of capsular contracture. Only two of the studies were the same as those analyzed by Wong *et al.* Only three of the studies involved silicone gel implants. The other four studies involved saline implants. One of the silicone gel studies involved submuscular insertion. It is well known that saline implants have a much lower capsular rate than silicone gel implants. It is also accepted that submuscular insertion results in a lower capsular contracture rate than subglandular placement (Wong *et al.*, 2006). Therefore, in these four studies, a statistical comparison with the silicone gel subglandular studies is not accurate. In addition, Barnsley's study suffers from the same shortcomings as the Wong study.

1.5.2 Current status of textured implants

Double-blind studies, that control all variables except texturing and have adequate numbers, are not available. Current studies of textured implants have provided conflicting results. However, certain findings have emerged from these studies. Textured surfacing appears to have no advantage with saline implants, whether they are inserted in the subglandular or the submuscular plane. Similarly, textured implants appear to have no advantage when silicone gel implants are inserted in the submuscular plane. Textured surfacing appears to have an advantage when silicone gel implants are inserted in the subglandular plane. However, that advantage has not been well elucidated. No difference has been demonstrated between Siltex and Biocell surface texturing, but no studies have compared these surfaces against each other.

Among the six recently quoted studies with gel implants, only two reported a follow-up of over 1 year. In both of those studies, blinding was broken after 1 year and there was significant attrition bias. Therefore, the preventative effect of texturing on capsular contracture has been confirmed to occur only over a short time period (1 year in most studies). In addition, it is unclear if texturization actually reduces the incidence or merely delays the onset of capsular contraction. Long-term studies are needed to see whether this advantage is maintained over time. Studies are also needed to elucidate the mechanism of prevention of capsular contracture.

In spite of the potential effect of textured gel implants on reducing capsular contracture, many plastic surgeons continue to use smooth surfaced gel implants. They have cited the studies with comparable capsular contracture rates. They are aware of the contour irregularities (wrinkling and palpable edges), which are more common with textured implants. They have also cited the theoretical increased risk of bacterial adherence, because of the greater surface area present in textured implants.

1.5.3 Moratorium

On January 6, 1992, Dr David Kessler, the then head of the FDA, announced a moratorium on the use of silicone gel breast implants (Kessler, 1992). This ban was also adopted in Canada. From 1963 until the moratorium on gel implants, about 95% of all breast implants inserted were silicone gel-filled. Only 5% were saline-filled. Since this time, in the United States, silicone gel implants have been available only for patients who are enrolled in the Special Adjunct Study, with an FDA approved protocol. By contrast, in Canada, silicone gel implants were approved for unrestricted use in anyone who requested them, on November 17, 2004.

In 1992, after the moratorium, implant manufacturers began developing fourth-generation gel implants, which had increased cross-linking to create a more viscous gel (cohesive gel). The cohesive nature of the gel was designed to restrict gel migration. The barrier layer of these implants was designed to reduce leakage of low molecular weight silicone oil. Almost in

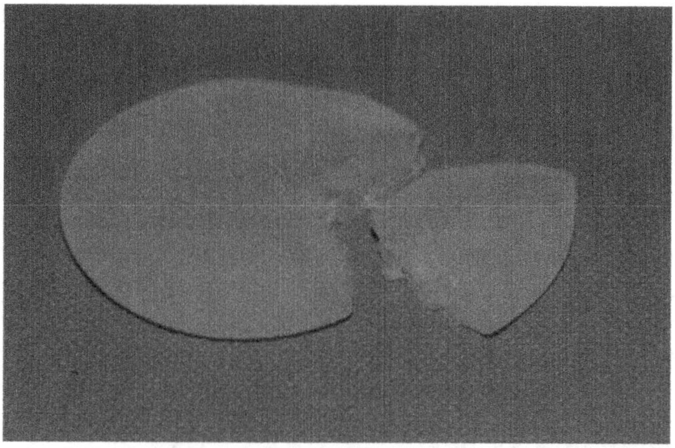

1.20 Fifth generation, contemporary, form stable, Mentor cohesive gel implant.

parallel to the fourth-generation implants, a fifth generation was also created, that had had a more cohesive, form-stable gel (Fig. 1.20). This technology allowed for the construction of anatomically shaped implants. Many of the changes in these implants remain proprietary. A variety of round and anatomic (contoured, teardrop) shapes are available. Anatomic implants are coated with a surface texturing, to restrict rotation. Round implants are available with smooth or textured surfaces. Fourth- and fifth-generation implants appear to have capsular contracture rates that are much lower than earlier implants (Heden *et al.*, 2001).

1.6 Inflatable implants

Like silicone gel-filled breast implants, there have been at least four 'eras', and a number of lesser variations, of inflatable implants (Middleton, 1993, 1998; Bondurant *et al.*, 1999). There was considerable overlap between these eras, depending on the manufacturer and model of the implant. The first era was characterized by the Simaplast implant, which was seamed. Second era saline implants (1968–1976) were made using a high-temperature vulcanized (HTV) platinum catalyzed process. They had a thinner shell than first era implants, and a correspondingly higher failure rate. After 1968, all shells made in the U.S. were seamless. They were formed by dipping a mandrel into a dispersion fluid. Third era saline implants (1976–1992) were made using a room temperature vulcanized (RTV) tin catalyzed procedure. These shells appeared to be stronger and more durable than the HTV shells (Middleton, 1993; Peters, 2002). After the FDA moratorium, fourth-generation saline implants were developed. Their exact formulation has remained proprietary.

1.6.1 Simaplast implants

Inflatable breast implants were introduced in 1965 by Dr Henri G. Arion. These implants were manufactured in Toulon, France, the birthplace of Brigitte Bardot. Arion stated that the Simaplast implant was the first one to produce a truly soft 'bouncy' breast. The initial Simaplast prosthesis consisted of a cream-colored elastomeric shell with a peripheral circumferential seam, with a seamed filling tube and valve permanently attached to one side (Fig. 1.21). The seam extended along the full length of the filler

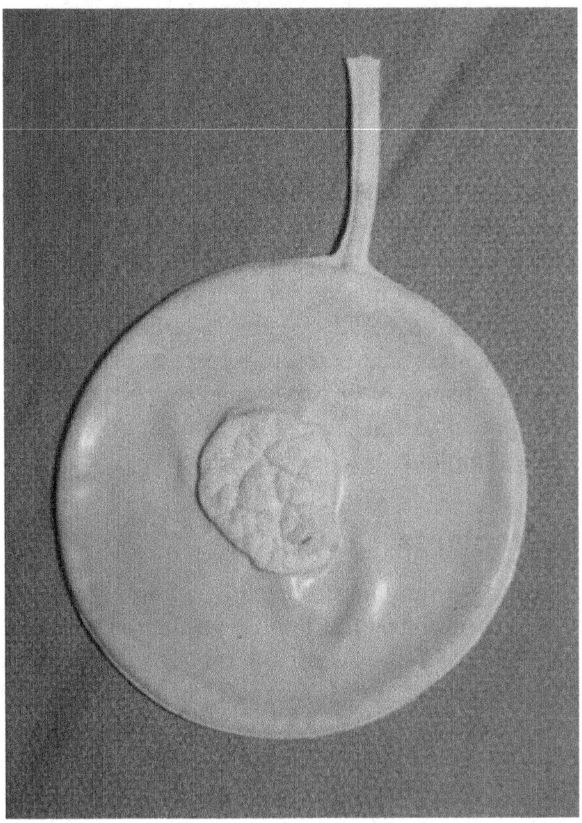

1.21 Simaplast breast implants were the first inflatable breast implants to be developed. This initial model (1965) was seamed, and had a cream-colored shell. The filling tube was also seamed. It was attached to one side of the implant. After filling, a Teflon plug provided a water-tight seal. The anterior surface of this implant has a central area of calcification.

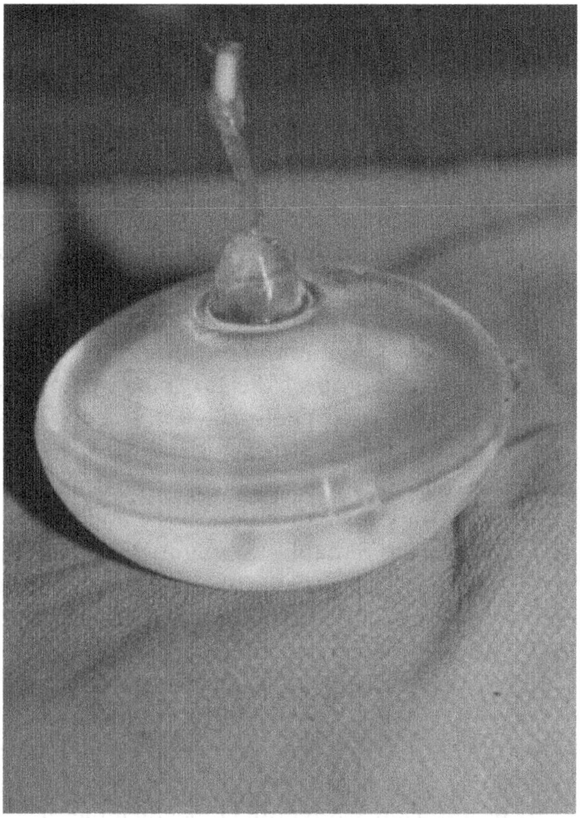

1.22 The second model of the Simaplast implant (1968) had a seamed clear shell with a seamless filling tube attached to the posterior surface of the implant. A Teflon plug provided a water-tight seal. The filling tube was buried into a pocket on the posterior surface of the implant.

tube. After filling, a Teflon plug was inserted into the filling tube to provide a watertight seal. Sometimes, this plug was tied with a suture. The initial model was introduced into North America in 1969. The implant shown in Fig. 1.21 was removed from a woman in 1999, 29 years after it was inserted. This implant had remained clinically intact for 29 years. The contralateral implant had deflated many years earlier.

In 1975, a second model of Simaplast inflatable implant was introduced. It had a clear, seamed, elastomeric shell with a seamless filling tube attached to the posterior surface of the implant (Fig. 1.22). The shell thickness of both models was 0.35 mm. After filling, a Teflon plug was inserted into the end of the filling tube, which was then buried into a pocket on the posterior surface of the prosthesis to conceal it. Initially, Arion suggested that the filling solution for these implants should be a hypertonic solution, consisting of 6% Dextran in normal saline. Subsequently, he recommended using saline alone.

The second model of Simaplast prostheses came in two sizes:100–250 cc and 200–350 cc. They were inserted in the subglandular plane, through a smaller incision than gel implants. They could be inflated to varying sizes, allowing a wider range of breast sizes. They were initially marketed by the Simaplast Company in Toulon, France. In 1966, they were also marketed in Yonkers, New York, Watertown, Massachusetts, and Montreal, Canada. It is interesting that the product information brochure for this implant recommended that if a patient became pregnant, then the prosthesis should be 'partially emptied in the second month of the pregnancy to minimize the cutaneous distention of the gravid state' (Peters, 2002). The prosthesis could then be refilled after weaning.

In 1967, the Simaplast Company was sold to the pharmaceutical firm Perdue Frederick. There are only a small number of published reports in the world literature describing the Simaplast implant (Wilson, 1969; Peters *et al.*, 1999). In 1969, Tabari described 30 cases of bilateral breast augmentation, with 10% of those implants undergoing early spontaneous deflation. By 1972, Williams reported a spontaneous deflation incidence for Simaplast implants of 76% within 3 years of implantation. Simaplast implants were then removed from the market. Only approximately 6000 pairs of Simaplast implants were sold worldwide (Arion, H.G., personal communication). In 1999, Peters and colleagues described two Simaplast implants that were removed after 23 years in situ. They were both clinically intact. The anterior surface of both implants had developed large areas of calcification, which appeared to develop after a surface abrasion to the surface of the elastomeric shell. One of the implants had undergone significant autoinflation.

The first inflatable implants manufactured in the United States were made by Heyer-Schulte in 1968 (Peters, 2002; Heyer-Schulte Corporation, 1974). They were designed by Dr Henry Jenny and were called the Jenny implant (Fig. 1.23). They were round and their shell was opaque and was 0.40 mm thick. They were the first RTV implants manufactured by Heyer-Schulte. Jenny initially implanted them in December 1968. After 1968, all implants manufactured in the United States were seamless. In 1971, clear round HTV implants were introduced. In 1972, the teardrop-shaped HTV implant became available. In 1973, a second teardrop-shaped HTV implant was introduced. Other models of round and teardrop implants followed. An optional Dacron backing could be ordered on many of these implants. Others came with a fenestrated patch, into which tissue could grow to anchor the implant. In 1974, Heyer-Schulte was acquired by American Hospital Supply. Mentor subsequently acquired this company in 1984. Mentor continued to manufacture the inflatable, silicone gel, and double

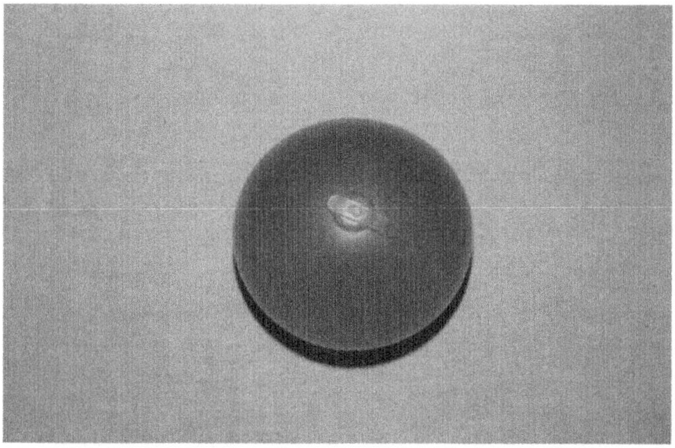

1.23 Jenny inflatable saline-filled implant (Heyer-Schulte, 1969) with a room temperature vulcanized opaque shell.

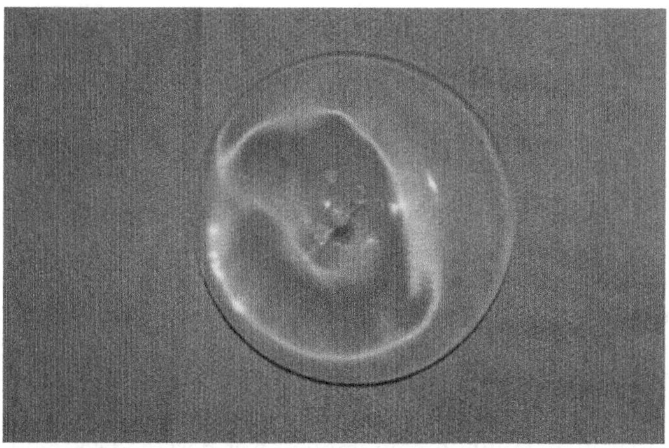

1.24 Contemporary Mentor inflatable implant with a diaphragm valve and a High Performance shell.

lumen models. In 1992, new models of these implants were introduced. Many of the specifications of these models are not known. A contemporary Mentor saline inflatable implant with a diaphragm valve and a High Performance shell is shown in Fig. 1.24.

Dow Corning produced their first inflatable breast implant in 1970 (Regnault *et al.*, 1972). Unfortunately, it had a deflation rate of 8% during the first year, forcing cancellation of the project. Dow Corning re-entered this area in 1977, with the development of the Varifil implant (Fig. 1.25). This was the first implant with the stronger 'High Performance' elastomeric shell. However, these implants also had a high leakage rate, which was probably

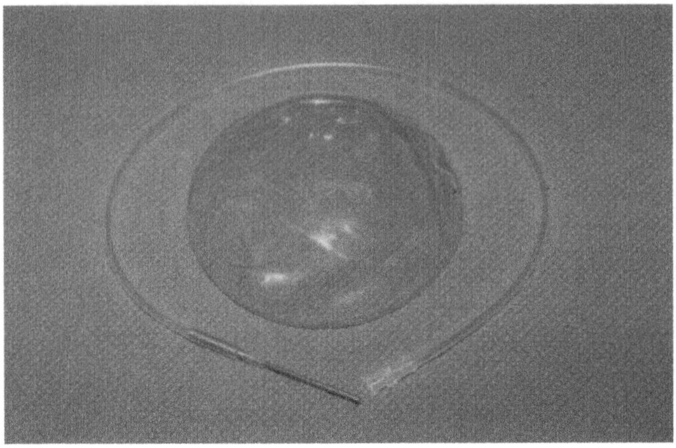

1.25 Varifil saline-filled implant (Dow Corning, 1977) with a leaflet valve and a High Performance shell. Throughout the history of inflatable implants, leaflet valves have been associated with high failure rates.

related to their leaflet valve. This forced Dow Corning to discontinue this implant in 1982.

By 1972, several types of saline implants had demonstrated spontaneous deflation rates of 76 to 88% during their first 3 years (Williams, 1972). Leaks were noted in seams, valve stems, and valve mechanisms. Many of these implants were therefore removed from the market. Most surgeons became discouraged with this high failure rate and began to use only silicone gel-filled implants. Heyer-Schulte subsequently became the dominant player in the inflatable implant market. It introduced the hydrocephalic valve (developed by Mr Schulte) that decreased the deflation rate significantly. Over the years, Heyer-Schulte developed several unique models of implants. For example, the Hartley double-lumen implant was designed so that the outer saline lumen could be deflated, in an attempt to reduce the firmness resulting from capsular contracture.

In 1980, Worton and coworkers described a 'new' mechanism for the late leakage of inflatable implants. This failure developed 6–7 years after insertion. In these patients, implants developed a small hole at the end of one of the wrinkles in the elastomeric shell. This was termed the 'fold flaw' leak and was thought to result from an 'internal abrasion' at a wrinkled (and presumably weakened), site in the shell. While this mechanism has not been scientifically proven, it seems logical. This type of leak would be expected to be more common in an implant that was under-inflated, which would allow more folds to develop. It would also be expected to be more common in saline implants than gel implants, because the more viscous nature of the gel would 'cushion' folds in the shell.

From 1963 through to 1991, about 95% of all implanted breast prostheses were filled with silicone gel, rather than saline. Following the moratorium on silicone gel breast implants in 1992, the use of inflatable saline implants escalated. In the early and mid-1990s there were deflation problems with certain models of saline implants, particularly those with leaflet valves (Peters, 1997). Subsequently, most saline implants incorporated diaphragm valves. In 2002, 95% of all breast implants inserted were saline-filled. Only 5% were gel-filled, and those were used only under the Special Access Guidelines in the United States and the Special Access Program in Canada (Peters, 2002).

1.7 Trilucent (*LipoMatrix*) implants – 1995 to 2000

One of the most important disadvantages of silicone gel-filled and saline-filled breast implants is that they are radiopaque on mammography (Fig. 1.26). This obscures varying amounts of breast parenchyma. By contrast, implants filled with triglycerides such as soybean oil (Trilucent, *LipoMatrix*, USA) are radiolucent (Fig. 1.27). This advantage stimulated clinical trials of Trilucent soybean oil-filled implants in the United Kingdom (Alcaraz *et al.*, 2001) and in North America (Young *et al.*, 1996). Between 1995 and 1999, over 18 000 women in the United Kingdom received Trilucent implants. The soybean oil in these implants was initially thought to be innocuous if the implants were to rupture. However, by 1999, several hundred patients had presented with acute unilateral breast enlargement following rupture. Potentially toxic aldehydes were found in some cases. In addition, the transponder on the implant was shown to interfere with MRI studies. Following this, the Medical Devices Agency of the United Kingdom released an emergency recall of all of these implants. Many Trilucent implants were also removed in North America. These implants have now been taken off the market.

The story of the evolution of breast implants has been a colorful one, extending over the past 50 years. Many different types of implants have come into vogue, and have then been discarded and replaced with newer products. Following the conclusive findings that silicone gel-filled breast implants are not related to the development of medical disease (Bondurant *et al.*, 1999), breast augmentation surgery has now become more popular than ever. In fact, it is currently the most common type of aesthetic plastic surgery done in North America.

Since the inception of fourth- and fifth-generation implants, manufacturers have conducted prospective multi-center trials to examine their safety and efficacy (Stevens *et al.*, 2008; Cunningham and McCue, 2009). Examples include the Mentor Adjunct Study (1992), Mentor Contour Profile Gel Study (1993), and Mentor Core Gel Study (2000), and the corresponding

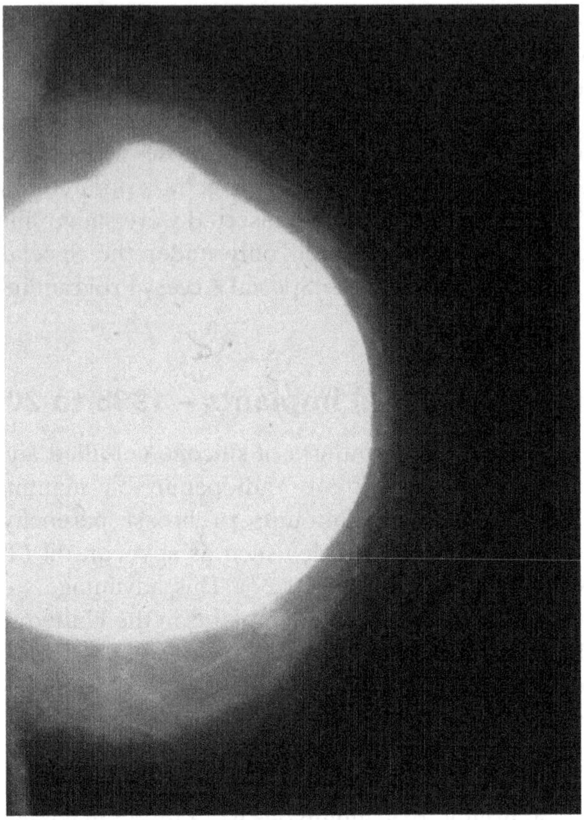

1.26 Silicone gel and saline-filled breast implants are radiopaque on film screen mammography. This can obscure imaging of breast tissue.

McGhan studies. Future research studies will likely concentrate on the following areas:

- The mechanism of failure of implants
- Further comparisons of round and anatomic implants to assess their advantages
- Analysis of patients' perceptions of their results
- Further studies on the etiology of capsular contracture
- Careful double-blinded studies comparing the rate of capsular contracture between smooth and textured implants. Most of the current studies in this area have had many limitations
- New designs in saline and silicone gel implants and other potential filler materials will be developed. However, this will be very slow because of the current very strict guidelines imposed by the FDA.

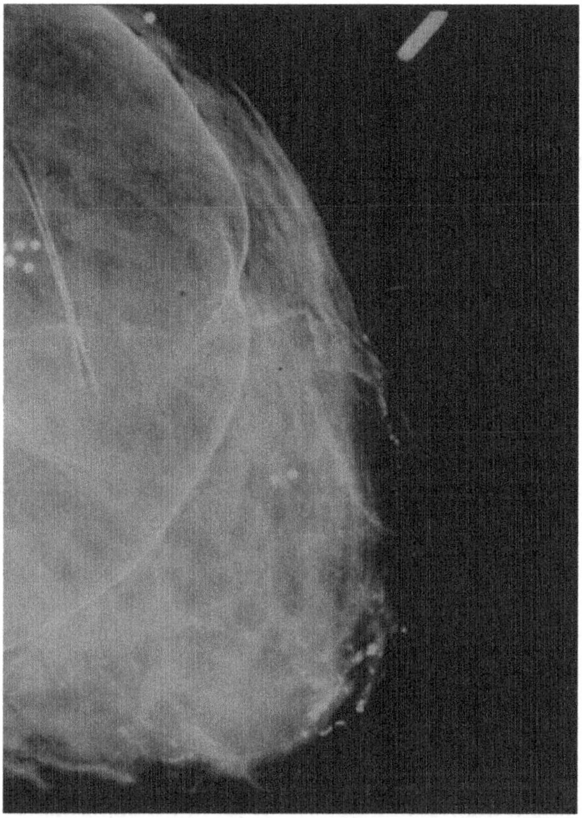

1.27 In contrast to Fig. 1.26, Trilucent (*LipoMatrix*) soybean oil-filled implants are radiolucent.

1.8 Acknowledgements

This study was funded by a grant from the Medical Research Council of Canada. The author is very grateful to Mr Jim Curtis, Technology Leader, Medical Device Operations, Dow Corning Corporation, for providing the Pangman Ivalon implant shown in Figs 1.7 and 1.8.

1.9 References

ACHAUER BM (1982), A serious complication following medical-grade silicone injections of the face, *Plast Reconstr Surg*, 71, 251–253.

AHN CY, KO CY and WAGAR EA (1995), Clinical significance of intracapsular fluid in patients' breast implants, *Ann Plast Surg*, 35, 445–457.

ALCARAZ JB, DOMINGUEZ ED and BUSQUESTS NM (2001), Rupture of Trilucent-type breast implants: A clinical case, *Aesth Plast Surg*, 24, 43–45.

ARION HG (1965), Presentation d'une prosthese retra mammaire, *J Soc French Gynec*, 2, 5–9.

ASHLEY FL (1970), A new type of breast prosthesis. Preliminary report, *Plast Reconstr Surg*, 45, 41–44.

ASHLEY FL (1972), Further studies on the Natural Y breast prosthesis, *Plast Reconstr Surg*, 49, 414–419.

ASPLUND O, GYLBERT L, JURREL G and WARD C (1996), Textured or smooth implants for submuscular breast augmentation: A controlled study, *Plast Reconstr Surg* 97, 1200–1206.

BARNSLEY GP, SIGURDSON LJ and BARNSLEY SE (2006), Textured surface breast implants in the prevention of capsular contracture among breast augmentation patients: a meta-analysis of randomized controlled trials, *Plast Reconst Surg*, 117, 2182–2190.

BARONE FE, PERRY L and KELLER T (1992), The biochemical and histopathic effects of surface texturing with silicone and polyurethane in tissue implantation and expansion, *Plast Reconstr Surg*, 90, 77–83.

BENOIT FM (1993), Degradation of polyurethane foam used in the Meme breast implant, *J Biomed Mater Res*, 27, 1341–1348.

BONDURANT S, ENESTER V and HERDMAN R (Editors) (1999), *Safety of Silicone Breast Implants*, Institute of Medicine. Washington, D.C., National Academy Press.

BURKHARDT BR (1984), Comparing contracture rates: Probability and theory and the unilateral contracture, *Plast Reconstr Surg*, 74, 527–532.

CAPOSSI A and PENNISI VR (1981), Clinical experience with polyurethane-covered gel-filled mammary prostheses, *Plast Reconstr Surg*, 68, 512–518.

CAPOZZI A (1991), Long-term complications of polyurethane-covered breast implants, *Plast Reconstr Surg*, 88, 458–461.

CHENG N, WANG Y, WANG J, ZHANG X and ZHONG H (2002), Complications of breast augmentation with injected hydrophilic polyacrylamide gel, *Aesthetic Plast Surg*, 26, 375–382.

CHENG NX, XU SL and DENG J (2006), Migration of implants: A problem with injectable polyacrylamide gel in aesthetic plastic surgery, *Aesthetic Plast Surg*, 30, 215–225.

CHINESE STATE FOOD AND DRUG ADMINISTRATION (2006), Polyacrylate hydrogel, China announces ban on polyacrylamide hydrogel breast implants. Press release.

CHRISTENSEN LH, BREITING VB and AASTED A (2003), Long-term effects of polyacrylamide hydrogel on human breast tissue, *Plast Reconstr Surg*, 111, 1883–1890.

CHRISTENSEN L, BREITING V and JANSEN M (2005), Adverse reactions to injectable soft tissue permanent fillers, *Aesthetic Plast Surg*, 29, 34–48.

CHRISTENSEN LH and BREITING V (2006), Management of postoperative complications of breast augmentation by injected polyacrylamide hydrogel, *Aesthetic Plast Surg*, 30, 132–133.

COLEMAN SR (2001), Injectable silicone returns to the United States, *Aesthetic Surg*, 21, 576–578.

COLEMAN DJ, SHARPE DT, NAYLOR IL, CHANDES CL and CROSS SE (1993), The role of the contractile fibroblast in the capsules around tissue expanders and implants, *Br J Plast Surg*, 46, 547–555.

COLLIS N, COLEMAN D, FOO IT and SHARPE DT (2000), Ten year review of a prospective randomized controlled trial of textured versus smooth silicone gel implants, *Plast Reconstr Surg*, 106, 786–792.

CONWAY H and DIETZ GH (1962), Augmentation mammaplasty. *Surg Gynec & Obst*, 114, 573–577.

CRONIN TD and GEROW FG (1964), Augmentation mammaplasty: A new natural feel prosthesis, *Transactions of the Third International Congress of Plastic Surgery*, Amsterdam, Excerpta Medica Foundation, pp 41–49.

CUNNINGHAM B and MCCUE J (2009), Safety and effectiveness of Mentor's Memory Gel Implants at 6 years, *Aesth Plast Surg*, 33, 440–444.

DUFFY DM (1998), Injectable Liquid Silicone: New Perspectives In: Klien AW, ed., *Tissue Augmentation in Clinical Practice* 1st ed. New York, Marcel Dekker Inc, pp 237–267.

EDGERTON MT and MCCLARY AR (1958), Augmentation mammaplasty: Psychiatric implications and surgical indications, *Plast Reconstr Surg*, 21, 279–305.

EDWARDS BF (1963), Teflon silicone breast implants, *Plast Reconstr Surg*, 32, 519–523.

FOOD AND DRUG ADMINISTRATION (1991), Current and Useful Information on Collagen and Liquid Silicone Injections, FDA Backgrounder, BG91-2.0.

FOOD AND DRUG ADMINISTRATION PRESS RELEASE (1992), Physicians to stop Injecting Silicone for Cosmetic Treatment of Wrinkles, 92–95.

FOOD AND DRUG ADMINISTRATION PRESS RELEASE (1994), 11/07/1994.

GERSUNY R (1903), Harte and weiche Paraffinprothesen, *Zentralbl Chir*, 30, 1–3.

GRINDLAY JH and CLAGETT OR (1951), Plastic sponge which acts as a framework for living tissue, *Arch Surg*, 63, 288–297.

HAKELIUS and OHLSEN L (1997), Tendency to capsular contracture around smooth and textured gel-filled silicone mammary implants: A 5-year follow-up, *Plast Reconstr Surg*,100, 1566–1572.

HANDEL N, JENSEN JA and BLACK Q (1995), The fate of breast implants: A critical analysis of complications and outcomes, *Plast Reconstr Surg*, 96, 1521–1533.

HARRIS HI (1961), Survey of breast implants from the point of view of carcinogenesis, *Plast Reconstr Surg*, 28, 81–83.

HEDEN P, JERNBECK and J HOBER M (2001), Breast augmentation with anatomical cohesive gel implants, *Clin Plast Surg*, 28, 531–552.

HESTER JR. TR, FORD NF and GALE PJ (1997), Measurement of 2,4-toluenediamine in urine and serum samples from women with Meme or Replicon breast implants, *Plast Reconstr Surg*, 100, 1291–1298.

HEYER-SCHULTE CORPORATION (1974), Product Information Binder, Santa Barbara, California.

INDEPENDENT REVIEW GROUP (1998), Silicone Gel Breast Implants, *The Report of the Independent Review Group*, Cambridge, U.K.

KESSLER DA (1992), The basis of the FDA's decision on breast implants, *N Engl J Med*, 326, 1713–1715.

KOLLE FS, *Plastic and Cosmetic Surgery*, New York, 1911.

LIU LW and TRUONG LD (1996), Morphologic characterization of polyvinyl sponge (Ivalon) breast prosthesis, *Arch Pathol Lab Med*, 120, 876–878.

MASTRUCERIO DN and PESQUEIRA MJ (1996), Severe granulomatous reaction and facial ulceration occurring after subcutaneous silicone injection, *J Am Acad Dermatol*, 34, 849–852.

MATTON G (1985), The history of injectable biomaterials and the biology of collagen, *Aesthetic Plast Surg*, 9, 133–140.

MIDDLETON MS (1998), Magnetic resonance evaluation of breast implants and soft-tissue silicone, *Top Magn Reson Imaging*, 9, 92–137.

MIDDLETON MS (1993), *Mammary Implant Product List 1962–1968*, UCSD Magnetic Resonance Institute, San Diego, CA.

MILOJEVIC B (1982), Complications after silicone injection therapy in aesthetic plastic surgery, *Aesthetic Plast Surg*, 20, 267–276.

NASO A (1953), Mastectomy and aesthetic reconstruction of the mammary region with polyethylene sponge, *Rioforma Med*, 675, 662–665.

ORENTREICH DS (2000), Liquid injectable silicone: techniques for soft tissue augmentation, *Clin Plast Surg*, 27, 595–612.

PANGMAN WJ and WALLACE RM (1955), The use of plastic prosthesis in breast plastic and other soft tissue surgery, *West J Surg Obstet Gynecol*, 63, 503–512.

PENNISI VR (1990), Long-term use of polyurethane breast prostheses: A 14-year experience, *Plast Reconstr Surg*, 86, 368–371.

PETERS W (1997), Failure properties of leaf valve inflatable saline breast implants, *Can J Plast Surg*, 5, 241–245.

PETERS W (2000), Current status of breast implant survival properties and the management of the woman with silicone gel breast implants, *Can J Plast Surg*, 8, 54–67.

PETERS W (2002), The evolution of breast implants, *Can J Plast Surg*, 10, 223–236.

PETERS W (2009), Complications from injectable materials used for breast augmentation, *Can J Plast Surg*, 17, 89–96.

PETERS W and LUGOWSKI S (2002), Survival properties of third-generation silicone gel breast implants, *Can J Plast Surg*, 10, 109–112.

PETERS W and SMITH DC (1981), Ivalon breast prostheses: Evaluation 19 years after implantation, *Plast Reconstr Surg*, 67, 514–518.

PETERS W, SMITH DC and LUGOWSKI S (1996a), Failure properties of 352 explanted silicone gel breast implants, *Can J Plast Surg*, 91, 828–834.

PETERS W, SMITH DC and LUGOWSKI S (1996b), Silicon capsule assays with low-bleed silicone gel breast implants, *Plast Reconstr Surg*, 97, 1311–1312.

PETERS W, SMITH DC and LUGOWSKI S (1999), Simaplast inflatable breast implants: Evaluation after 23 years in situ, *Plast Reconstr Surg*, 104, 1539–1544.

PICKRELL K (1962), *An evaluation of Etheron as an augmentation material in plastic and reconstructive surgery. A long-term clinical experimental study*, Presented at the Annual Meeting of the American Society of Plastic & Reconstructive Surgery, Hawaii.

POLLOCK H (1993), Breast capsular contracture: A retrospective study of textured versus smooth silicone implants, *Plast Reconstr Surg*, 91, 404–410.

QIAO Q, WANG X and SUN J (2005), Management for postoperative complications of breast augmentation by injected polyacrylamide hydrogel, *Aesthetic Plast Surg*, 29, 156–161.

RASO DS and GREENE WB (1997), Silicone breast implants: Pathology, *Ultrastructural Pathology*, 21, 263–271.

REGNAULT PC (1967), Indications for breast augmentation, *Plast Reconstr Surg*, 6, 524–529.

REGNAULT P, BAKER TJ and GLESON MC (1972), Clinical trial and evaluation of a proposed new inflatable mammary prostheses, *Plast Reconstr Surg*, 50, 220–226.

RIZKALLA M, DUNCAN C and MATTHEWS RN (2001), Trilucent breast implants: A 3-year series, *Br J Plast Surg*, 54, 125–127.

ROBINSON OF, BRADLEY EL and WILSON DS (1995), Analysis of explanted silicone implants: a report of 300 patients, *Ann Plast Surg*, 34, 1–7.

ROMM S (1992), *The changing face of beauty*, Mosby Year Book, pp 188–190.

SMAHEL J, SCHNEIDER and K DONSKI P (1977), Bizarre implants for augmentation mammaplasty: Long term human reaction to polyethylene strips, *Brit J Plast Surg*, 30, 287–290.

SPEAR SL, ELMARAGHY M and HESS C (2000), Textured-surface saline-filled silicone breast implants for augmentation mammaplasty, *Plast Reconstr Surg*, 105, 1542–1554.

STEVENS WG, PACELLA SJ and GEAR AL (2008), Clinical experience with a fourth-generation textured silicone gel breast implant: A review of 1012 Mentor MemoryGel breast implants, *Aesthetic Surg J*, 28, 642–647.

TABARI K (1969), Augmentation mammoplasty with Simaplast implant, *Plast Reconstr Surg*, 44, 468–470.

VASQUEZ G (2000), A ten-year experience using polyurethane-covered breast implants, *Aesth Plast Surg*, 23, 189–196.

VINNIK CA (1978), Silicone mastopathy, In: *Symposium on Aesthetic Surgery of the Breast*, Owsley JQ and Peterson RA, Eds, The C. V. Mosby Company pp 151–155.

WILLIAMS JE (1972), Experiences with a large series of Silastic breast implants, *Plast Reconstr Surg*, 49, 253–260.

WILKIE TF (1977), Late development of granuloma after liquid silicone injections, *Plast Reconstr Surg*, 60, 179–188.

WILSON CA (1969), Experiences with Arion's Simaplast inflatable prosthesis, *Southern Med J*, 62, 1107–1110.

WONG CH, SAMUEL M, TAK BK and SONG C (2006), Capsular contracture in subglandular breast augmentation with textured versus smooth breast implants: a systematic review, *Plast Reconstr Surg*, 118, 1224–1236.

WORTON EW, SEIFERT LN and SHERWOOD R (1993), Late leakage of inflatable silicone breast prostheses, *Plast Reconstr Surg*, 65, 302–306.

YOUNG VL, LUND H and DESTOUET J (1991), Effect of breast implants on mammography, *Southern Med J*, 84, 707–714.

YOUNG VL, LUND H and UEDA K (1996), Bleed of and biologic response to triglyceride filler used in radiolucent breast implants, *Plast Reconstr Surg*, 97, 1179–1193.

YU LT, LATORRE G and MAROTTA J (1996), In vitro measurement of silicone bleed from breast implants, *Plast Reconstr Surg*, 4, 756–764.

2 The development of breast implants

G. P. MAXWELL and A. GABRIEL,
Loma Linda University Medical Center, USA

Abstract: Female glandular hypomastia is a frequently encountered entity that occurs either developmentally or by postpartum involution. Historically, women have long sought breast enlargement to improve physical proportions, to foster a more feminine appearance, or to enhance self-image. This chapter explores the evolution of breast implants, and discusses saline-filled and silicone-filled implants. Silicone gel-filled implants have evolved from first-generation implants in the 1960s to the current fifth-generation devices and form-stable implants. Future trends indicate the increased use of acellular dermal products alongside implants.

Key words: breast implants, evolution, silicone, saline, breast augmentation.

2.1 Introduction

It is estimated that over 300 000 primary breast augmentations were performed in the United States in 2009, and therefore there are now over 3 million women with augmented breasts in this country.[1–3] Breast augmentation has become one of the most frequently performed operations in plastic surgery.[4] The popularity of the procedure is thought to be based on the satisfaction of the patients' results.[5] Women in general have been shown to have enhanced self-image, increased self-assurance, improved sexual functioning, and better interpersonal relationships after augmentation.[6]

2.1.1 History

The first report of successful breast augmentation appeared in 1895 in which Czerny described transplanting a lipoma from the trunk to the breast in a patient deformed by a partial mastectomy.[7] In 1954, Longacre described a local dermal-fat flap for augmentation of the breast.[8] Eventually, both adipose tissue and omentum were also used to augment the breast. However, the clinical results of using autogenous tissue for breast augmentation were often unpredictable and unacceptable.

During the 1950s and 1960s, breast augmentation with solid alloplastic materials was carried out using polyurethane, polytetrafluoroethylene

(Teflon), and expanded polyvinyl alcohol formaldehyde (Ivalon sponge). Ultimately, the use of these materials was discontinued after patients developed local tissue reactions, firmness, distortion of the breast, and significant discomfort.[9] Various other solid and semi-solid materials have been injected directly into the breast parenchyma for augmentation including epoxy resin, shellac, beeswax, paraffin, petroleum jelly and liquid silicone.

Liquid silicone (polydimethyl siloxane) was originally developed in the aeronautics industry during World War II. Because of its softness and inert nature, it attracted interest from the medical sector and was soon evaluated as an implantable medical device by plastic surgical researchers.[10,11] In 1961, Uchida reported the injection of liquid silicone into the breast for breast augmentation.[12] Unfortunately, injection of liquid silicone resulted in frequent complications including recurrent infections, chronic inflammation, drainage, granuloma formation and even necrosis.[13] Breast augmentation by injection of free liquid silicone was abandoned in most areas of the United States in light of these complications. Although none of these methods proved satisfactory, the introduction of the silicone gel breast implant in 1962 by Cronin and Gerow began the modern era of breast augmentation.[14] This is a two-component prosthetic device manufactured with a silicone elastomeric shell filled with a stable filling material, consisting of either saline solution or silicone gel.[14]

The silicone gel implants commercially available in the United States today are more refined and safer devices than their predecessors. The currently approved fourth-generation silicone implant devices are widely approved for patients over 22 years of age and the fifth-generation devices are currently under review by the Food and Drug Administration (FDA).

2.2 Breast implant evolution

2.2.1 Saline-filled implants

The use of inflatable saline-filled breast implants was first reported in 1965 by Arion in France.[15] The saline-filled implant was developed to allow the empty implant to be introduced through a relatively small incision. The implant was then inflated in situ.[16] Although the incidence of periprosthetic capsular contracture was lower with the saline-filled implants compared to the early silicone gel-filled implants, the deflation rate was initially quite high. The original saline-filled implants, manufactured by Simaplast in France, had a deflation rate of 75% at 3 years, and were subsequently withdrawn from the market. In 1968, the Heyer-Schulte Company introduced its version of the inflatable saline-filled breast implant (Mentor 1800) in the United States.

The thin, platinum-cured shell and the leaflet-style retention valve were two features of the early saline-filled implants that contributed to their high deflation rate.[17] The silicone elastomeric shell of the saline-filled implant has been improved by making it thicker and by employing a new room-temperature vulcanization (RTV) process. The original Heyer-Schulte saline-filled implant shell had a leaflet-style retention valve through which the implant was inflated.[18] A more reliable diaphragm valve was developed and is currently incorporated into the shell of all modern saline-filled breast implants.

Saline-filled implants are manufactured with a range of recommended fill volumes. Minimal breast asymmetry may be corrected by taking advantage of this range of fill volumes during placement of the implants. Under-filling saline-filled implants may lead to increased deflation rates due to folding or friction subjected to the implant shell, and is not recommended. Under-filling saline-filled implants may also lead to a wrinkled appearance or rippling with the breast in certain positions. Saline-filled implants have historically performed better when slightly overfilled, and when placed under thicker soft tissue coverage. Although these implants may be slightly overfilled, aggressive overfilling may lead to a more spherical shape and scalloping along the implant edge, with knuckle-like palpability and unnatural firmness. Another potential disadvantage of saline-filled implants is that the consistency of these implants on palpation is similar to that of water, compared to the more viscous feel of natural breast tissue. Several saline-filled breast prostheses are available from both manufacturers in the United States with different surface textures, shapes, and degrees of projection.

2.2.2 Silicone-filled implants

Silicone chemistry

Silicone is a mixture of semi-inorganic polymeric molecules composed of varying length chains of polydimethyl siloxane [$(CH_3)_2$-SiO] monomers. The physical properties of silicones are quite variable depending on the average polymer chain length and the degree of cross-linking between the polymer chains.[19] Liquid silicones are polymers with a relatively short average length and very little cross-linking. They have the consistency of an oily fluid and are frequently used as lubricants in pharmaceuticals and medical devices. Silicone gels can be produced of varying viscosity by progressively increasing the length of the polymer chains or the degree of cross-linking. The consistency of silicone gels may vary widely from a soft, sticky gel with fluid properties to a firm, cohesive gel exhibiting shape retention or form-stability, depending upon the polymer chain length and the degree of cross-linking. Extensive chemical cross-linking of the silicone gel polymer will produce a solid form of silicone referred to as an elastomer with a flexible, rubber-like quality. Silicone elastomers are used for the manufacture of facial implants, tissue expanders, and the outer shell of all breast prostheses. The versatility of these compounds has made them indispensable in aerospace engineering, medical devices and the pharmaceutical industry.

Silicone gel-filled implants

The first-generation silicone gel-filled implant was introduced in 1962 by Cronin and Gerow and was manufactured by Dow Corning Corporation[14]. The shell of the first-generation implant was constructed using a thick, smooth silicone elastomer as a two-piece envelope with a seam along the periphery. The shell was filled with a moderately viscous silicone gel. The implant was anatomically shaped (teardrop) and had several Dacron fixation patches on the posterior aspect to help maintain the proper position of the implant. Unfortunately, these early devices had a relatively high contracture rate that encouraged implant manufacturers to develop second-generation silicone gel-filled implants.

In the 1970s, the second-generation silicone implants were developed in an effort to reduce the incidence of capsular contracture with a thinner, seamless shell and without Dacron patches incorporated into the shell. These implants were round in shape (non-anatomical) and filled with a less viscous silicone gel to promote a natural feel. However, the second-generation breast implants were plagued by diffusion or bleed of small silicone molecules into the periprosthetic intra-capsular space, due to their thin permeable shell and less viscous silicone gel filler. This diffused silicone may be encountered as an oily, sticky residue surrounding the implant within the periprosthetic capsule during explantation of older silicone-filled implants. Microscopic silicone particles have been demonstrated within the periprosthetic tissues, and even within the draining lymphatics and axillary lymph nodes.[20] The phenomenon of silicone bleed has not been shown to create significant local or systemic problems.[21] However, long-term device failure issues have plagued these second-generation devices due to the thin weak shells.

The development of the third-generation silicone gel-filled implants in the 1980s focused on improving the strength and integrity of the shell in order to reduce silicone gel bleed from intact implants, and reducing implant rupture and subsequent gel migration. The former Inamed Corporation developed a multi-layer implant shell in which a patented barrier-coat material is sandwiched between two layers of silicone elastomer (Intrashiel®). The former Mentor Corporation also developed a shell for their silicone gel-filled breast implants, which consists of a multi-layered silicone elastomer. These third-generation prostheses reduced gel bleed to an almost immeasurable level and significantly lowered device shell failure rate.

After the FDA required the temporary removal of third-generation silicone gel implants from the American market in 1992, the fourth-generation gel devices evolved for their market re-introduction. These silicone gel breast implants were designed under more stringent ASTM (American Society for Testing Methodology) and FDA-influenced criteria for shell thickness and gel cohesiveness. Furthermore, the fourth-generation devices were manufactured with improved quality control.

With the evolution of the fifth-generation silicone gel implants, the concept of anatomically shaped implants was carried to the next level. Allergan (former Inamed) Corporation developed the BioDimensional® Planning System in which a matrix of 12 possible combinations of implant height and projection are available for the specific needs of the individual patient. These anatomically shaped (Style 410) implants are available only to investigators in the United States, with a range of volumes and any of the twelve combinations of low, moderate, and full height with low, moderate, full and extra projection. These implants are available to all plastic surgeons in Canada, without any restrictions. The Contour Profile® Gel (CPG) implant has been designed by the Mentor Corporation with a more rounded and projecting lower pole and a flatter, more sloping upper pole to yield a more natural breast shape in breast augmentation and reconstruction.

It is thought that as the gel flows inferiorly with gravity, the upper portion of the implant collapses due to its relatively reduced volume. To combat this characteristic of silicone gel implants, efforts have been made to develop fifth-generation devices containing more cohesive silicone gel, which exhibits less flow and more form-stability. The development of these fifth-generation devices has resulted from advances in the technology of silicone gel.

2.3 Alternative types of implant and safety aspects

2.3.1 Alternative filling materials

Manufacturers of breast implants have developed alternative filler materials in response to concerns about the safety of silicone gel.[22] In 1991, the Bioplasty Corporation introduced the MistiGold implant that uses polyvinylpyrrolidone (PVP) as the filling material. The PVP filling material is described as a bio-oncotic gel and is thought to be more radiolucent than silicone. NovaMed acquired Bioplasty and still markets the PVP-filled implant under the name NovaGold outside the United States. The PIP Corporation in France developed breast implants filled with a hydrated polysaccharide gel (hydrogel). However, there have been reports of swelling of hydrogel and PVP-filled implants postoperatively, due to the osmotic pressure gradient.[22] In December 2000, the British Medical Devices Agency issued an alert, citing a lack of studies that demonstrate the safety of these implants. In 1994, the LipoMatrix Corporation developed the Trilucent implant that was filled with a triglyceride derived from soybean oil. However, problems have developed with oil bleed, tissue irritation, and a foul rancid odor.[22] These implants were withdrawn from the market in 1999, and none of the alternative filling material implants is currently available in the United States.

2.3.2 Textured surface implants

Early attempts at augmentation with polyurethane sponge were not successful, but in 1970, Ashley reported the favorable use of a silicone gel implant covered with a thin layer of polyurethane foam.[23] Although the foam was placed on the implant primarily to maintain its position, clinical use seemed to show a decreased incidence of capsular contracture.[24] Throughout the 1980s, increasing numbers of plastic surgeons found polyurethane-covered silicone gel implants to produce aesthetically pleasing results with low capsular contracture rates.[25–28] The polyurethane surface adhered to the surrounding tissues, subsequently delaminated, and created a relatively non-contractible capsule.[29] Unlike smooth-surfaced implants that had to be mobile within their pocket, polyurethane-covered implants could be immobile yet soft. These devices had reached a zenith of popularity by 1990, when questions of the safety of polyurethane foam breakdown products caused Bristol-Myers Squibb, which owned Surgitek (the company manufacturing the implants), to withdraw from the breast implant market.[27]

The favorable clinical outcomes and commercial success of polyurethane-covered implants led American implant manufacturers to develop textured silicone surfaces in the hope of achieving similar results. In 1986, McGhan Medical (now Allergan) introduced Biocell textured implants and expanders, and Mentor introduced Siltex textured implants. These remain the two textured surfaces available in the United States today. Dow Corning subsequently introduced its Micro Structured Implant (MSI) in 1990, but the company withdrew from the market in 1992.

Biocell is an aggressive open-pore textured silicone surface composed of irregular pores having an average density of 3.1 pores/mm^2 with a mean pore size of 389 μm (range, 300 μm to 600 μm), and an average height of 500 μm to 800 μm. Created by a lost-salt technique, these interconnected pores promote adherence to the surrounding, developing capsule through an 'adhesive effect'.[30–32] This tissue adherence, which is clinically similar to that seen with the polyurethane foam surface, differs in that there is no delamination of the texturing, which occurs with polyurethane. The adhesive effect and tissue adherence are enhanced in Biocell-covered expanders; these have the added mechanical advantage of expansion pressure, which pushes the textured surface into the developing capsule and imparts its mirror image into the surrounding tissue.[33] Whereas adherence may not occur around the entire device or with all Biocell breast implants, there is a high friction coefficient around these devices, making them relatively immobile. Like polyurethane implants, Biocell implants are also characterized by 'immobility with softness'. Prospective clinical studies have demonstrated that Biocell textured silicone gel implants have a significantly lower incidence of capsule contracture than their smooth counterparts.[34] The results with saline implants are less definitive.[35,36]

Siltex is a less aggressive textured silicone surface created as a negative contact imprint of texturing foam. It is characterized by a raised, dense pattern of irregularities ranging in height from 65 μm to 150 μm and in width from 60 μm to 275 μm.[30,31] Siltex does not adhere to the surrounding tissue and is also not characterized by immobility with softness, as are polyurethane and Biocell.[31] Whereas Siltex-covered implants thus move within their surrounding pocket similar to smooth-walled implants, some prospective clinical studies have shown a significantly lower incidence of capsule contracture compared with their silicone gel smooth counterparts.[37] The results with saline implants are not as convincing.[35]

2.3.3 Enhanced cohesive gel implants

All silicone gel implants are cross-linked to maintain a gel consistency, and thus all silicone gel has cohesive properties. As the cross-linking is increased, the consistency or firmness of the 'liquid-feeling' gel changes to that of a soft cheese. The enhanced cohesive nature of these implants makes them 'form stable'. This refers to the implant's maintaining its shape in all positions (shape maintenance). These implants are designed in various anatomic dimensions in addition to round shapes and are collectively referred to as cohesive silicone gel implants. These form-stable implants are currently popular worldwide[38] and undergoing FDA-approved clinical trials in the United States.[39,40]

2.3.4 Safety

Interestingly, silicone-containing compounds are ubiquitous in everyday life. The general public has been exposed to them for over 50 years in consumer products such as hairsprays, suntan lotions, and moisturizing creams. Silicones are extremely resistant to the action of enzymes when implanted into living tissue largely due to their hydrophobic nature.[19] This makes silicone compounds extremely stable and inert. Silicones are often used in the consumer safety testing industry as the standard to which all other products are compared for biocompatibility.[19] While elemental silicon and silicone particles are detected in the periprosthetic tissues, the biological significance of this finding remains undetermined and uncharacterized.[41] In one study, no significant difference was found in levels of anti-silicone antibodies between patients who had silicone elastomer tissue expanders and control subjects.[42]

Several clinical studies have shown no difference in the incidence of autoimmune diseases in mastectomy patients receiving silicone gel implants compared to patients who had reconstruction with autogenous tissue.[43–47] Even meta-analysis research combining data from over 87 000 women has revealed no association between silicone breast implants and connective tissue diseases.[48–50] In the modern era of evidence-based medicine, it seems that the only exception to the rule of science is in the use of silicone gel-filled breast implants where lawsuits and hysteria supersede science. Notably, virtually all industrialized nations in the world – except the United States – use silicone gel implants almost exclusively for breast augmentation.

2.4 Future trends

Breast augmentation is the most common aesthetic procedure performed in the United States and perhaps in the world. As plastic surgeons, we strive to achieve perfection and continue to improve our surgical techniques to achieve the aesthetic breast form. Despite advances in implant technology and surgical techniques, undesired outcomes are encountered leading to revisionary surgeries.

The use of acellular dermal products (ADM) has been popularized in both breast and abdominal wall reconstructions.[51–61] In reconstruction cases, ADMs have been used to replace tissue, extend existing tissue or act as a tissue supplement. In aesthetic revisions, the ADM essentially becomes an outer conforming, regenerative layer of the implant. ADMs have been used to correct implant rippling and displacement, ptosis and capsular contracture.[62–64] ADMs are used as an alternative to other autologous tissue methods of coverage. They provide camouflage, to decrease rippling and increase soft tissue padding.[65] We have also used them for the treatment of capsular contracture (G. P. Maxwell, A. Gabriel and L. C. Perry, unpublished observations, 2009).

The rising demand for the use of ADM coupled with good outcomes in breast reconstructions, has spurred tremendous interest in its use for aesthetic breast surgery patients. We have used ADM for primary and revisionary aesthetic and reconstructive breast cases coupled with silicone implants and believe that intimate engagement of the implant with the

ADM is critical for the predictable long-term outcomes. With such advances in breast adjunctive materials, the future in implant technology remains bright.

2.5 References

1. MAXWELL, G.P. and A. GABRIEL, The evolution of breast implants. *Clin Plast Surg*, 2009, **36**(1): 1–13, v.
2. SPEAR, S.L. *et al.*, Inamed silicone breast implant core study results at 6 years. *Plast Reconstr Surg*, 2007, **120**(7 Suppl 1): 8S–16S; discussion 17S–18S.
3. CUNNINGHAM, B. and J. MCCUE, Safety and effectiveness of Mentor's MemoryGel implants at 6 years. *Aesthetic Plast Surg*, 2009, **33**(3): 440–4.
4. TERRY, M.B. *et al.*, The estimated frequency of cosmetic breast augmentation among US women, 1963 through 1988. *Am J Public Health*, 1995, **85**(8 Pt 1): 1122–4.
5. HETTER, G.P., Improved patient satisfaction with augmentation mammoplasty: the transaxillary subpectoral approach. *Aesthetic Plast Surg*, 1991, **15**(2): 123–7.
6. BANBURY, J. *et al.*, Prospective analysis of the outcome of subpectoral breast augmentation: sensory changes, muscle function, and body image. *Plast Reconstr Surg*, 2004, **113**(2): 701–7; discussion 708–11.
7. CZERNY, V., Plastic replacement of the breast with a lipoma. *Chir Kong Verhandl*, 1895, **2**: 216–8.
8. LONGACRE, J.J., Correction of the hypoplastic breast with special reference to reconstruction of the 'nipple type breast' with local dermo-fat pedicle flaps. *Plast Reconstr Surg*, (1946), 1954, **14**(6): 431–41.
9. BONDURANT S., ENESTER V. and HERDMAN R. (Editors), *Safety of Silicone Breast Implants*, Institute of Medicine. Washington, D.C.: National Academy Press, 1999.
10. BLOCKSMA, R. and S. BRALEY, The Silicones in Plastic Surgery. *Plast Reconstr Surg*, 1965, **35**: 366–70.
11. BROWN, J.B. *et al.*, Silicones in plastic surgery; laboratory and clinical investigations, a preliminary report. *Plast Reconstr Surg*, (1946), 1953, **12**(5): 374–6.
12. UCHIDA, J., Clinical application of crosslinked dimethylpolysiloxane, restoration of the breast, cheeks, atrophy of infantile paralysis, funnel-shaped chest. *J Plas Reconstr Surg,* 1961, **4**: 303–6.
13. ORTIZ-MONASTERIO, F. and I. TRIGOS, Management of patients with complications from injections of foreign materials into the breasts. *Plast Reconstr Surg*, 1972, **50**(1): 42–7.
14. CRONIN, T.D. and R.O. BRAUER, Augmentation mammaplasty. *Surg Clin North Am*, 1971, **51**(2): 441–52.
15. ARION H.G., Presentation d'une prosthese retra mammaire. *J Soc French Gynec*, 1965, **2**: 5–9.
16. REGNAULT, P. *et al.*, Clinical trial and evaluation of a proposed new inflatable mammary prosthesis. *Plast Reconstr Surg*, 1972, **50**(3): 220–6.
17. YOUNG, V.L. and M.E. WATSON, Breast implant research: where we have been, where we are, where we need to go. *Clin Plast Surg*, 2001, **28**(3): 451–83, vi.
18. LAVINE, D.M., Saline inflatable prostheses: 14 years' experience. *Aesthetic Plast Surg*, 1993. **17**(4): 325–30.

19. BRODY, G.S., Silicone technology for the plastic surgeon. *Clin Plast Surg*, 1988, **15**(4): 517–20.
20. BARNARD, J.J. *et al.*, Distribution of organosilicon polymers in augmentation mammaplasties at autopsy. *Plast Reconstr Surg*, 1997, **100**(1): 197–203; discussion 204–5.
21. THOMSEN, J.L. *et al.*, Histologic changes and silicone concentrations in human breast tissue surrounding silicone breast prostheses. *Plast Reconstr Surg*, 1990, **85**(1): 38–41.
22. SPEAR, S.L. and S. MARDINI, Alternative filler materials and new implant designs: what's available and what's on the horizon? *Clin Plast Surg*, 2001, **28**(3): 435–43.
23. ASHLEY, F.L., A new type of breast prosthesis. Preliminary report. *Plast Reconstr Surg*, 1970, **45**(5): 421–4.
24. ASHLEY, F.L., Further studies on the natural-Y breast prosthesis. *Plast Reconstr Surg*, 1972, **49**(4): 414–9.
25. HERMAN, S., The Meme implant. *Plast Reconstr Surg*, 1984, **73**(3): 411–4.
26. HESTER, T.R., JR. *et al.*, A 5-year experience with polyurethane-covered mammary prostheses for treatment of capsular contracture, primary augmentation mammoplasty, and breast reconstruction. *Clin Plast Surg*, 1988, **15**(4): 569–85.
27. HESTER, T.R., JR., J.B. TEBBETTS, and G.P. MAXWELL, The polyurethane-covered mammary prosthesis: facts and fiction (II): a look back and a 'peek' ahead. *Clin Plast Surg*, 2001, **28**(3): 579–86.
28. MELMED, E.P., Polyurethane implants: a 6-year review of 416 patients. *Plast Reconstr Surg*, 1988, **82**(2): 285–90.
29. SINCLAIR, T.M., C.L. KERRIGAN, and J. SAMPALIS, Biodegradation of polyurethane foam, revisited, in the rat model. *Plast Reconstr Surg*, 1995, **96**(6): 1326–35.
30. BARONE, F.E. *et al.*, The biomechanical and histopathologic effects of surface texturing with silicone and polyurethane in tissue implantation and expansion. *Plast Reconstr Surg*, 1992, **90**(1): 77–86.
31. DANINO, A.M. *et al.*, Comparison of the capsular response to the Biocell RTV and Mentor 1600 Siltex breast implant surface texturing: a scanning electron microscopic study. *Plast Reconstr Surg*, 2001, **108**(7): 2047–52.
32. MAXWELL, G.P. and D.C. HAMMOND, Breast implants: smooth versus textured. *Adv Plast Reconstr Surg*, 1993, **9**: 209–14.
33. MAXWELL, G.P. and P.A. FALCONE, Eighty-four consecutive breast reconstructions using a textured silicone tissue expander. *Plast Reconstr Surg*, 1992, **89**(6): 1022–34; discussion 1035–6.
34. HAKELIUS, L. and L. OHLSEN, Tendency to capsular contracture around smooth and textured gel-filled silicone mammary implants: a five-year follow-up. *Plast Reconstr Surg*, 1997, **100**(6): 1566–9.
35. BURKHARDT, B.R. and C.P. DEMAS, The effect of Siltex texturing and povidone-iodine irrigation on capsular contracture around saline inflatable breast implants. *Plast Reconstr Surg*, 1994, **93**(1): 123–8; discussion 129–30.
36. BURKHARDT, B.R. and E. EADES, The effect of Biocell texturing and povidone-iodine irrigation on capsular contracture around saline-inflatable breast implants. *Plast Reconstr Surg*, 1995, **96**(6): 1317–25.
37. MALATA, C.M. *et al.*, Textured or smooth implants for breast augmentation? Three year follow-up of a prospective randomised controlled trial. *Br J Plast Surg*, 1997, **50**(2): 99–105.

38. HEDEN, P. *et al.*, Long-term safety and effectiveness of style 410 highly cohesive silicone breast implants. *Aesthetic Plast Surg*, 2009, **33**(3): 430–6; discussion 437–8.
39. BENGTSON, B.P. *et al.*, Style 410 highly cohesive silicone breast implant core study results at 3 years. *Plast Reconstr Surg*, 2007, **120**(7 Suppl 1): 40S–8S.
40. CUNNINGHAM, B., The Mentor Study on contour profile gel silicone MemoryGel breast implants. *Plast Reconstr Surg*, 2007, **120**(7 Suppl 1): 33S–9S.
41. SCHNUR, P.L. *et al.*, Silicon analysis of breast and periprosthetic capsular tissue from patients with saline or silicone gel breast implants. *Plast Reconstr Surg*, 1996, **98**(5): 798–803.
42. ROHRICH, R.J., J.B. ROBINSON, JR., and L.H. HOLLIER, JR., Determining the safety of the silicone envelope: in search of a silicone antibody. *Plast Reconstr Surg*, 1997, **99**(5): 1472.
43. EDWORTHY, S.M. *et al.*, A clinical study of the relationship between silicone breast implants and connective tissue disease. *J Rheumatol*, 1998, **25**(2): 254–60.
44. GABRIEL, S.E. *et al.*, Risk of connective-tissue diseases and other disorders after breast implantation. *N Engl J Med*, 1994, **330**(24): 1697–702.
45. GABRIEL, S.E. *et al.*, Risk of connective tissue disorders (CTDs) among women with breast implants. *Life Sci*, 1995, **57**(19): 1737–40.
46. PARK, A.J. *et al.*, Silicone gel-filled breast implants and connective tissue diseases. *Plast Reconstr Surg*, 1998, **101**(2): 261–8.
47. SCHUSTERMAN, M.A. *et al.*, Incidence of autoimmune disease in patients after breast reconstruction with silicone gel implants versus autogenous tissue: a preliminary report. *Ann Plast Surg*, 1993, **31**(1): 1–6.
48. KARLSON, E.W. *et al.*, Association of silicone breast implants with immunologic abnormalities: a prospective study. *Am J Med*, 1999, **106**(1): 11–19.
49. SANCHEZ-GUERRERO, J., Autoantibody testing in patients with silicone implants. *Clin Lab Med*, 1997, **17**(3): 341–53.
50. SANCHEZ-GUERRERO, J. *et al.*, Silicone breast implants and the risk of connective-tissue diseases and symptoms. *N Engl J Med*, 1995, **332**(25): 1666–70.
51. BINDINGNAVELE, V. *et al.*, Use of acellular cadaveric dermis and tissue expansion in postmastectomy breast reconstruction. *J Plast Reconstr Aesthet Surg*, 2007, **60**(11): 1214–8.
52. BREUING, K.H. and S.M. WARREN, Immediate bilateral breast reconstruction with implants and inferolateral AlloDerm slings. *Ann Plast Surg*, 2005, **55**(3): 232–9.
53. BREUING, K.H. and A.S. COLWELL, Inferolateral AlloDerm hammock for implant coverage in breast reconstruction. *Ann Plast Surg*, 2007, **59**(3): 250–5.
54. COTHREN, C.C. *et al.*, Chest wall reconstruction with acellular dermal matrix (AlloDerm) and a latissimus muscle flap. *Plast Reconstr Surg*, 2004, **114**(4): 1015–7.
55. GARRAMONE, C.E. and B. LAM, Use of AlloDerm in primary nipple reconstruction to improve long-term nipple projection. *Plast Reconstr Surg*, 2007, **119**(6): 1663–8.
56. GLASBERG, S.B. and R.A. D'AMICO, Use of regenerative human acellular tissue (AlloDerm) to reconstruct the abdominal wall following pedicle TRAM flap breast reconstruction surgery. *Plast Reconstr Surg*, 2006, **118**(1): 8–15.
57. KIM, H., K. BRUEN, and D. VARGO, Acellular dermal matrix in the management of high-risk abdominal wall defects. *Am J Surg*, 2006, **192**(6): 705–9.

58. NAHABEDIAN, M.Y., Secondary nipple reconstruction using local flaps and AlloDerm. *Plast Reconstr Surg*, 2005, **115**(7): 2056–61.
59. PATTON, J.H., JR., S. BERRY, and K.A. KRALOVICH, Use of human acellular dermal matrix in complex and contaminated abdominal wall reconstructions. *Am J Surg*, 2007, **193**(3): 360–3; discussion 363.
60. SALZBERG, C.A., Nonexpansive immediate breast reconstruction using human acellular tissue matrix graft (AlloDerm). *Ann Plast Surg*, 2006, **57**(1): 1–5.
61. SPEAR, S.L. *et al.*, Acellular dermis-assisted breast reconstruction. *Aesthetic Plast Surg*, 2008, **32**(3): 418–25.
62. DUNCAN, D.I., Correction of implant rippling using allograft dermis. *Aesthet Surg J*, 2001, **21**(1): 81–4.
63. BAXTER, R.A., Intracapsular allogenic dermal grafts for breast implant-related problems. *Plast Reconstr Surg*, 2003, **112**(6): 1692–6; discussion 1697–8.
64. COLWELL, A.S. and K.H. BREUING, Improving shape and symmetry in mastopexy with autologous or cadaveric dermal slings. *Ann Plast Surg*, 2008, **61**(2): 138–42.
65. GAMBOA-BOBADILLA, G.M., Implant breast reconstruction using acellular dermal matrix. *Ann Plast Surg*, 2006, **56**(1): 22–5.

3
The chemistry and physical properties of biomedical silicones

M. A. BROOK, McMaster University, Canada*

Abstract: Silicone polymers are used in a variety of biomaterials applications. This chapter reviews the chemical composition of silicones, and their structure as polymers based on a repeating dimethylsiloxane unit, then describes the production of silicones using the Rochow–Müller or Direct Process. The chemical structure of silicones is discussed, highlighting how this affects the physical properties of silicones and their uses. The formation of silicone elastomers is examined, along with methods such as high-temperature and room-temperature vulcanization (HTV, RTV) and platinum-cured hydrosilylation. The use of silicone materials in the manufacture of breast implants is reviewed. A discussion of the perceived chemical risks associated with breast implants is provided.

Key words: silicones, polymers, breast implants, elastomers and gels by hydrosilylation, silica, bleed.

3.1 Introduction

3.1.1 Silicones in society

Silicones have been known since the early 1900s, although they were only commercialized in the early 1940s when viable processes for their preparation were independently developed during World War II in both Germany and the United States.[1,2,3] These polymers possess very unusual properties, which are not matched by alternative materials, including organic polymers. As a consequence, they touch almost all aspects of modern life in developed societies, and it is virtually impossible to go through a day without coming into contact with them. Humans are commonly exposed to silicones by a variety of routes:

*The author provided information on the chemical nature of the platinum in silicone breast implants at the FDA panel hearing on breast implants April 2005 on behalf of Inamed Corporation (now Allergan). He was also a member of a Health Canada regulatory advisory panel considering applications by Mentor Corporation and Inamed Corporation for new breast implant models in March and September 2005.

- topically, e.g. personal care products, bathroom sealants, furniture polish,
- through ingestion of food additives, e.g. defoamers in 'antacid' formulations,
- through inhalation, e.g. personal care products and, in some cases,
- by injection – glass syringes are usually lubricated with silicone fluids.

Silicones have found broad utility in medical devices used both externally and internally. For example, silicones are used to coat the electrical leads of pacemakers, in shunts and, among other things, in breast implants, the subject of this book.

The safety of silicone breast implants was challenged in the early 1990s, which led to a decade and a half of extensive litigation and many studies on the impact of silicones in the body, both through biological research studies and epidemiological assessment.[4,5] Although there remain concerns that a small number of patients with relatively rare diseases may be affected by silicone, the record of safety of implanted silicones has been shown to be extremely good. For a very clear narration of the entire silicone breast implant story, the reader is directed to *Science on Trial*,[4] and for a symposium presenting both sides of the debate, *Immunology of Silicones*.[5]

3.1.2 Chemical composition of silicones

Silicones are made up, for the most part, of four chemical elements: silicon, oxygen, carbon and hydrogen. Chemists make the distinction between things that are, or could be, constituents of living things, and those that are not. Organic chemicals always contain carbon and hydrogen, and frequently other elements like nitrogen and sulfur (in proteins), and phosphorus (in genetic material like DNA and RNA). Things that do not contain carbon are inorganic or metallic. Because of the presence of carbon, silicones are technically 'organometallic' polymers.

A polymer is generally comprised of a repeating unit ('mer') that – when linked together – forms a long chain ('polymer'). Polymer properties are always affected both by their chemical constituents and their chain length: further differences arise when the polymer chains are branched and, even more, when crosslinked into elastomers/rubbers (see below). Although in principle it is possible to make myriad types of silicones with different organic groups, most commercial silicones have methyl (Me = CH_3) substituents and are based on a dimethylsiloxane ('D', Me_2SiO) repeat unit (an Si-O bond is a 'siloxane' as shown in Fig. 3.1). The most important non-methyl substituents are hydrido (~H) and vinylgroups (~$CH{=}CH_2$, where the '~' is the bond that joins the group to the rest of the silicone), which are used for crosslinking, and phenyl 'Ph' (~C_6H_5) groups that convey thermal stability to the polymer. In practice, small quantities of different siloxane

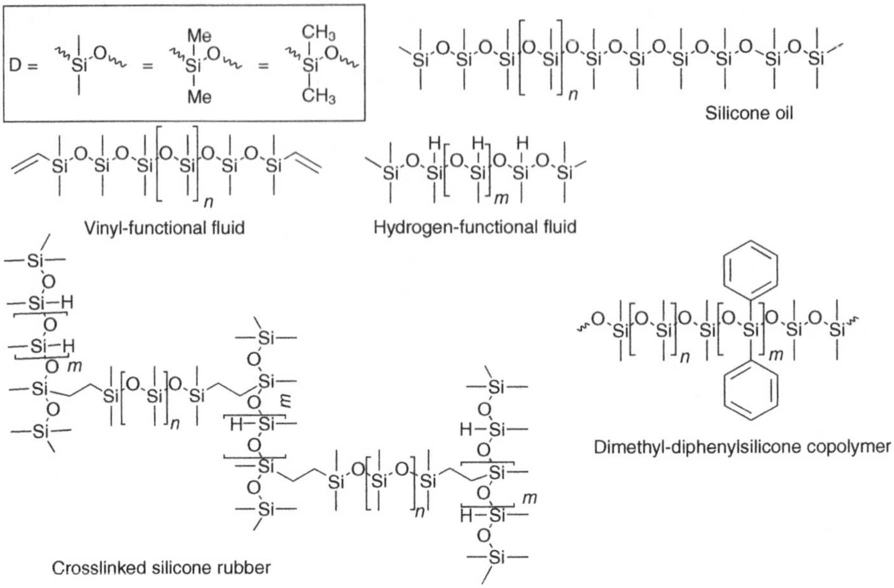

3.1 Typical silicone structures.

units within or at the end of the dimethylsiloxane chains allow the polymer chemist to introduce both subtle and profound changes in properties of the polymer. For example, silanols groups (SiOH) at chain ends can be used to increase the length of the chain.

3.1.3 The production of silicones

There is no reliable evidence suggesting that organic silicon (containing Si-C and C-H bonds) compounds exist in nature:[6] organic silicon compounds result from human intervention. Naïvely, one would imagine that silicones should be very inexpensive because the starting materials for their preparation are primarily sand and methanol. However, silicones are typically more expensive than most organic polymers because of the energy expended in their synthesis.

The constituents

The organic component of silicones comes from methanol (H_3COH) that is converted by hydrochloric acid into chloromethane (H_3CCl). The inorganic component comes from silica. The earth's crust is made up of about 80% silica (SiO_2) or silicates, which can be crystalline or amorphous. Various forms of crystalline silica include beach sand and gem stones like amethyst.

A crystal has well-defined shapes and facets because the atoms are packed into very regular patterns. Amorphous silica has the same molecular formula (SiO_2), but because the atoms are more randomly organized, they do not form crystals. Certain animal and plant organisms, such as diatoms and rice, respectively, use amorphous silica as a reinforcing agent or for protection; window glass is a form of amorphous silica that contains other constituents. The differences between these types of silica, when considering breast implants, are further discussed in Section 3.3.2.

The first step of the silicone manufacturing process requires temperatures of about 2000 °C, which imposes a significant cost on their manufacture. Silica is converted to elemental silicon in the presence of a source of carbon such as wood chips, with concomitant production of CO and CO_2. The resulting silicon 'metal' can be used, for example, to create computer chips, or further reacted to give organic silicon compounds.

The Direct (Rochow–Müller) Process for making silicones

The most commercially viable process for introducing carbon onto silicon involves the 'Direct Process,' also known in North America as the Rochow Process, and in Europe as the Müller Process (or occasionally as the Müller–Rochow Process) for their respective inventors in the 1940s.[1] Although in principle many different organic compounds, in the form of organic chlorides, could be used, the Direct Process is only efficient in combining chloromethane (H_3CCl) with silicon and, on average, two molecules of chloromethane react with each silicon atom to give mostly dichlorodimethylsilane (Fig. 3.2).[7] This is the key feedstock for the silicone industry.

Manufacturing of silicone

When water is added to dichloromethane, the chloride groups are replaced by oxygen to give a series of low molecular weight cyclic/ring and linear silicones (Fig. 3.3). Thus, in the silicone synthesis process, one starts with a silicon atom possessing four bonds to oxygen and converts it to a silicon atom with two bonds to oxygen and two bonds to methyl groups.

The linear and cyclic silicones may be used in their own right. For example, D_5 ($(Me_2SiO)_5$) is commonly used in a variety of personal care products.

$$MeCl + Si \xrightarrow[\Delta]{Cu} Me_2SiCl_2 + MeSiCl_3 + MeHSiCl_2 + SiMe_4 + SiCl_4$$

Major product >85% | Minor products | Very minor products

3.2 The Direct Process.

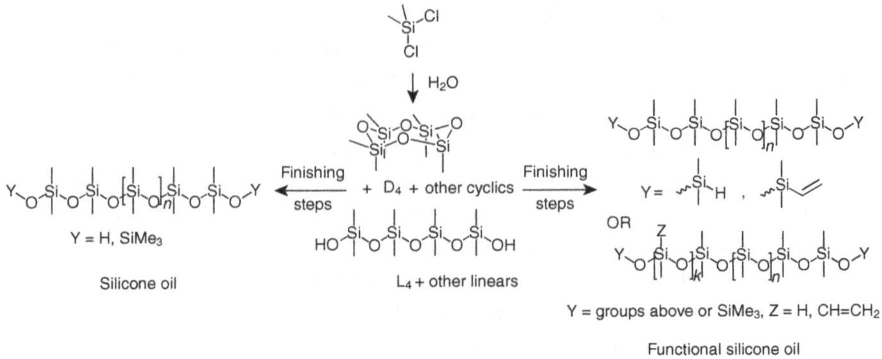

3.3 Conversion of chlorosilanes into silicone products.

However, longer silicone chains are commonly needed and are produced by increasing the size (molecular weight) using both linear and cyclic products as feedstocks (Fig. 3.3). These simple linear chains with Me_3Si groups on the end, usually known as silicone oils, are used in a wide variety of products: of particular relevance for this chapter is their use as part of the gel in silicone gel breast implants.

Functional silicones are required to make rubbers (see Section 3.3.2). For some rubbers (including the rubbers used as bathroom sealants), it is sufficient to create linear silicone oils with silanol groups on the end (SiOH, Y=H, Fig. 3.3): these undergo condensation with small molecules to give networks.[8] Alternatively, linear silicones containing SiH groups are combined with other linear silicones containing vinyl groups. Silanol, SiH and vinyl-containing polymers are normally created from small dimethylsilicones that are 'equilibrated' with the appropriate functional groups (Z = H, $CH{=}CH_2$, Fig. 3.3).[9]

3.2 Properties of silicones

3.2.1 The differences between silicones and organic polymers

There are constitutional differences between silicones and organic polymers, primarily involving the presence of silicon in the former. In organic polymers such as polyethylene, polypropylene, polystyrene, and others, the chains have localized zig-zag patterns. Adjacent chains interact through a variety of means including crystallization and interchain entanglement (like spaghetti). With the average bond angles of 109° the polymer behaves very much like a linked metal chain, which 'kinks' when chains are bent. By forcing interchain interactions, such kinks help solidify polymer chains. These types of interactions are quantified by glass transition temperatures

(T_g, a softening temperature) and melting points (T_m, where the polymer becomes a fluid). For the three polymers mentioned, the T_gs range from about –10 to 100 °C and T_ms are all over 100 °C. The very different properties of silicone polymers are associated with their molecular structure. Key factors include the high polarization of the Si-O bond (the way in which the two atoms share electrons), the longer length of the Si-O bond compared to a C-C bond, the presence of only two groups on each oxygen, and the presence of two CH_3 groups on each silicon atom.[5] The bond angles around the oxygen atoms are much more open (~145°) than around carbon in organic polymers (~109°). In addition, each silicon atom bears two methyl groups, which makes it difficult for one chain to associate with another. The comparatively high linearity of the Si-O-Si angle and the very low torsional energy required to twist the silicone chains results in highly mobile polymers. Unlike more rigid, kinked organic polymers, dimethylsilicones can readily reptate (undergo snake-like thermal motion) below their melting points. As a consequence, crystallization of silicones is relatively unusual: dimethylsilicones (PDMS, poly(dimethylsiloxanes)) have a T_g of about –123°C and T_m of –55 °C. That is, silicones are fluids at room temperature irrespective of the chain length or average molecular weight.[10]

The combination of high flexibility, mobility, hydrophobicity of the methyl groups and polarization of Si-O bonds leads to polymers with very interesting properties. Silicones are highly thermally stable, only starting to undergo decomposition above about 300 °C.[11] They are also excellent electrical insulators. The most important property of silicones (in the author's view) is their hydrophobicity (water repellency), which is higher than all organic polymers except fluorocarbon polymers such as Teflon®. Unlike fluorocarbon polymers, however, which are rigid materials at room temperature, silicones are fluids and can migrate to interfaces. The surface activity of silicones is the basis of their uses, depending on structure, as foaming agents, defoamers, adhesives, and anti-fog agents, among a very long list of applications.[12,13]

3.2.2 The biocompatibility of silicones

Silicones have a long history of use in biomedical applications. They are widely used in the form of elastomers (rubbers) and oils. For example, most glass syringes used to deliver drugs are lubricated with silicone oils; silicone oil is contained in food and antacid formulations as a defoamer (anti-gas agent); silicone elastomers are used in baby bottle nipples, in pacemakers, in shunts, and in testicular and breast implants.

Primarily because of fervent scientific activity associated with breast implants in the two decades following 1990, a wealth of data about the health and safety of silicones has been accumulated. Initially, it was speculated that silicones, particularly in patients with silicone gel breast implants, could be affiliated with increased rates of cancer in general and breast cancer in particular, and in a variety of autoimmune and other diseases. (Litigators looked extensively for a link between silicones and human disease. When no such link was evident, the pseudo-disease siliconesis was created, which manifested in non-measurable outcomes.[2]) At the time of writing, there remains concern that there may be weak associations between silicone breast implants and suicide, and also with the rare disease anaplastic large cell lymphoma (ALCL).[14] Overall, however, there seems to be no firm link between systemic disease in humans and silicones: their use in many applications, including breast implants, continues to be approved by health regulatory agencies around the world.[15]

3.2.3 Silicones and the environment

The behavior of dimethylsilicones in the environment has been relatively well studied. Volatile compounds, particularly cyclic siloxanes, mostly partition to air where they undergo facile oxidation, typically within about 2 weeks.[16–19] Longer chain polymers are non-volatile and essentially insoluble in water. When found in waste water, the polymers do not affect the biological operation of the waste water plants;[20] the silicone ends up primarily in sludge that is normally spread on agricultural fields. Silicones on soil undergo efficient depolymerization (degradation) to dimethylsilanediol ($Me_2Si(OH)_2$), catalyzed by clay, providing the soil is not too wet. This compound then undergoes degradation to innocuous silica.[21] Thus, the studies suggest that irrespective of the type of methylsilicone, the final degradation product is amorphous silica, similar to the silica initially used in the synthesis of silicon metal. Thus, the silicon loop – from sand to silicon to silicones to sand – is a closed loop.

Environmental agencies, at the time of writing, are examining the cyclic silicones D_4 and D_5 in detail.[22] The accumulated data suggests that, at high concentrations, some organisms in sediment are negatively affected by the presence of high concentrations of these compounds. Regulators are concerned that these cyclic compounds may accumulate in sediment at elevated concentrations. However, it is rather difficult to achieve such concentrations because the cyclic compounds partition first to water, then air, and then degrade.

3.3 The main forms of silicones/siloxanes

3.3.1 Silicone oils

Silicone oils are simply long chain polymers made up of multiple D units (Me_2SiO). As the chain length and molecular weight increases, the mobility goes down and the viscosity goes up (viscosity is resistance to flow: there is an increase in viscosity as one goes from cooking oil, to motor oil and axle grease). Other relevant silicone oils include those that have mixed methyl/phenyl units, e.g. Me_2SiO + MePhSiO and/or Ph_2SiO. Compounds with fluorocarbon side chains are of historical relevance for breast implants ($F_3CCH_2CH_2SiMeO$). Oils may be non-functional ($OSiMe_3$ end groups), or functionalized with SiH, Si-vinyl, OH or other groups that permit the oils to be converted into elastomers.

3.3.2 Silicone elastomers

An elastomer or rubber is a material that, when stretched, returns back (essentially) to its original shape – an elastic response. We are all familiar with rubber bands. The process of making a rubber involves crosslinking polymer chains into a network. When the material is stretched, the chains uncoil until they are fully extended and then 'recoil' when the force is released. As a general rule, the larger the number of crosslinks in a given volume (crosslink density), and the shorter the distance between crosslink sites, the more rigid is the rubber and the 'bouncier' it is. Eventually, of course, when the crosslink density gets too high, the material loses elasticity and become brittle. One can imagine the effects of crosslink density changes by comparing the behavior of a mosquito net with a fish net: the latter with larger chain lengths between crosslinks has a lower crosslink density and is much more flexible.

Silicone oils are turned into elastomers by a variety of means. The process involves linking chains of silicone together (the silicone oils described above) until a three dimensional network is formed. Traditionally, in commerce, three methods are used to do this: radical chemistry, condensation cure (moisture cure) room temperature vulcanization, and platinum-cured hydrosilylation (or hydrosilation – addition cure).[6] Although all of these have previously been used in breast implants, only the latter two are commercially relevant at the present time. These are discussed in turn in more detail.

Radical cure (high-temperature vulcanization (HTV))

Radicals are atoms or molecules with an unpaired electron. They react vigorously and, typically, not selectively. Radical processes are used for certain applications to create crosslinked silicones, although this process has become much less important for silicone breast implants.

Initiators (Y_2, Fig. 3.4) are heated to high temperature and decompose to give radicals ($Y^{\bullet}$) that react with the methyl groups on silicones to generate carbon-based radicals. These can either (re)combine in a relatively

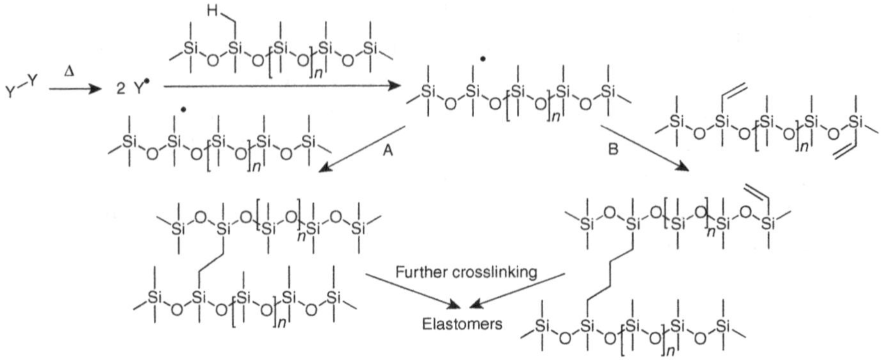

3.4 Radical crosslinking.

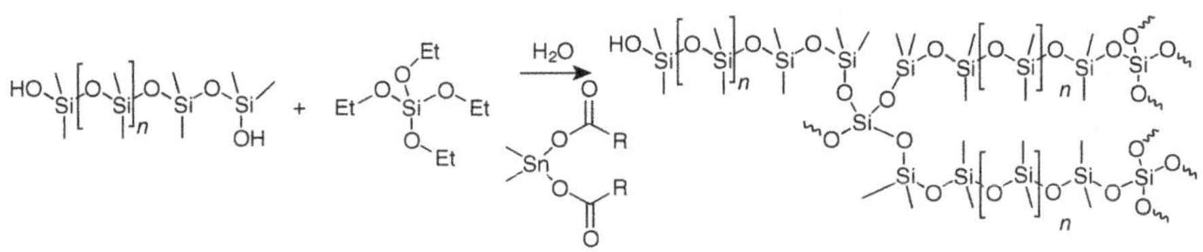

3.5 RTV silicone crosslinking.

inefficient process (due to low concentrations of radicals) or, under milder conditions, react with vinyl groups present to create three carbon spacers between silicone chains (Fig. 3.4 A vs B). There is little control over where the radical reactions occur, unlike the other types of crosslinking used for silicones.

Condensation cure (room-temperature vulcanization (RTV))

Small silane molecules with either three or four (replaceable) functional groups are readily available. These react efficiently in the presence of a tin- or titanium-derived catalyst with silanol-terminated silicone oils: one of the co-constituents of the process is water. There are currently environmental concerns in Europe (the REACH program) about the fate of tin catalysts. This curing process is frequently referred to as room temperature vulcanization (Fig. 3.5). It is therefore possible to formulate these silicones as a 'one pot' system that only starts to react once water from the atmosphere is present. This chemistry is used for silicone sealants in bathrooms and is one that most readers will be familiar with: the vinegary smell when the silicone cures is a signal that the crosslinking reaction is occurring. This process is typically used to form the shells/envelopes (see below) in saline breast implants.

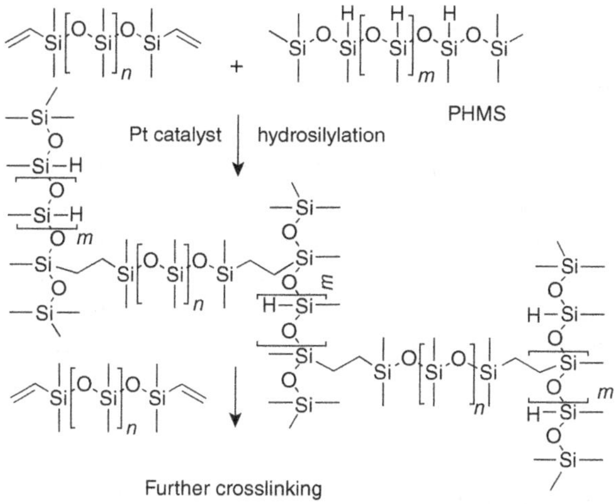

3.6 Platinum-catalyzed silicone crosslinking (PHMS, polyhydromethylsiloxane).

Addition cure

Silicone gel breast implants benefit from platinum-catalyzed crosslinked silicones in two different forms: the chemistry used to create both the external shell and the internal gel is identical. The differences in the materials properties are a consequence of the other additives in the respective formulations. When vinyl-containing silicone oils are combined with hydrogen-containing silicone oils in the presence of a catalyst, typically based on platinum, a 'hydrosilylation' reaction occurs that links the chains with a two-carbon bridge. The crosslink density is controlled by the number of functional groups on the respective types of oils and different network structures, resulting from different distributions of functional groups on the chain, can be used to tune the elastomer properties (Fig. 3.6).[6]

3.3.3 Silicone gels

The last type of silicone we will discuss is a gel. The formal definition of a gel is a network, including a polymeric network, swollen with a mobile solvent/fluid.[23] Gelatin desserts are an example of gels consisting of cross-linked proteins (gelatin) swollen with water. Silicone gels used in breast implants are comprised of silicone elastomers, normally formed by addition cure, that are swollen with silicone oils. By controlling the crosslink density and viscosity of the silicone oil it is possible to prepare gels with a wide variety of viscosities/cohesivities ranging from the viscosity of motor oil to that of 'gummy bear' candies.

3.3.4 Formulation of silicones

Reinforcement with silica

Silicone elastomers are mechanically weak. They are easy to tear, particularly if they have been cut or nicked. The weakness can be addressed in large measure by adding 'fillers', which are normally small particles of silica.[24] As discussed below, silicone gel breast implants are filled with amorphous rather than crystalline silica. The additional surface area of the particles and the high affinity of silicone oils for the silica significantly strengthens the silicone. Silica is not used to reinforce the gel component of breast implants.

3.4 Silicones in breast implants

Detailed descriptions of the construction of breast implants are provided elsewhere in this book (See Chapter 2). We include this simplified section to correlate the materials described above with their use in silicone breast implants. Note that the different generations of implants vary mostly in the details of the devices: the materials have changed over the decades but, with respect to chemistry, in only relatively minor ways. By way of contrast, the performance of the devices has changed and improved significantly.

3.4.1 Structural elements

All silicone breast implants consist of a silicone elastomer outer envelope, which comes into contact with the biology of the chest wall region after implantation, and a core that gives the device its 'feel' (Fig. 3.7). In principle, the aesthetic feel should approximate mammary tissue as closely as possible. Medical devices based on silicone are made from 'medical grade' silicone. The difference between this quality of material and normal silicone is that the silicones have undergone extensive testing after manufacture to demonstrate that they do not contain biological entities and they do not elicit an abnormal biological response.

3.4.2 Saline implants

The 'core' in saline implants is salt water: the saline has an ionic strength that is isotonic with that found in the body. The saline solution is added after the envelope has been implanted, and the physician can choose the level to which the device is filled. Typically, the envelopes used for saline implants are created from silicone elastomers cured using condensation chemistry.

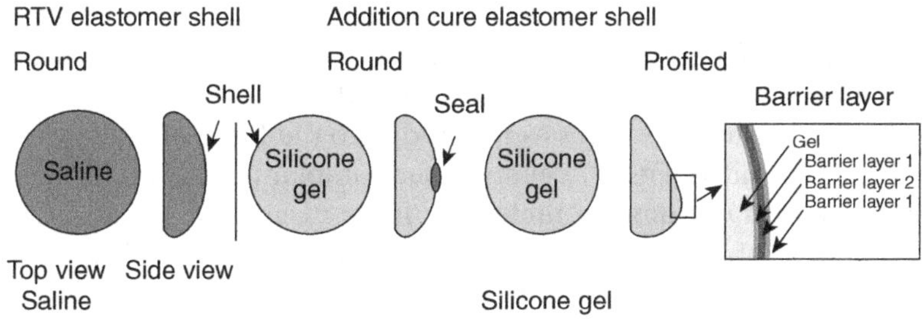

3.7 Structure of silicone breast implants. Left side: saline with RTV elastomer shell. Right side: silicone gel showing round and profiled styles and an expansion of the shell showing multiple layers.

3.4.3 Silicone gel implants

Silicone gel breast implants (Fig. 3.7) are composed of a silicone elastomer envelope normally cured by platinum-catalyzed addition chemistry. However, the actual base materials used for the elastomer have evolved historically, and may also be distinct by manufacturer.

Early implants had pure dimethylsiloxane elastomer shells, cured by platinum, that were reinforced with silica. However, these envelopes had a tendency to 'bleed' (to allow silicone oil to migrate from the gel in the core to the outside of the device; see also Section 3.9). To mitigate bleed, manufacturers developed multilayer envelopes (see expansion, Fig. 3.7). Each layer was based on different silicone elastomers that had to adhere well to one another, but which also had to repel the dimethylsilicone oil found in the gel. The principle 'like dissolves like' dictates that the dimethylsilicone oils in the gels should not swell efficiently into silicones with a lower Me_2SiO content. Different manufacturers developed silicone layers for shells based on mixtures of Me_2SiO, Ph_2SiO and $CF_3CH_2CH_2SiMeO$ monomers. For example, some currently available devices have a tri-layer envelope consisting of an inner layer with $(Me_2SiO)_{95\%}(Ph_2SiO)_{5\%}$; a middle layer of $(Me_2SiO)_{85\%}(Ph_2SiO)_{15\%}$; and an outer layer of $(Me_2SiO)_{95\%}(Ph_2SiO)_{5\%}$ copolymers. Platinum is used to cure all three layers, each of which is reinforced with amorphous silica. These envelopes are associated with significantly reduced levels of gel bleed compared to elastomers based on (Me_2SiO) monomers alone.

The core of a silicone gel breast implant is, not surprisingly, a silicone gel, although in very early devices fluids were used. The viscosity/cohesivity of the gels have changed considerably over the decades. Typical gels in commercial devices are comprised of about 15% of a silicone elastomer network swollen with 85% silicone oil. The viscosity of the silicone oil can vary. However, a more important parameter for aesthetic feel/performance is the crosslink density of the elastomer, which is primarily responsible for the firmness of the final implant. In most of the world, two devices are currently available commercially, mobile gels (round, Fig. 3.7, if one holds the device in the air, its shape changes as it sags due to the force of gravity), and cohesive gels (profiled, Fig. 3.7, 'gummy bear' implants; they are firm, hold their shape and do not deform under the force of gravity; see also Chapter 4). At the time of writing, cohesive implants were only available in the United States for patients who elect to participate in a clinical trial. The manufacture of gel implants involves forming an envelope on a mold. After removal, there is an opening in the envelope that must be sealed with a 'patch'. A needle is inserted into the patch, the gel is injected, and after removal of the needle, a small drop of silicone is placed on the needle entry point, sealing the device. The patch is often made of silicone elastomer prepared by condensation cure.

3.4.4 Issues with silicone breast implants

As will be discussed elsewhere in this book, the toxicity of silicones was initially brought into question during the litigation involving silicone breast implants in the 1990s and 2000s (Chapter 1 and Chapter 2). Initially, it was inferred that all the constituents (silicones per se, mobile silicones, silica and platinum) were toxic, and key players in a putative association between silicone gel breast implants and disease. Detailed studies of each of the constituents subsequently showed these hypotheses to be incorrect. The data developed now paints a picture that fits in with general experience: the safety of silicones in humans is very good, regardless of the routes of exposure, which include topical contact, inhalation, ingestion, injection and implantation.

Silicone breast implants can undergo rupture. Manufacturers perform a series of tests to quantify the robustness of the devices prior to implantation and have extensively examined devices that rupture. These tests are described elsewhere in this book (Chapter 7). We examine here three other issues that are associated with the chemistry of the implants: gel bleed, the chemistry of platinum, and silica.

Leachables

There is evidence that both silicone oil[13] from the gel and platinum,[25] probably from the shell but possibly also from the gel, can migrate from the implant to the adjacent biological environment. Regulators (and litigators) have examined the implication of such 'bleed' on patient health. As noted below, the consensus is that the magnitude and type of bleed from currently regulated devices does not impact on the health of patients.

Gel bleed

Current barrier layer envelopes are comprised of silicones that are chemically distinct from the dimethylsilicones that are found in the gel. The larger the difference in chemical composition of shell and gel, the lower the propensity of dimethylsilicone oils to swell the shell and then migrate from the inside to the outside of the device. However, even though multi-layer barrier envelopes are used in current devices, a small amount of gel bleed still occurs. As a general rule (and not including degradable polymers), larger polymer structures tend to stay localized in vivo at the site of implantation (except in the GI tract) and become walled off in a fibrous capsule as part of normal wound healing responses. However, lower molecular weight materials are more mobile in the body. Regulatory agencies are particularly concerned with silicones of molecular weights below about 1500 g/mol (approximately $(Me_2SiO)_n$ $n < 20$).[26] Calculations based on in vitro release studies suggest that less than 1% of weight will be lost over the lifetime of an implant: measurements on explanted devices showed essentially no weight change within the error of the experiment. This information was presented at the FDA Panel on Silicone Gel Breast Implants held in April 2005. While the information was publicly presented, it is apparently not currently on the FDA website.

Biological studies of the small cyclic silicone D_4 in mammals including humans shows that it is mobile in the body, and is mostly exhaled, with the residue excreted after oxidation/hydrolysis in the liver. That is, D_4 is dealt with by the body in an analogous way to other hydrophobic materials, including lipids. Much less data is available for other silicones, although one can speculate that mobility in the body will decrease with increasing molecular weight; loss via exhalation will similarly decrease with increasing molecular weight/decreasing volatility. It should also be noted that various biological entities such as macrophages have been identified as agents that facilitate migration of higher molecular weight silicones throughout the body, for example, to lymph glands.

Platinum chemistry

Concern was raised that the platinum, used to cure the silicone into elastomers and gels, was toxic.[27,28,29] It was asserted that the platinum in implants is, or was transformed into, an ionic form. Such ionic platinum compounds can have high biological activity and may be associated with an allergic response: some ionic platinum compounds are used as anti-cancer agents, and are associated with significant side effects.[30]

A more detailed analysis of this proposal showed it to be inconsistent with both scientific precedent and good science.[31,32] The paper was ultimately brought into question by the editors of the journal.[33] The general consensus among scientists, an opinion with which the FDA is affiliated,[20] is that platinum found in breast implants is in the form of platinum metal, a form known to have good biocompatibility.

Amorphous vs crystalline silica

There are many forms of silica (SiO_2), but we focus only on pure amorphous and crystalline silicas. Quartz is the crystalline silica that may be found as sand on any beach. As noted above, in a crystal, atoms are arrayed in well-defined units that stack together to give a three dimensional crystal. By contrast, amorphous silica, which is often the product of small organisms including diatoms and sponges, has no long-range order. Silicosis is a fibrotic disease of the lungs associated with breathing air containing small particles of crystalline quartz over extended periods of time. No similar association has been made between amorphous silica and silicosis.[34,35,36]

At one time, it was proposed that the silica used as a reinforcing agent in breast implants was detrimental to patient health. In part, this was based on an erroneous suggestion that silicones are oxidized, under biological conditions, to the crystalline silica. This proposal has been largely discredited not least of which because amorphous, not crystalline, silica is used to reinforce the silicone elastomers used in the shells of breast implants.

3.5 References

1. ROCHOW, E. G. *J. Am. Chem. Soc.* 1945, 67, 693.
2. ROCHOW, E. G. *US Patent* 2380995 (to General Electric), 1941.
3. MÜLLER, R. *German Patent* C57411, 1942.
4. ANGELL, M. *Science on Trial*, Norton: New York, 1995.
5. *Immunology of Silicones*, Potter, M.; Rose, N. R., Eds., Springer: Berlin, 1996.
6. *Silicon Biochemistry*, Evered, D.; O'Connor, M., Eds., (Ciba Foundation Symposium 121), Wiley: Chichester, U.K., 1986.
7. LEWIS, L. N. *Recent Advances in the Direct Process*, In *The Chemistry of Organic Silicon Compounds,* Rappoport, Z.; Apeloig, Y., Eds., Wiley: Chichester, U.K., 1998, Vol. 2, p. 1581.
8. BROOK, M. A. Silicones, In *Silicon in Organic, Organometallic, and Polymer Chemistry*, John Wiley & Sons, Inc.: New York, 2000, p. 256.
9. THOMAS, D. R. *Crosslinking of Silicones*, In *Siloxane Polymers*, Clarson, S. J.; Semlyen, J. A.; Eds., Prentice Hall: Englewood Cliffs, NJ, 1993.
10. NOLL, W. *Chemistry and Technology of Silicones*, Academic Press: New York, 1968.
11. *Ibid.* ref. 7, pp. 439–440.
12. OWEN, M. J. Surface Chemistry and Application. In *Siloxane Polymers*, Clarson, S. J.; Semlyen, J. A., Eds. Prentice Hall: Englewood Cliffs, 1993; p. 309.
13. OWEN, M. J. Siloxane Surface Activity. In *Silicon-Based Polymer Science: A Comprehensive Resource*, Zeigler, J. M.; Fearon, F. W. G., Eds. American Chemical Society: Washington, D.C., 1990; pp. 705–739.

14. www.fda.gov/MedicalDevices/ProductsandMedicalProcedures/Implantsand-Prosthetics/BreastImplants/ucm239995.htm
15. *Safety of Silicone Breast Implants*. Institute of Medicine, National Academy Press: Washington, 2000.
16. BUCH, R. R.; INGEBRIGTSON, D. N. *Envir. Sci. Technol.* 1979, 13, 676.
17. LEHMANN, R. G.; VARAPRATH, S.; ANNELIN, R. B.; ARNDT, J. L. ENVIR. *Toxicol. Chem.* 1995, 14, 1299.
18. LEHMANN, R. G.; FRYE, C. L.; TOLLE, D. A.; ZWICK, T. C. *Water, Air & Soil Pollution* 1995, 83, 1.
19. CARPENTER, J. C.; CELLA, J. A.; DORN, S. B. *Environ. Sci. Technol.* 1995, 29, 864.
20. WATTS, R. J.; KONG, S.; HALING, C. S.; GEARHART, L.; FRYE, C. L.; VIGON, B. W. *Water Res.* 1995, 9, 2405.
21. LENTZ, C. W. *Ind. Res. Dev.* 1980, 139.
22. REISCH, M. S. Storm Over Silicones, *Chem. Eng. News* 2011, 89 (18, May 2), 10–13.
23. IUPAC. Compendium of Chemical Terminology, 2nd ed. (the 'Gold Book'). Compiled by McNaught, A. D.; Wilkinson, A. Blackwell Scientific Publications, Oxford, 1997. XML on-line corrected version: http://goldbook.iupac.org; Nic, M.; Jirat, J.; Kosata, B., updates compiled by Jenkins, A. 2006, (ISBN 0-9678550-9-8. doi:10.1351/goldbook.
24. CLARSON, S. J.; MARK, J. E. *Siloxane polymers*, PTR Prentice Hall, Englewood Cliffs, NJ, 1993, 637.
25. www.fda.gov/MedicalDevices/ProductsandMedicalProcedures/Implantsand-Prosthetics/BreastImplants/ucm064040.htm
26. www.fda.gov/MedicalDevices/DeviceRegulationandGuidance/GuidanceDocuments/ucm071228.htm#44
27. FLASSBECK, D.; PFLEIDERER, B.; KLEMENS, P.; HEUMANN, K. G.; ELTZE, E.; HIRNER, A. V., *Anal. Bioanal. Chem.* 2003, 375, 356–362.
28. MAHARAJ, S. V. M. *Anal. Bioanal. Chem.* 2004, 80, 4–89.
29. LYKISSA, E. D.; MAHARAJ, S. V. M. *Anal Chem.* 2006, 78, 2925–2933.
30. NIEZBORALA, M.; GARNIER, R. *Occup. Environ. Med.* 1996, 53, 252–257.
31. LAMBERT, J. M. *J. Biomed. Mater. Res. Part B* 2006, 78B, 167–180.
31. BROOK, M. A. *Anal. Chem.* 2006, 78, 5609–5611.
33. MURRAY, R. W.; *Fenselau,* C. C. *Anal. Chem.* 2006, 78, 5233.
34. PASTERIS, J. D.; WOPENKA, B.; FREEMAN, J. J.; YOUNG, V. L.; BRANDON, H. J., *Amer. Mineral.* 1999, 84, 997–1008.
35. PASTERIS, J. D.; WOPENKA, B.; FREEMAN, J. J.; YOUNG, V. L.; BRANDON, H. J. *Plast. Reconstruct. Surg.* 1999, 103, 1273–1276.
36. MERGET, R.; BAUER, T.; KÜPPER, H.; PHILIPPOU, S.; BAUER, H.; BREITSTADT, R.; BRUENING, T. *Arch. Toxicol.* 2002, 75, 625–634.

4
Cohesive gel breast implants

P. HEDÉN, Akademikliniken, Sweden

Abstract: Breast augmentation surgery has been revolutionised with the advent of more controllable breast shaping based on dimensional planning and measurements. Previously only non-form stable implants filled with responsive gel were available and thus breast augmentation was more arbitrary, based on evaluation of adequate volume rather than a careful measurement of the biological conditions.

The foundation for this new era was the introduction of form stable implants in the mid 1990s and the development of a wide range of implant shapes, both anatomical with varying height and projections and round with variable projection. Breast augmentation has thereby become much more customised in relation to patients' desires and biological prerequisites. To achieve superior results with these new implants it is important to understand the fundamental differences that exist in choosing, planning and executing the surgery compared to traditional breast augmentation techniques. This chapter will describe how this is done in detail.

Key words: high cohesive form stable silicone gel, dimensional planning, breast shaping, sharp atraumatic technique, submammary fold approach.

4.1 Introduction

In 1994, the first anatomical form stable breast implant, the Style 410 FM breast implant, was introduced by the McGhan Corporation (later called Inamed, and now Allergan). The fact that the advent of these form stable implants would result in a paradigm shift was probably not fully understood by the industry or doctors at the time. The fundamental differences between form stable and non-form stable filling material are still not well understood by many plastic surgeons. What is then the fundamental difference between traditional breast augmentation techniques and this 'new era' of form stable implants? Much of the discussion in the literature has focused on anatomical breast implant shape versus round implant shape. The introduction of anatomically shaped implants has been heralded as a major event in breast augmentation surgery. However, this is not just a question of shape: other implant characteristics are of even greater importance. Thus a round implant filled with saline will behave considerably differently to a round one filled with high cohesive silicone gel. The same is obviously true for anatomical implants, but the degree of filling of the implant will also influence its characteristics as will the degree of silicone gel cohesiveness. This can be noted during a so-called tilt test, whereby a form stable implant is turned vertically and the stability of the upper pole is noted. It is the author's opinion that the differences in breast implants today are not related to anatomical or round shape, but to the huge selection of form stable versus non-form stable breast implants.

In breast augmentation surgery, a pocket is created, which has certain dimensions, widths and heights and can be expanded ventrally. There are fundamental differences in how the different types of implant behave in these implant pockets. For instance, if a non-form stable breast implant with greater base width than the implant pocket is selected, then these implants can be deformed and stuffed into the breast implant pocket, whereby the implant pocket expands ventrally. On the other hand, if a form stable breast implant with a base exceeding the implant pocket is selected, these implants cannot be deformed to fit the implant pocket. Thus form stable breast implant requires new and radically different surgical implant selection techniques. Form stable implants are more demanding and difficult to use compared to non-form stable breast implants.

So why is the use of form stable breast implants currently growing so rapidly? The reason is that a prerequisite for good control of the shape of the new breast is to have control of the shape of the implant, and this requires control of the shape of the filling material. High cohesive silicone gel implants retain their shape and form, even when cut and under pressure. With form stable devices, the shape of the breast can be controlled to a much higher degree than ever before. Breast augmentation has become more customised and individualised in relation to patients' desires and biological prerequisites. The benefit of this is seen for instance in asymmetric cases, where different shaped implants can be used on different sides. This is the best alternative in thoracic asymmetries. With glandular size differences, the alternative is to use similar sized implants and to reduce the larger side (Fig. 4.1). If the size differences between the breasts are large, this provides the best long-term stability, for example, during weight gain. The same type of augmentation should according to the author be used more in breast reconstructive procedures, where it is common that implants are used on the mastectomy side and reductions on the remaining breast. If an augmentation on the remaining breast was considered more frequently it is likely that there would be better long-term stability of the results.

The difference between this 'new era' of breast augmentation surgery and traditional breast augmentation is that this new surgery involves breast shaping as opposed to the traditional old breast-stuffing procedure. With form stable implants, the days of choosing implants arbitrarily out of thin air must be over. A prerequisite for shaping of the breast in relation to patients' biological prerequisites and desires is to have a wide variety of

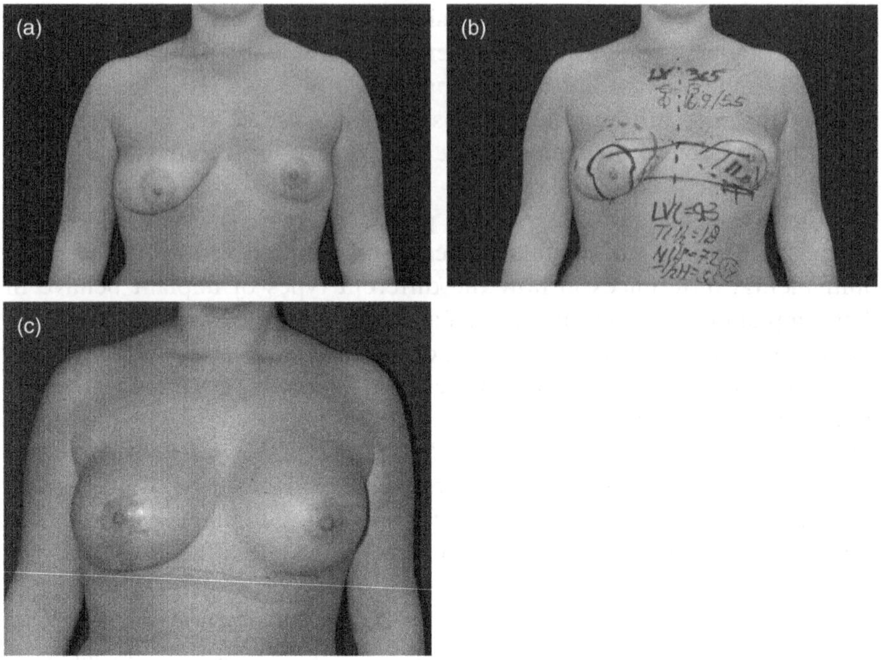

4.1 (a) Pronounced breast asymmetry and (b) preoperative markings. A reduction augmentation was planned for the right side, and for the left a Puckett procedure to spread the gland in the lower pole and augmentation with the same type of low height, extra projecting implants as on the other side. (c) Six months postoperative. Note fullness in upper pole in spite of low height anatomical implants.

implant shapes. The Allergan Corporation has by far the widest range of form stable breast implants, with 20 basic different shapes currently available. Several hundred different implants can by variations in width of these 20 shapes thus be selected to individualise the breast augmentation procedure. This makes breast augmentation surgery much more customised than before. Obviously this is better as patient desire, thoracic shape and amount of glandular tissue vary greatly. With the use of form stable implants, we have also come to realise that breast augmentation surgery is much more about dimension and proportions than volume. In spite of this, it is still difficult to get patients, nurses and plastic surgeons to stop thinking about the volume as the first and most important thing in selecting a breast implant for a procedure.

4.2 Available form stable breast implants

Since McGhan/Inamed/Allergan's pioneering introduction of form stable implants in the early 1990s, many implant manufactures have produced

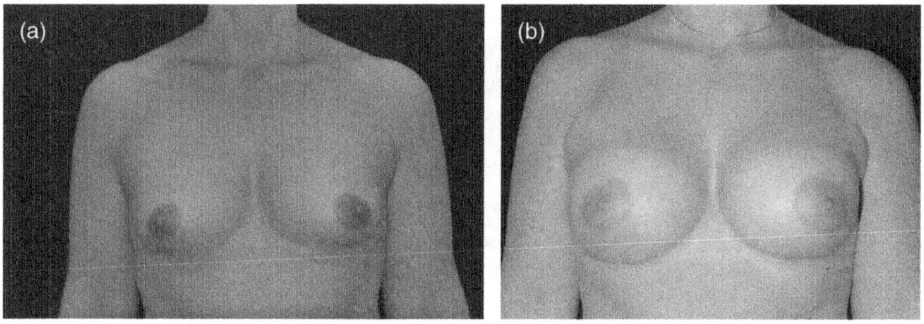

4.2 (a) Before and (b) after breast augmentation with a low height anatomical implant. Round implants are not suitable in these type of patients as they produce too much upper pole fullness, pushing down the nipple areola complex, or else they will be located too far distally in relation to the inframammary fold. This produces a higher risk of irregularities or the creation of double bubble deformities in the lower pole.

form stable devices, and currently both anatomical and round form stable breast implants are available. Allergan provides the largest number of implants with a matrix system of anatomical implants with 15 different cells in the Nartelle® Style 410 and Style 510 range. The difference between Style 410 and 510 implants is that the 510 implants have variable cohesiveness within the implant. The ventral part is firmer to provide more projection. The edge of the 510 is also more tapered and the base is concave to fit the thoracic surface better. However 510 implants are only available in three different shapes. The 410 implants have 12 different cells. Form stable breast implants are also available as round devices and Allergan currently provides five different models. Round implants may not be suitable in patients with short lower pole (Fig. 4.2) as it may be located well below the existing submammary fold and produce a double bubble (see implant selection below). The Inspira models are available in four different projections: TSL–low projection, TSM–moderate projection, TSF–full projection and TSX–extra full projection. All Allergan implants have recently been renamed Natrelle® and the different silicone cohesiveness under the generic name True Form®, where True Form I is equal to the low cohesive not form stable or responsive standard gel and III represents the firmer gel in the standard Style 410 implants.

Mentor Corporation also provides a relatively wide range of form stable breast implants called the Cohesive Memory Gel implant, the so-called DCTG300 series. These are available in five different anatomical shapes with varied width, height, and projection. Outside the US, the Silimed and Polytech Corporations are the only companies providing form stable

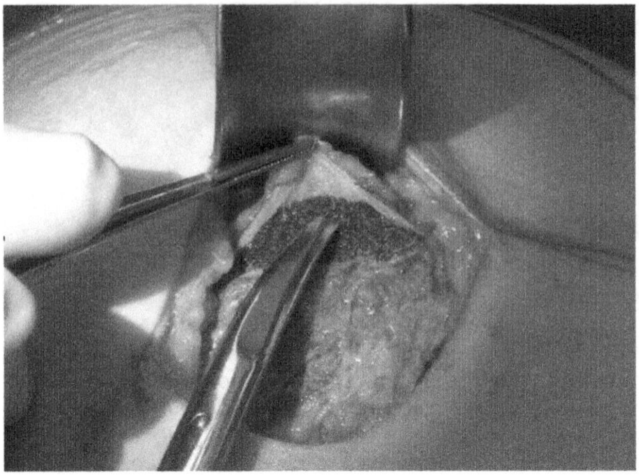

4.3 Textured implant surface with a pore size >300 μm permits tissue in-growth and thus fixation.

implants with a polyurethane cover, which may be considered in severe capsular contraction. Other implant manufacturers also provide form stable breast implants, but it is beyond the scope of this publication to review all of these. For the consumer and surgeon, it is important to emphasise that there are differences in the firmness of the high cohesive silicone gel and thereby variations in the degree of form stability. The surface technology of these implants also varies. It has been documented that the pore size of textured implants should be larger than 300 μm to provide for tissue in-growth and fixation of the implant.[1] Without fixation to the tissue, an anatomical form stable implant may rotate and provide an unnatural appearance. The Biocell® surface of the Allergan implant has surface texturing (Fig. 4.3) with pore size larger than 300 μm whereas the Siltex® surface of Mentor implants has a pore size smaller than 300 μm. It is important to underline that the majority of implants without tissue fixation do not experience rotational problems. In the author's experience, rotational problems of form stable implants are uncommon and account for only 1% of reoperations. Recently much discussion has focused on the quality of different implants, especially relating to medical authorities banning the use of PIP implants[2,3] because of their high rupture frequency rate, and their filling with industry grade silicone instead of the accepted medical grade products. The US Food and Drug Administration (FDA) have strict control of production facilities and have only approved the use of implants from the Allergan and Mentor Co. The FDA do not govern the use of implants outside the United States, but it is clear that the CE marking of implants does not provide the same strict regulation as offered by the FDA.

4.2.1 Advantages of form stable breast implants

The customisation of the breast augmentation and control of the final shape of the breast are probably the most important advantages of form stable breast implants. Other advantages of these devices are that the filling material minimises gel bleed through the shell and that the consistency of the filling material minimises movement of the implant shell. Because of this, the wear of the envelope is likely to be minimised and it is possible that form stable implants could provide a much longer life span compared to implants with liquid or low cohesive filling material. A reduced rupture rate has also been confirmed in a magnetic resonance imaging (MRI) study after long-term implantation of form stable breast implants. Patients with Allergan Style 410 implants implanted between 5 and 9 years had a confirmed rupture rate of only 0.3% and another 0.7% of indeterminate rupture.[4] Other MRI studies investigating non-form stable breast implants with standard responsive silicone gel filling have shown a rupture frequency between 5–10%,[5] and this may indicate that risk for rupture after up to 10 years of implantation time is at least five times higher with standard silicone gel breast implants compared to form stable breast implants. Another advantage of form stable breast implants is that any ruptured material is much easier to remove, compared to implants filled with standard low cohesive silicone gel. The concept of a non-liquid material is also very appealing to patients. Many European patients have expressed their confidence in a material that does not spontaneously leak out through a ruptured shell (Fig. 4.4). Form stable devices are less prone to deform during capsular contractions. Much less force is needed to deform a low cohesive filling material into a deformed shape, compared to form stable breast implants; also the high degree of cohesiveness of the filling material minimises rippling and irregularities, but it should be underlined that even form stable implants can be buckled or wrinkled. However, more force is needed to deform implants in this way. When comparing similar types of breasts with implantation of round and anatomically shaped breast implants, it is obvious that anatomical breast implants provide a more natural upper pole and shape of the breast (Fig. 4.5).

4.2.2 Applications

Form stable breast implants have the same applications as non-form stable devices. They are equally beneficial for aesthetic breast augmentation and in reconstructive procedures. The form stability of the extra projecting implants is also very suitable for use in tuberous or tubular breasts (Fig. 4.6). They provide good expansion of the contracted lower pole, and the extra projecting shape improves the poor transition between the implant

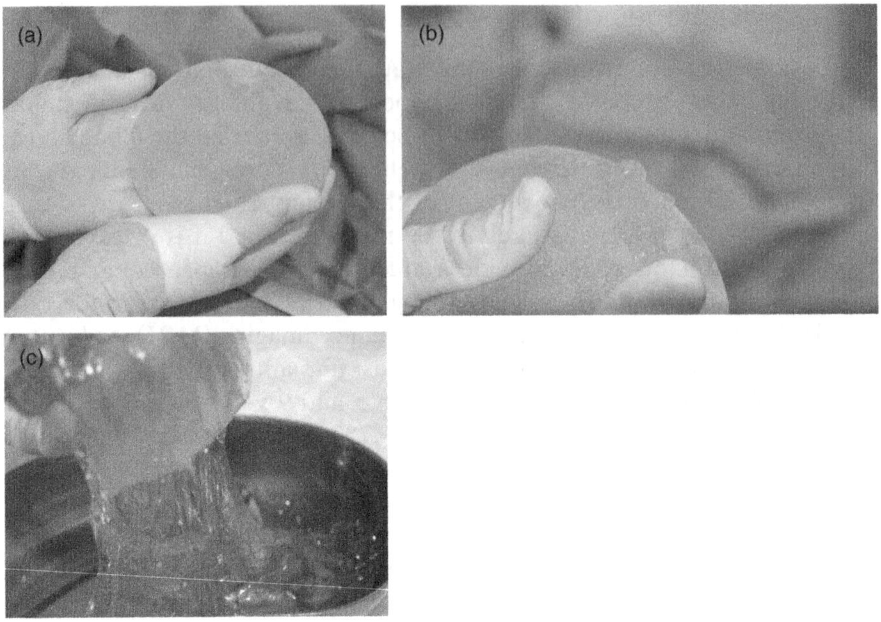

4.4 (a) A small asymptomatic hole in a form stable implant noted at implant exchange for other reasons 5 years after the primary operation. (b) Only when the implant is compressed does material migrate through the centimetre-sized rift. (c) A ruptured responsive older type of implant. Most of the silicone filling, which is sticky and difficult to remove, has migrated out of the envelope.

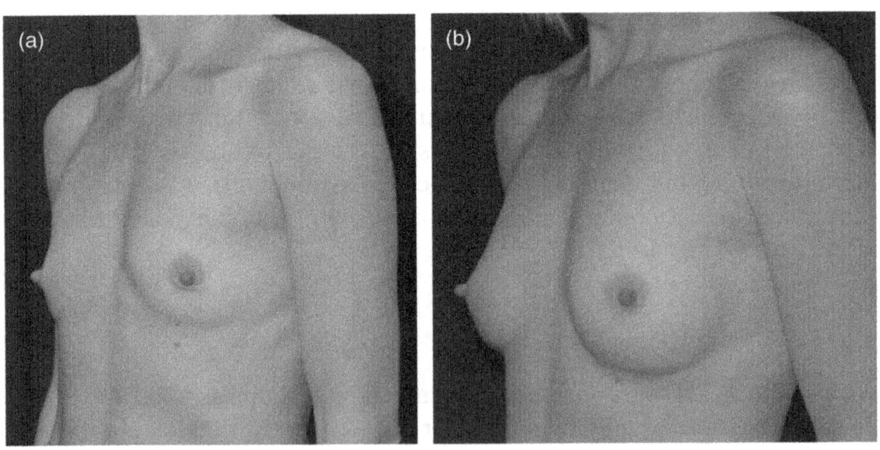

4.5 (a) Before and (b) after breast augmentation with a low projecting anatomical 125 cc implant. The patient desired to have a very natural appearance, mainly to restore the shape present before pregnancy and breast feeding.

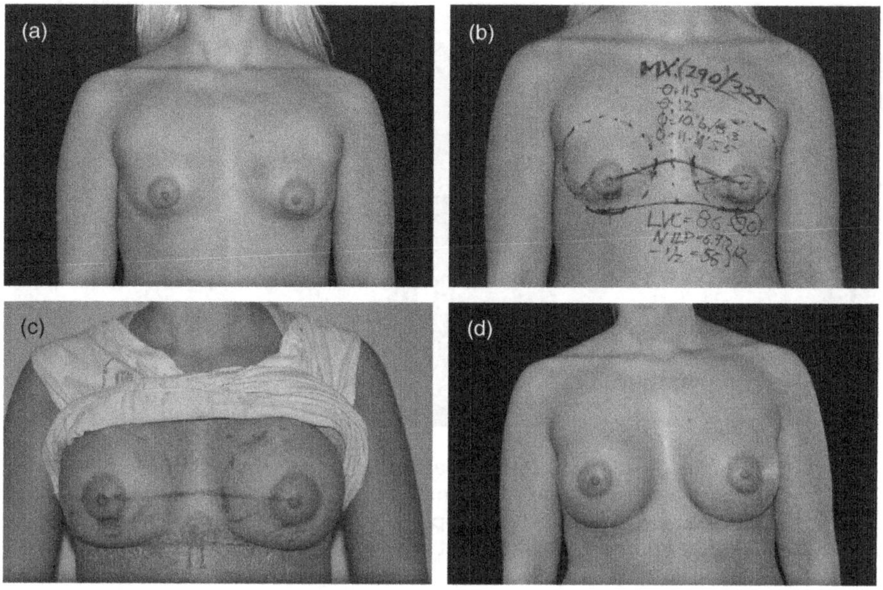

4.6 (a) Patient with constricted lower pole tubular breast. (b) The preoperative planning for an anatomical moderate extra projecting implant, including spreading of the gland in the lower pole with unfolding of the gland in the lower pole of the breast and suturing it down to the empty lower part. Even if a moderate height implant would come more distal to the lower existing submammary fold than a low height implant, this was selected to get good upper pole fullness as requested by the patient. (c) At dismissal from the clinic four hours after the procedure. Note elevation of NS-line compared to the situation preoperatively shown in (b). (d) Six months postoperative.

and glandular tissue, minimising the risk of a double bubble deformity. Form stable implants can also be used in mastopexy-augmentation cases (Fig. 4.7).

There are situations, however, where non-form stable responsive silicone gel implants or saline filled implants are better alternatives to form stable devices. These include patients with a recurrent rotational problem of an anatomical implant. It should be pointed out that with appropriate surgical techniques and implant selection this is an uncommon situation. In our first evaluation of form stable Style 410 implants the frequency was only 0.42%.[6] As most form stable breast implants are more expensive, it may also be an economical consideration for the patient to select a non-form stable device. In selected secondary cases, non-form stable implants may also be advantageous, as form stable implants do not deform and mould into the dead space of an old implant pocket. This is especially true in severe unilateral capsular contracture with glandular atrophy in front of the old contracted implant.

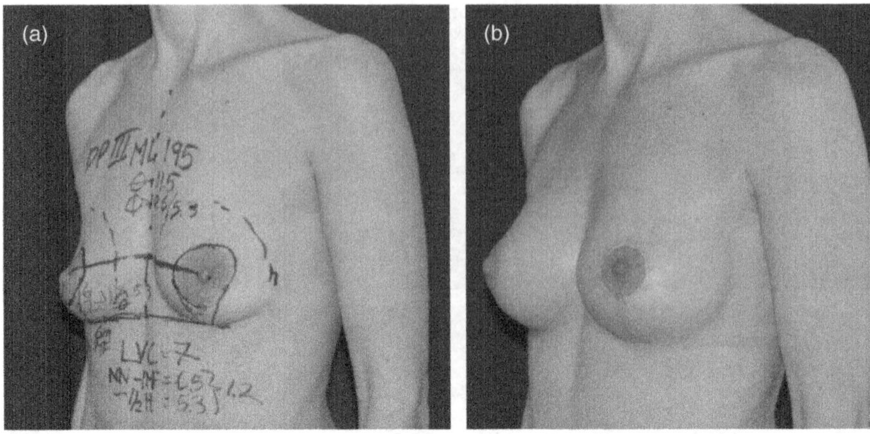

4.7 (a) Before and (b) after breast augmentation with low projection implants and reduction of the nipple areola complex and the skin envelope with a vertical mastopexy, in a patient who desires breast rejuvenation and reshaping but only a discreet augmentation.

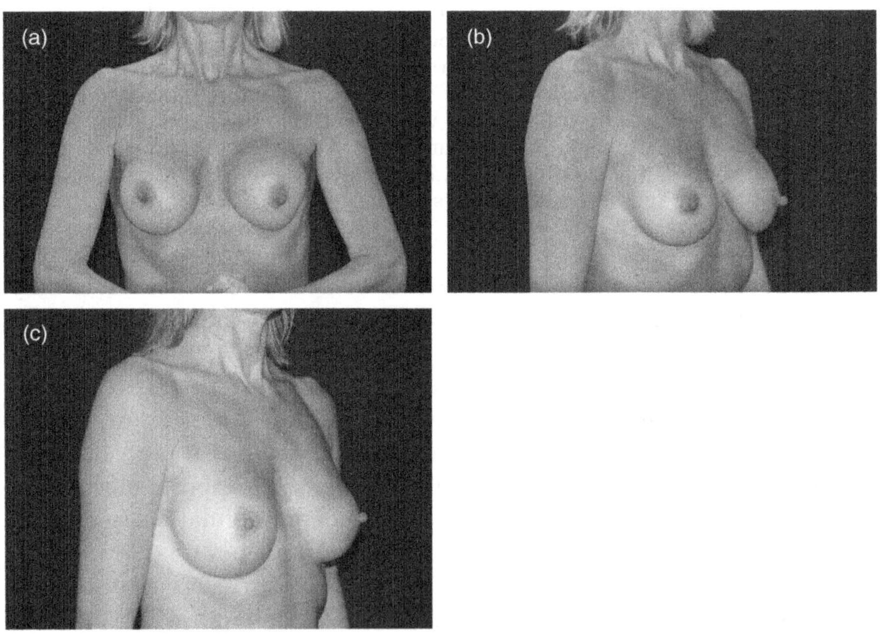

4.8 (a) Before (frontal view muscle tightening), (b) relaxed side view and (c) after implant exchange, site change from a subglandular to a submuscular pocket and a simultaneous mastopexy to reduce the expanded envelope.

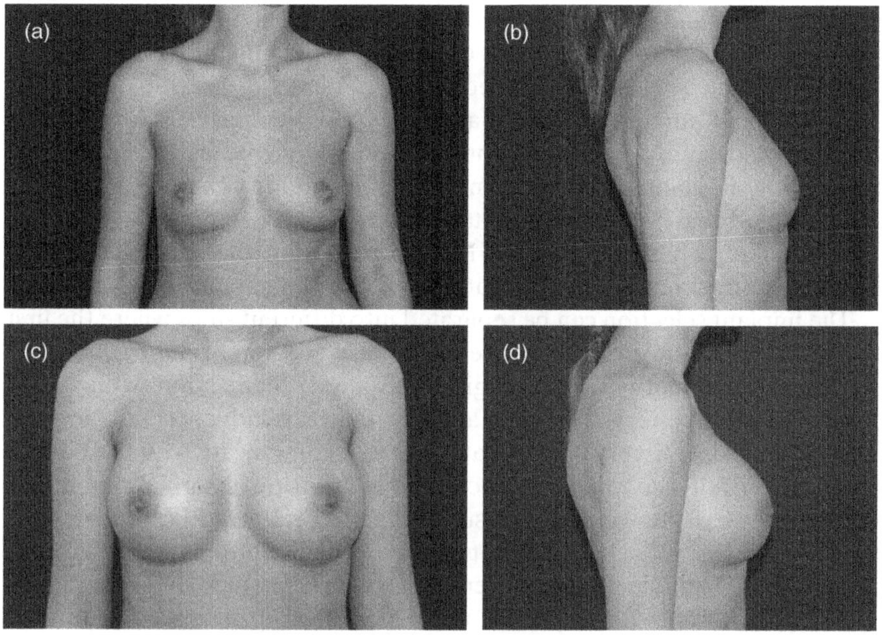

4.9 (a) Frontal view and (b) side view before breast augmentation in a patient who specifically requested a more rounded appearance in the upper slope, after viewing estimated and different results in 3D imaging prediction. (c) Frontal view after the operation with round form stable moderate projecting implants, and (d) the side view. It is only the side view that is likely to clearly show the difference between anatomical and round implants. If full or extra projection implants had been selected this difference would be even greater.

Many secondary breast augmentations can, however, be favourably treated with form stable implants, provided that specific measures are undertaken (Fig. 4.8). Patients who prefer a more unnatural rounded appearance may also favour a round device (Fig. 4.9). Overfilled saline implants and form stable round implants provide the most rounded unnatural upper pole compared to responsive gel in non-contracted situations and anatomical implants which both provide a more anatomical breast appearance.

4.3 Selection of the appropriate form stable breast implant

During a conventional breast augmentation consultation, commonly a suitable implant volume is estimated, based on the surgeon's experience. This type of implant selection is no longer appropriate when it comes to selection of form stable breast implants, because the dimensions and proportions of the implant and the patient's biological prerequisites need to be considered. The consultation should first define the ideal implant base, width and implant height. This is then related to the patient's desire, biological prerequisites, and amount of glandular tissue. A projection of the implant is then selected. Knowing the appropriate implant dimensions will finally help provide the implant's volume from the manufacturer's charts. This type of form stable breast implant consultation is reversed compared to the standard volumetric implant selection. Necessary tools in implants selection are a tape measure, a calliper, and charts from the manufacturer.

The implant selection can be separated into different steps where the first step is to define the patient's desires. Obviously it is important to underline for the patient what type of biological limitations she has, but within these limitations, the patient can select a breast that is relatively small, large or moderate in size. A very appropriate way to communicate with the patient is to have a full size mirror and to stand in front of this pointing out the width of the existing glandular tissue and appropriate width of the desired new breast. This makes the patient aware of the limitations when it comes to size. The glandular tissue and envelope characteristics should be taken into consideration when selecting implants. Measuring the distance between the nipple and the inframammary fold during maximal tension will provide information on appropriate implant dimensions for filling the envelope (see Section 4.4). If the envelope is too lax for the implant projection desired by the patient, a mastopexy-augmentation may be necessary. When a patient requests a relatively large augmentation, it should be pointed out that a tight envelope will need to expand and relax and that the breast, at least initially, will be tight. In front of the mirror, asymmetries in submammary fold, nipple position and so on should also be examined and pointed out to the patient. Thoracic asymmetries and the shape of the upper thorax should be examined as this may influence selection of appropriate implant height. Another important tool for implant selection is to use implant sizers in a tight-fitting sports bra (Fig. 4.10). These should not, however, be used to select an appropriate implant size, but rather to let the patient see what type of change the recommended implant is likely to produce. An important tool in the analysis of breast shapes is 3D imaging (Fig. 4.11). Today this permits analysis of the existing breast shape, but new reliable and accurate systems for prediction of the outcome of a breast augmentation using different shaped implants are also under development. This could be an extremely valuable tool, not only for the planning of a breast augmentation, but also for informing the patient before surgery.

The most important step in the selection of an appropriate form stable implant is deciding the width. If implants are selected without respecting biological conditions such as chest and thoracic width, the breast would at best look unnatural with too wide an intramammary distance or much

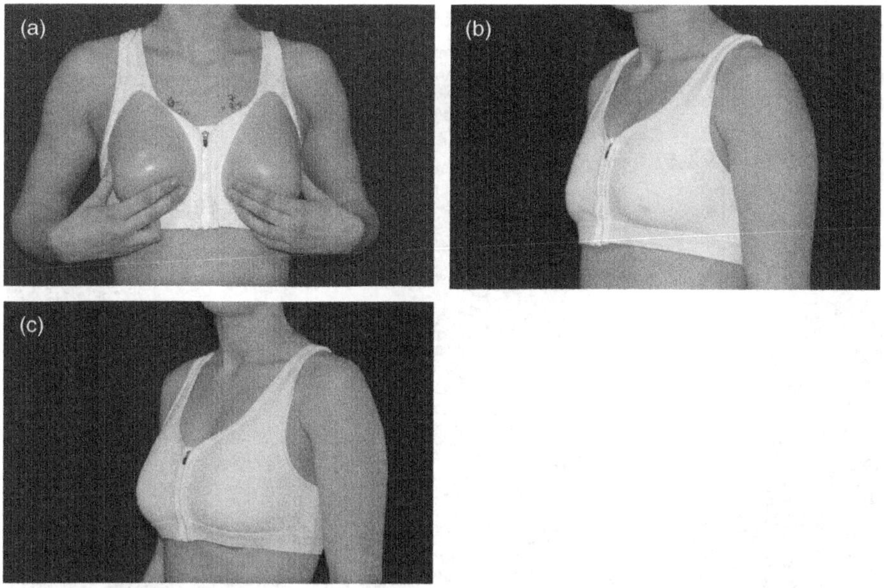

4.10 (a) Sizers of these types are a more accurate guide when placed in a sports bra than the implant itself because the implant underestimates the new breast width as it is on top of the breast when testing and under after the operation. (b) Patient with sports bra only and (c) a sizer of adequate volume in the bra giving a realistic impression of the outcome.

worse develop severe complications, e.g. synmastia (Fig. 4.12). If an implant does not exceed the existing glandular tissue, the risk of implant palpability and visibility is minimised. Therefore, existing glandular tissue should be measured with a calliper (Fig. 4.13). Usually a proportional and natural appearance of the augmented breast leaves an inframammary distance of 2–3 cm, and does not go laterally to the anterior axillary line. Taking the measurement of ideal breast width, measured with a calliper, and subtracting the tissue cover provides information on the ideal implant width. The tissue cover is measured with a pinch test at the medial border of the breast and at the lateral axillary line. Adding these two pinch measurements and dividing them by two will provide information about the tissue cover. Sometimes the selected implant must exceed the width of the existing breast to provide a natural appearance. This is the case in contracted lower pole breasts, where the base width is usually very narrow. For patients desiring a large and wide breast, the existing width of the glandular tissue may be exceeded by 0.5 cm to 1.0 cm, underlining for the patient that this will give somewhat more implant visibility and palpability. The decision of ideal

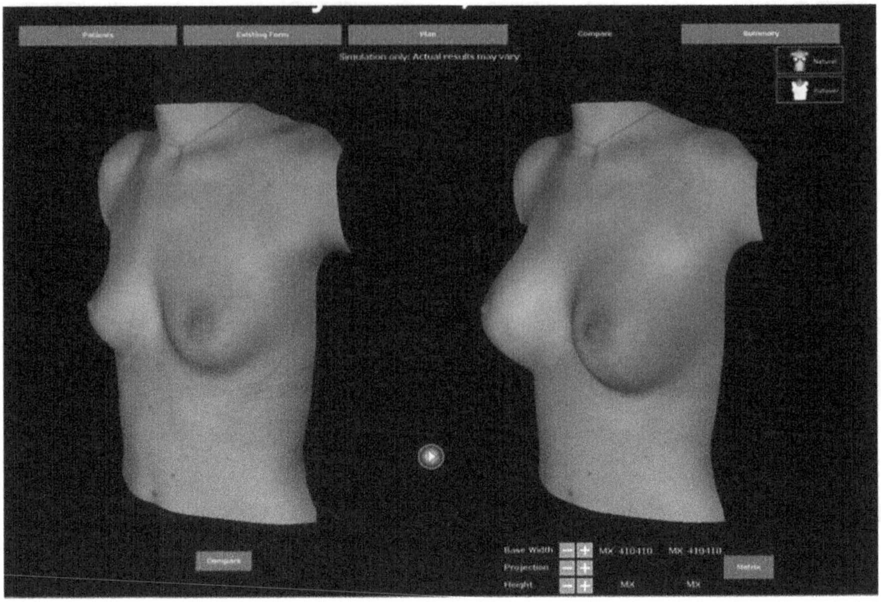

4.11 3D imaging prediction with a Canfield Vectra II camera and Precision Light software. The predicted outcome of a breast augmentation with anatomical moderate height extra projecting Natrelle Style 410 implants.

implant width is probably the most important part in selection of form stable breast implants.

Following this the ideal implant height should be decided. Both the pre-operative upper and lower pole appearance is of great importance for the implant height selection. Measurements must be made to determine the location of the lower and upper pole of the implant. This should be compared to the upper pole shape and how the implant correlates to the existing submammary fold and the lower pole appearance of the breast. The author has found that elevation of the arms to 45° above the horizontal plane provides an accurate estimate of where the nipples will be positioned after a proportionate breast augmentation (Fig. 4.14). After the ideal implant width is decided, the height of different implants can be easily found in the manufacturer's charts. With the patient's arms elevated to 45° (with the arms on top of the head) the author has demonstrated that the postoperative nipple position can be predicted. It is easy to measure where the lower and upper pole of different implants will be located as 50% of an anatomical and 50–55% of a round implant height is recommended to be placed distal to the new nipple position (Fig. 4.15). Remember that implants that fall within the borders of the existing breast minimise the risk of complica-

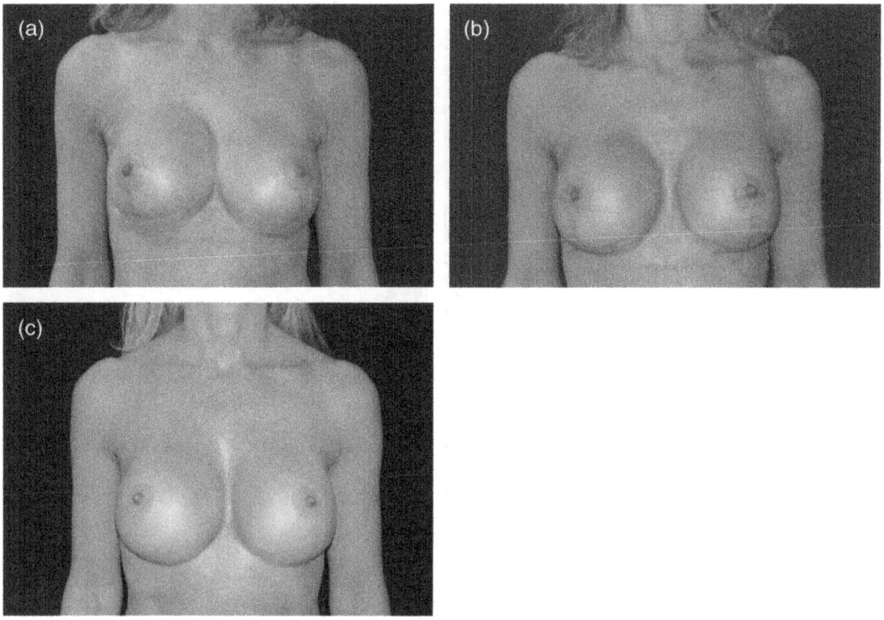

4.12 (a) Synmastia without remaining intramammary distance due to selection of too wide an implant. The surgeon had let the patient decide the implant volume without checking how the width would suit the chest wall. (b) Six months after correction with a neo-submuscular pocket technique and 1 cm narrower implant which was the maximum accepted width even if the patient requested wider. Due to the large implant in this thin and small patient, the implant edge is clearly visible, something the patient was warned about and accepted. (c) One year after 100 cc of fat transplantation to the upper and medial pole to cover implant edges.

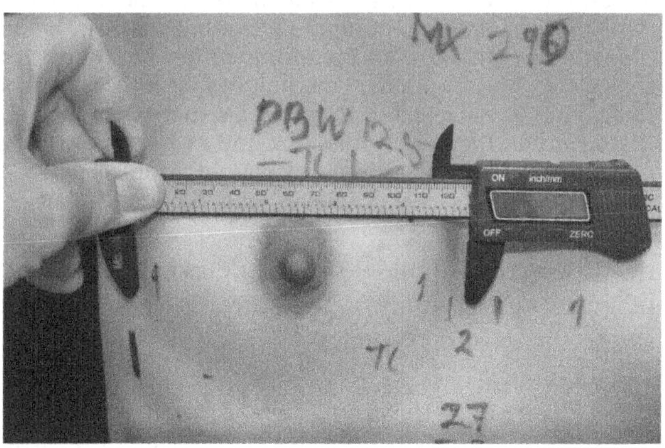

4.13 The width of the existing breast is measured with a calliper.

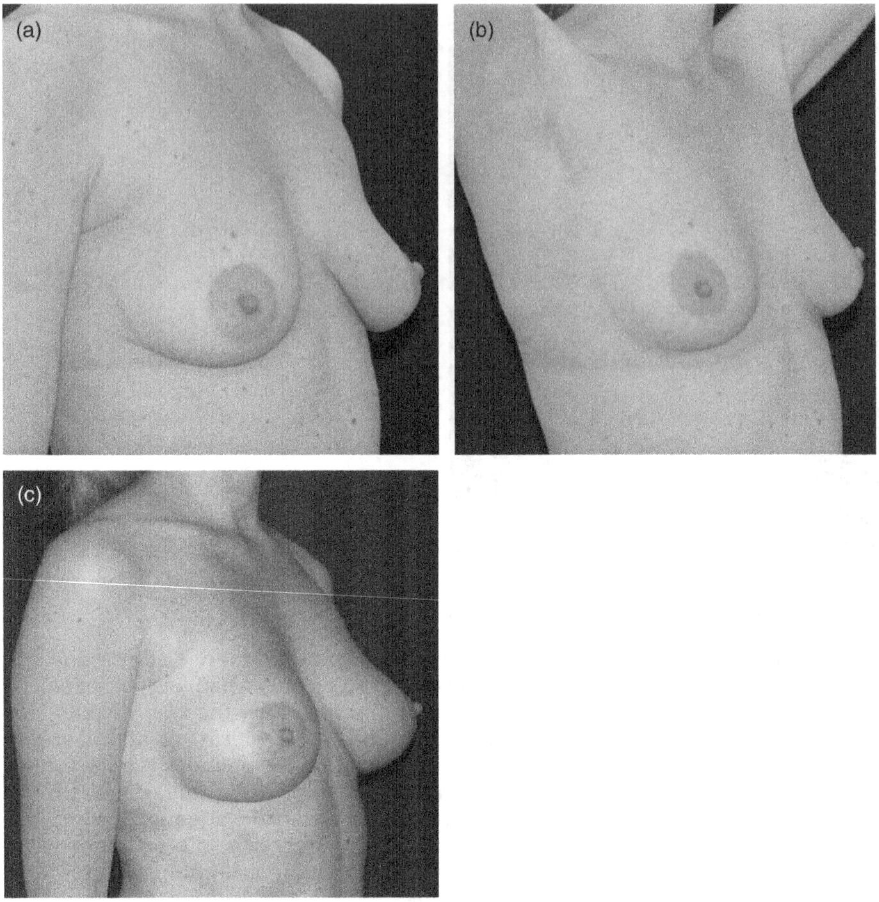

4.14 (a) Ptotic breast before augmentation with arms hanging. (b) Before augmentation with arms elevated 45° above the horizontal plane predicting the amount of nipple elevation that can be achieved with a breast augmentation. (c) Six months after augmentation with Natrelle® Style 410 LX implants. Low height implants give less upper pole fullness, but were selected to minimise the risk of a double bubble deformity in the lower pole. If round or full height implants had been selected and placed higher to avoid double bubble deformity, the nipples would not have been elevated.

tions such as the lower pole double bubble deformity. The risk of this complication increases considerably if the lower pole of the implant is located well distal to the existing submammary fold, especially if the gland is firm and well defined.

The final implant decision is the implant projection. Obviously knowledge about the implant dimensions and shape will provide information on the selected volume and not vice versa. Implant projection is greatly related

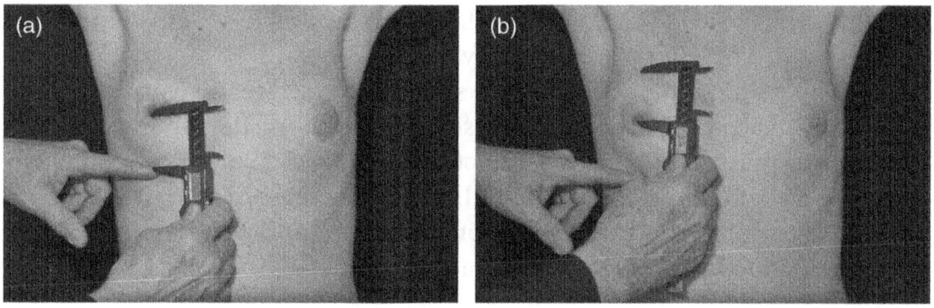

4.15 (a) With the patient's arms elevated 45° above the horizontal plane (with the arms on top of the head) the postoperative nipple position is predicted. Knowing the height of different implants it is thus easy to measure the location of the lower and upper pole of different implants in relation to the existing submammary fold and (b) also to estimate how the upper implant slope correlates to the upper chest wall and breast shape.

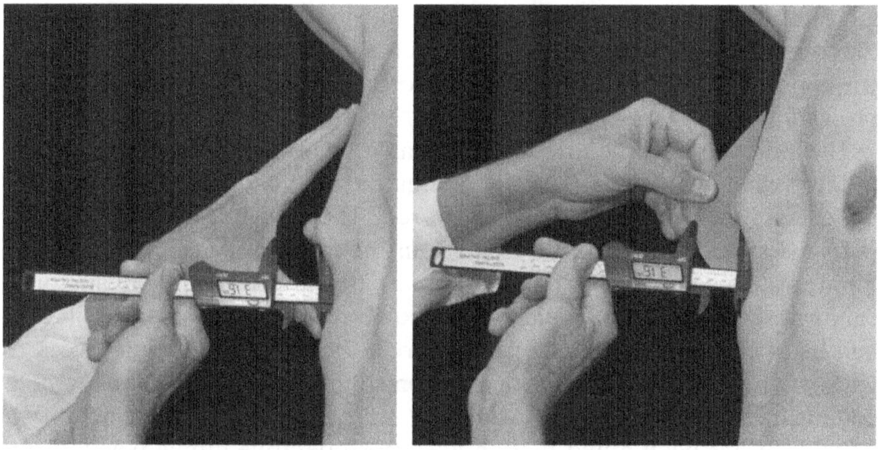

4.16 The projection of different implants is demonstrated in front of the mirror for the patient with her hands on her head. A calliper is pushed into the gland to simulate implant compression of the gland.

to patient desires. A good way to analyse this is to stand in front of the mirror obliquely, showing the expected outer border of the augmented breast with a cupped hand or a paper cut-out (Fig. 4.16). When demonstrating the projection of different implants, a calliper can be pushed into the glandular tissue to simulate the compression effect of the implant on the gland. Patients can usually easily discriminate if they prefer the low or extra projecting spectrum of implants. One should remember also that the selected implant projection must be selected in relation to the laxity of the envelope as described above. When selecting implant projection it is necessary to consider the envelope characteristics, as loose envelopes may need more projection or a mastopexy.

Anatomical implants with varying shapes permit greater variability but the implant selection process has also become more demanding for surgeons. As a meticulous implant selection minimises the risk of complications, the patient satisfaction rate is likely to increase. The extra effort in implant selection is therefore well worth the time, and with experience this way of selecting implants becomes quick.

4.4 Preoperative planning

As described in the introduction, form stable breast implants necessitate fundamentally different techniques and this applies both to the selection of implants, the preoperative planning and the surgical technique. Even if the use of form stable implants has opened our eyes to the necessity of considering implant dimensions, it is amazing that we have performed breast augmentation for nearly 50 years without giving much consideration to these issues. Before the current measurement techniques were used, there was a poorer understanding of the importance of implant base width and projection.

The author's technique for preoperative markings and measurement follows what we call the Akademikliniken method (AK method). Two important questions should be answered. The first question is how the implants should be vertically located on the chest wall in relation to the nipple areola complex. For a natural breast appearance, half of an anatomical form stable implant should be located above the nipple areola complex and half below. This can be adjusted in relation to personal preferences. A properly performed breast augmentation should elevate the nipple areola complex. In a careful clinical evaluation on several hundred augmentation patients, it has been noted that an ideal postoperative nipple position can be preoperatively simulated by an arm elevation 45° above the horizontal plane. A simple way to simulate the nipple position is to ask the patient to clasp her hands on top of her head. With this position a line is drawn from the nipple to the sternum, the so-called NS-line. Measurements in the midline are preferable as these are done on fixed tissue and in an area where the convexity of the breast can be disregarded. In the midline, half of the implant height is measured from the NS-line and distally. At the distal point of this line a horizontal line is extended indicating the implant's lower pole (ILP-line).

After the ideal vertical implant position has been located, the second question to answer is how much skin is needed between the nipple and the new inframammary fold. The new nipple–inframammary fold distance is influenced by the width and projection of the implant and the amount of glandular tissue and the characteristics of the envelope. The ideal amount of skin between the nipple and the inframammary fold is equal to the lower ventral curvature (LVC) of the implant plus the distance that has to be added for the amount of glandular tissue that the patient has. The lower ventral curvature of the implant is equal to the distance between the ideal nipple projection sites on the implant ventral surface, measured down to the implant lower border. Unfortunately no implant manufacturer provides this information, but it can easily be measured on a piece of paper with two perpendicular millimetre scales. On the vertical axis the tape measure is placed on the distance equal to the projection of the implant, and on the horizontal axis the other end of the tape is placed on half of the implant's height. The curved measurement with a tape measure provides information on the lower ventral curvature of the implant. If the patient were completely flat without any covering glandular tissue, this lower ventral curvature (LVC) measurement would be equal to the length of skin needed between the nipple and the new inframammary fold. However, as most patients have a certain amount of glandular tissue, this should also be taken into consideration. There are different ways to calculate how much the length between the nipple and the new submammary fold will have to be elongated in relation to the amount of covering glandular tissue:

- The simplest way is to estimate how much the LVC distance has to be elongated in relation to the size of the breast. In a very small breast, <1 cm is required, in a moderately sized breast, 1.0 cm to 1.5 cm is required, and in a large breast, >1.5 cm but very seldom >2.5 cm is added to the LVC value.
- A simple and much more accurate way to estimate this distance is to measure the lower breast pole pinch with a calliper and divide this value by 2.
- The most accurate way to calculate the elongation of the LVC value in relation to the amount of covering glandular tissue is done by measurements between the nipple and the previously described ILP-line, once again with the patient's arms on top of her head. Subtracting half the implant height from this measurement of the convexity of the breast will provide information on the length of skin that has to be added in relation to the amount of glandular tissue. The formula the LVC (lower ventral curvature of the implant) plus N-ILP (nipple to implant lower pole line measured with arms elevated) minus $\frac{1}{2}$ H (half the implant height) provide information on the length between the nipple and the new inframammary fold. When marking this distance on the breast, the envelope's characteristics should be taken into consideration. This means that the skin between the nipple and the new inframammary fold should be maximally stretched when marking this distance on the skin.

In most standard breast augmentation cases, the vertical implant location NS-ILP measurements and measurements on the ideal amount of skin between the nipple and the new inframammary fold falls into line. However, in ptotic breasts the amount of skin in the lower pole is often excessive and in these cases the ILP-line frequently is below the measurement of the ideal amount of skin in the lower pole. Conversely, in individuals with tight skin who request larger implants, it is common that the ILP-line ends up greater than the measurements for the ideal amount of skin between the nipple and the inframammary fold. In this situation, we recruit skin from the thoracic wall to the lower pole of the breast, as opposed to the procedure for the slightly ptotic breast where we pull down the lower pole of the breast to the ILP-line. If the distance between the ideal submammary incision point (= length of skin between nipple and submammary fold calculated as described above) and the ILP (ideal implants lower pole location) exceeds 1–2 cm, then the selected implant may be unsuitable or the patient may have too much ptosis for correction with breast augmentation alone.

The measurements and markings described above have been developed for the use of form stable devices, but they are equally important considerations when using non-form stable breast implants. Even if breast augmentation formerly was much more arbitrary, these new type of measurements can provide valuable information to minimise the risk of complications and reoperation.

4.5 Incisions and surgical technique

Form stable breast implants can be inserted through periareolar, axillary and submammary fold incisions. The umbilical incision is not applicable for these devices. It should be understood that the length of incision for form stable implants usually has to be somewhat larger than for non-form stable breast implants, as they cannot be deformed to the same degree. Usually a form stable breast implant of approximately 200 cc can be inserted through an incision of 4.5 cm length, a 300 cc implant needs about 5.0 cm to 5.5 cm, and an implant volume of 400 cc or more usually needs a 6.0 cm incision. These are relatively long incisions in the axilla, but they are well hidden in the relatively long submammary fold. Historically the submammary fold has had a relatively bad reputation, mainly because the incision has not been placed exactly in the new fold. The obvious reason for this has been that there were no measuring techniques telling us exactly where to place the incision, but with the above described preoperative measurements, the exact location of the new fold can be calculated and this adds to improvement of the final scar. A scar located on the lower pole of the breast is always more conspicuous than a scar located exactly in the fold (Fig. 4.17). There are several advantages to incisions in the submammary fold: there is

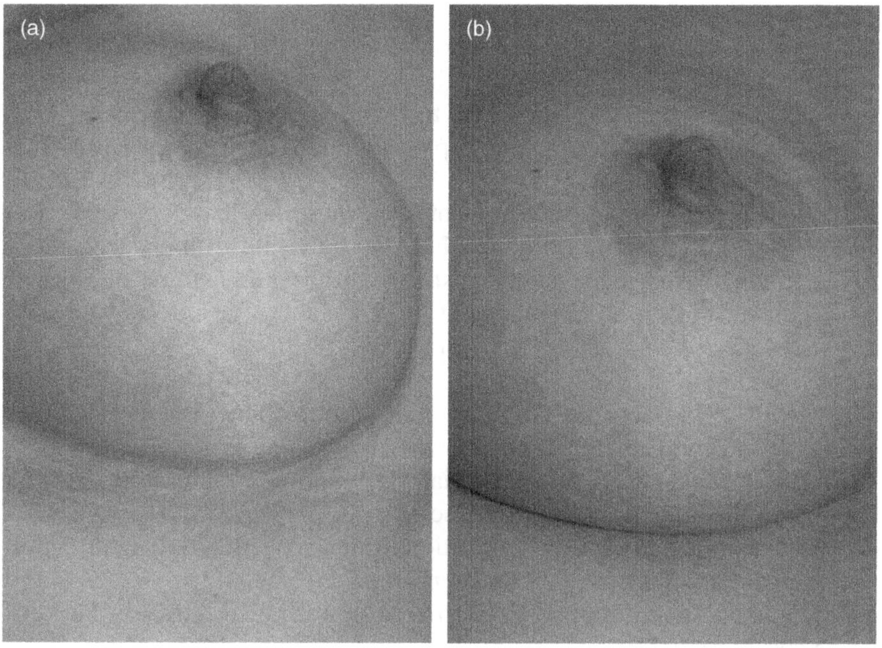

4.17 (a) A submammary scar which had its location calculated with the Akademikliniken method 2 years after breast augmentation, the arm is stretched above the head. (b) The same scar with the arm hanging.

less risk for sensory changes in the breast compared to the axillary and periareolar incisions, contamination is also minimised, and possible influence on sentinel node biopsy is minimised compared to axillary incision. The implant pocket dissection is more precise through inframammary fold, and the division of the pectoralis major origin and the dual plane surgical technique are also better facilitated through the inframammary fold incision. These advantages are the reasons why we favour the use of the new submammary fold or AK incision, when we use form stable implants. This is an exact calculation of the location of the incision and emphasises the fold by the suturing technique described below.

4.5.1 Surgical technique

1. Preoperative markings and measurements according to the AK technique.
2. Local anaesthesia with adrenaline in all cases (even under general anaesthetic).
3. Tegaderm covering the nipple areolar complex (NAC) to minimise contamination with *Staphylococcus epidermidis* usually present in the ducts.

4. Scalpel skin incision.
5. Vertical electrocautery dissection (Force FX®, Valleylab and Colorado® tip).
6. Dissection along thoracic fascia to ILP-line, distal or proximal.
7. Subglandular dissection to or past nipple areola complex for dual plane II-IV implantation.
8. Identification of lateral border of pectoralis muscle.
9. Elevations of lateral border with forceps division with electrocautery parallel to ribcage leaving the distal pectoralis muscle fibres on ribcage.
10. Exposure of sub muscular plane.
11. Leave loose connected tissue on ribs.
12. Dissect medial first.
13. Divide pectoralis muscle horizontal sternum and obliquely, always stop 1–2 cm distal to NS-line.
14. Follow proximately in the medial part and sweep lateral in between pectoralis major and minor muscles.
15. Use sharp electrocautery dissection. Blunt dissection only in direction of axilla for sensory nerve preservation.
16. Distal glandular division in constricted lower pole breasts or 'Puckett' procedure.
17. Subglandular dissection or subfascial elevation in patients with sufficient tissue cover positioning (>3 cm at upper border of implant). Submuscular placement (dual plane II–IV) in >90% of cases.
18. Irrigate implant pocket to remove debris (saline and/or antibiotic solution).
19. Implant insertion: use sterile 'no-touch' technique.
20. Lubricate implant (saline and/or antibiotic solution sufficient in most cases).
21. Place at 90° angle and rotate the tip of the implant into place first.
22. Control vertical position by indicator by palpation of indicator dots or line.
23. Palpate around implant to check appropriate size of pocket. Do not exceed implant width and height more than 0.5 cm, control that the pocket is sufficiently wide to minimise buckling and irregularities.
24. Close Scarpa's fascia to thoracic fascia at ILP-line. Deep dermal ridge suturing and subcutaneous closure.

If the preoperative planning and markings have been performed as described, it will greatly facilitate the surgery and maximise a favourable outcome. Before commencing the procedure and during the preoperative markings, the implant position in relation to the pectoralis major muscle is decided. Submuscular implantation provides better tissue cover and less visibility of implant edges and irregularities. Submuscular positioning of implants also results in less tendency for ptotis over time. In addition, implants under the muscle are less likely to put pressure on the glandular tissue, minimising glandular atrophy. It also provides a faster surgical dissection. The subglandular positioning has the advantage that the breast implant moves less with pectoralis activity and the risk of irregularities along the medial part of the inframammary fold is minimised. It is also easier to achieve a more natural appearance in the ptotic breast. The risk of double bubble deformity in the lower pole of the breast is also minimised if implants are placed subglandularly. Final decision on implant placement in relation to the pectoralis major muscle depends on the amount of covering glandular tissue. If the pinch test measured with a calliper at the upper pole of the implant is less than 2–3 cm, submuscular placement is recommended. When the pinch test measures tissue cover of more than 3–4 cm, it is usually better to choose subglandular or subfascial implant positioning.

Before commencing the operative procedure, with the patient lying prone on the operating table, the measurements of the markings are controlled and the distance between the nipple and the new inframammary fold is once again checked with the ruler. Local anaesthesia is also infiltrated around the borders of the implant pocket, 0.25% Xylocaine with adrenaline ($5\ \mu g\ ml^{-1}$) can be used and up to 80 cc per breast provides an accurate haemostasis and long-lasting pain reduction. Local anaesthesia is favoured even if patients receive general anaesthesia, as this minimises the anaesthesia depth and speeds up the postoperative recovery. It has been demonstrated that the effect of local anaesthesia is very long-lasting.

To facilitate the surgical dissection, good illumination is of paramount importance. Light retractors or a fibre optic head light can be used for this purpose. A lightweight fibre optic xenon head light is favoured as the light focal points parallel to the vision of the surgeon. The preoperatively marked incision is incised with a size 15-scalpel blade through the dermis, followed by electrocautery dissection with tungsten (Colorado®) tip. The author favours the Force FX® Valleylab cautery, but radiofrequency dissectors can also be useful even if these are somewhat slower. The dissection is carried on vertically straight down, through the Scarpa's fascia and to the thoracic fascia. This is then followed distally or proximally to the ILP-line where suture fixation will be performed in the end of the procedure. The electrocautery dissection is then continued proximally until the distal border of the pectoralis major is encountered. The dissection follows past this distal border and up to the level of the nipple areola complex. If a dual plane II positioning is planned, then the muscle is then divided distally, but one must remember to divide 2–3 cm above the ILP line, as good support for the scar fixation to the thoracic wall then is left in place. In dual plane III or IV dissection, the subglandular dissection is carried on past the level of the nipple areola complex. In dual plane II and III dissection the muscle is then divided distally a couple of centimetres above the incision in the submammary fold.[7] Muscle division is started at the lateral border of the pectoralis major muscle, elevating this vertically off the chest wall with forceps. It is recommended that the muscle is divided parallel to the ribcage to weaken the distal border of pectoralis major muscle, which provides a good transition between the subglandular and submuscular part of the implant. The dissection is carried out horizontally and medially in the direction of the sternum. When entering under the pectoralis major muscle, a loose submuscular connective tissue layer is encountered. Inserting the retractor under the muscle and pulling it ventrally away from the chest wall will provide easy dissection under the muscle. The loose connective tissue is dissected free from the muscle, leaving this intact on the ribcage. This minimises postoperative pain, seroma and bleeding. Blunt dissection with fingers should be avoided and dissection is continued with the tungsten tip electrocautery dissection. Insulated forceps can also be used for parts of this dissection when larger muscle fibres and small vessels are encountered.

Dissecting in the medial part of the pocket first is recommended, to avoid elevation of the origin of the pectoralis minor muscle, which in its distal parts may fuse with the pectoralis major origin. Sweeping in the upper part of the implant pocket in a lateral dissection will easily enter the space between the pectoralis major and minor muscles. The implant pocket dissection is then continued laterally with the electrocautery except for in the direction of the axilla, where limited blunt dissection may be recommended to minimise the risk of sensory affection to the nipple areola complex. The implant pocket is finalised by dividing the inferior medial origin of the pectoralis muscle, curving the medial muscle division cranial and up to the level of the nipple areola complex. The preoperatively marked NS-line should always be respected and muscle division should always be 1–2 cm distal to this line. The NS-line is of particular value in the ptotic breast where it is easy to divide too much of the inferior medial origin of the pectoralis major muscle. In dual plane IV dissection, the subglandular part of the implant pocket is much larger and passes well above the level of the nipple areola complex. Almost a full subglandular pocket is created. The pectoralis muscle is divided higher laterally, almost at the level of the nipple areola complex and the muscle division is done along a straight line going in the direction of a point 1–2 cm distal to the preoperatively marked NS-line. The muscle should be reattached, e.g. with a running Quill Monoderm 2/0 suture, to the overlying glandular tissue before inserting the implant. Dual plane IV dissection is a good choice for more ptotic breasts and tuberous or tubular breast deformities. It is also the method of choice for body builders (Fig. 4.18). These types of cases would have a better

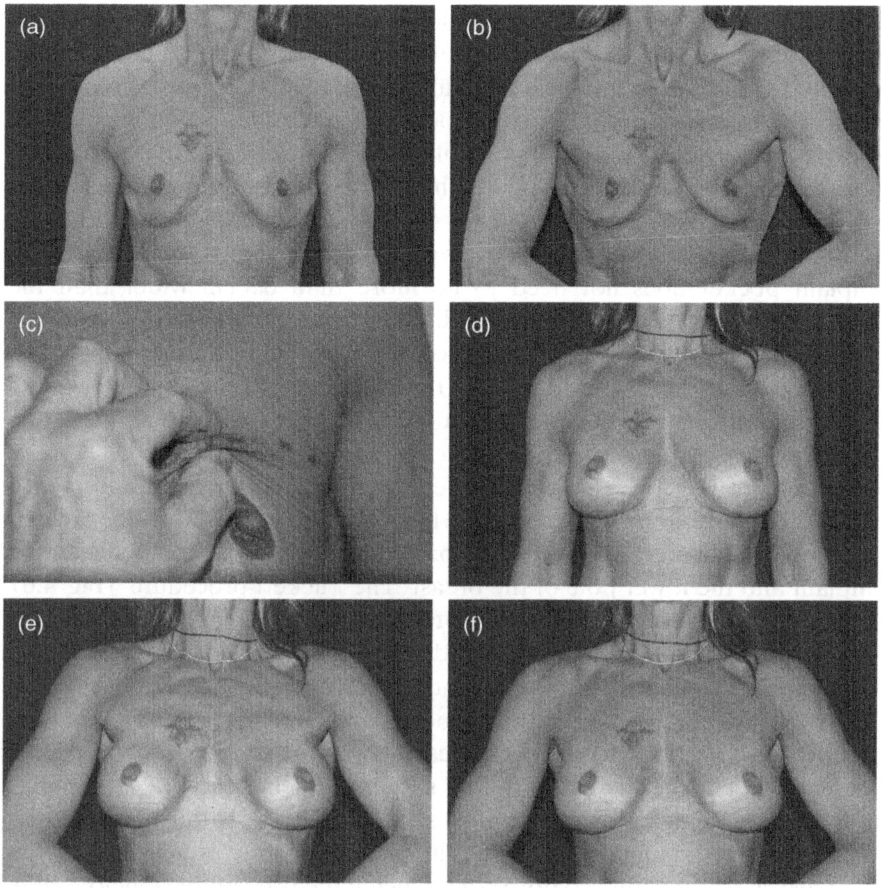

4.18 (a) Before breast augmentation with a dual plane IV submuscular technique in bodybuilder who in her youth underwent a breast reduction. (b) During preoperative pectoralis tightening. (c) The subcutaneous pinch thickness at the calculated upper border of the implant. (d) Six months postoperative. (e) During pectoralis muscle tightening and (f) in same position relaxed. Note minimal animation in spite of a very strong muscle and that the patient had not noted any loss in muscle strength.

chance of a more natural appearance with subglandular implantation as mentioned above, but if the tissue cover in the upper pole is insufficient with a pinch test less than 2–3 cm, dual plane IV positioning is favoured instead. The benefit of dual plane IV positioning is also that the lower pole of the implant has a true subglandular placement without adhesion of the posterior implant capsule to the ribcage.

If a subglandular position is planned, then the dissection is done in a cranial direction. The author favours inclusion of the pectoralis muscle fascia (subfascial placement) to provide a better tissue cover in the upper pole of the implant. The fascia is thin, but can easily be included in the elevated gland. Most important in subglandular implant positioning is to measure the height of the implant pocket, as under-dissection may add to the risk of buckling of the upper pole of the implant. A ruler should be inserted into the pocket to check the height before finalising the dissection, and the height of the implant pocket should exceed the implant with 1 cm to provide good draping of the upper pole of the implant. The width of the implant pocket does not need to be more than 0.5 cm wider than the implant on each side. In breasts with constricted lower pole or tuberous deformity, the glandular tissue in the lower pole should be modified. Moderate constriction can be addressed by radial division of the glandular tissue from the nipple areola complex down to the level of the submammary fold. Usually three radial incisions are carried out through the gland. If more expansion of the lower pole is needed, then a horizontal division is also added. For more severe tuberosities, a flap of glandular tissue can be created and unfolded in a distal direction to provide a good transition between the implant and the lower pole of the breast 'The Puckett procedure' (Fig. 4.6).

After completing the dissection of the implant pocket, haemostasis is checked. In primary cases, when the described procedure is used, bleeding is minimal. This has also minimised the use of drains and many primary breast augmentation patients do not receive drainage. During implant insertion a 'no-touch technique' is used. A clean sterile drape is placed underneath the breasts and only the surgeon touches the breast implants after having changed his or her gloves (powder-free). To further minimise the risk of contamination problems, the patient also receives IV antibiotics administrated 20 minutes before commencing the procedure (Flucloxacillin 2 g); no further antibiotic treatment is needed or recommended. During implantation of a form stable breast implant, it is important to have an incision that is not too short. This may create a fracture of the form stable silicone gel. Lubrication of the implant is recommended and the author favours saline solution padded into the textured surface. The reason for this is that this is the most natural of products. Some surgeons favour antibiotic solution, others Betadine®, but also sterile silicone gel has been used without reported problems. Implantation of form stable anatomical devices is facilitated if the thinner top of the implant is rotated into place first. This is done by holding an anatomical implant at a 90° angle at the border of the incision, first pushing the top into the pocket. This is then followed by wriggling the left, right, top and bottom sides, until the implant is in place. This is then followed by careful control of the implant position, palpating marking lines or dots in the implant to see that the vertical axis of the implant is aligned according to the desired position. The implant borders are also palpated with the index finger and it is important that implant pockets are not excessively big as this may increase the risk of rotation. However, under-dissection of the pocket is also unfavourable as this may buckle the edges of the implant. Thus, the implant should be lying flat on the chest wall with approximately 0.5 cm space on each side and approximately 1.0 cm space in the top of the implant. Finally the lower border of the implant is adjusted and pulled down or up to the preoperative marked ILP-line.

When using the above discussed 'new inframammary fold incision' or AK-incision, the suturing technique is of great importance. A good suture bite of the thoracic fascia is taken parallel to the ILP-line at the lower border of the implant. The suture is then passed through the Scarpa's fascia at the lower border of the incision, and then back into the thoracic fascia. A barbed suture (Quill® PDO no: 0) is favoured as it speeds up the suturing and creates a steady and long-lasting anchoring of the deep part of the scar. The suture is first placed in the central part of the incision. One end runs laterally and the other medially. In the end of the incision the suture is turned and the Scarpa's fascial of upper border of the incision is pulled down to the thoracic fascia in a running fashion until the midline of the incision is reached.

This suture fixation minimises migration of the scar away from the submammary fold during later arm elevation and improves the appearance of the inframammary fold scar. The Scarpa's fascia fixation is then followed by deep dermal relaxing ridging sutures with good strong bites, far away from the wound edge averting the dermis and creating a good deep dermal relaxation. The third layer of suture is a subcuticular running suture line with the other end of the barbed 2/0 Monoderm® suture. Only the suture end in each end of the incision is sticking out through the skin. This three-layered closure is usually done with absorbable stitches (Monocryl or Monocyn 3/0). Finally the wound is covered with Micropore® tape and a sports bra is applied as a support garment for 3 weeks postoperatively. The patient is recommended to avoid strenuous exercise that would move the implant and reduce the chance for good tissue adhesion into the implant surface.

4.6 Problems and complications

All complications reported for non-form stable implants can also be encountered when using form stable breast implants. These include surgical complications such as infections and bleeding, implant malposition and implant visibility. The risk of these problems can be minimised, by antibiotic prophylaxis and a careful surgical dissection in combination with a careful preoperative planning. Patient dissatisfaction is also a complication that could be encountered after any type of breast augmentation, and the risk of these problems is minimised with good and careful patient communication and preoperative information. In fact, all of the above complications and risks are no more frequent with form stable breast implants than with non-form stable implants.[8] The risk of these complications is not higher with anatomically shaped implants than with non-form stable implants. The only specific risk that is related to form stable anatomically shaped implants is rotation. However, the frequency of this complication has been low in our experience and with a careful meticulous preoperative planning of surgical techniques, this should be a minimal problem. There are several possible explanations for implant rotation. It may be related to secondary implantation into an old implant pocket, especially if a smooth walled implant was previously used. It may also be related to a poor surgical technique, with the creation of a pocket that is too large. In addition, blunt dissection could result in a seroma and postoperative bleeding. Another reason for rotation may be a low-grade infection with the creation of a biofilm that prevents tissue adhesion on the implant. Excessive early movement of the implant may result in an intracapsular rupture and creation of a double capsule.

The problem of double capsules is a relatively new phenomenon in breast augmentation surgery. This is defined as an inner implant adherent capsule free from the surrounding outer part of the capsule. Thus the implant can move and possibly rotate. A recent study by Hall-Findlay indicated that 14 of 105 Biocell implants were shown to have double capsules, in patients who were undergoing secondary breast implant surgery.[9] This finding was seen only with Biocell implants, and was not seen with other types of smooth or textured implants. This is however not surprising; as demonstrated by Danino *et al.*[1,10] a pore size >300 μm was needed for tissue ingrowth, thus other textured anatomically shaped implants (with smaller pore size) can not have tissue fixation and will thus have a higher risk of movement and rotation. With the right implant selection and surgical technique and postoperative recommendation rotational problems with the Biocell surface has been low (<1%) in frequency.[4]

Capsular contraction also occurs around form stable breast implants, but due to the resistance to spherical deformation, Baker grade IV contraction has been very uncommon. In a long-term evaluation of Style 410 implants no capsular contraction of Baker IV grade was detected whereas Baker III capsular formation was encountered in 5.6% of cases.[2] With a meticulous, tension-free suture closure and preoperative antibiotic coverage, infection problems have almost been nil in primary augmentations. In mastopexy augmentations, the frequency of minor postoperative infections not leading to implant extrusion has been approximately 1%. With sufficient muscle cover implant palpability has not been a reported problem in the upper medial pole, but for thin patients the implant in the lower and lateral pole of the breast may be palpated. Form stable implants also have fewer irregularities and rippling than non-form stable breast implants. In a long-term follow up evaluation, 98% had no visible creases or irregularities of the implant, and strong rippling and irregularities were not seen in any of the patients evaluated.[11] Beginning in 1995 and up until mid 2010, >14,000 form stable implants have been inserted in our unit. The patient satisfaction rate surpasses previously used techniques and 97% of patients feel that these procedures are advantageous after a long-term implantation time.[2] The complication rate has been low and the outcome more predictable than in our previous experience with non-form stable breast implants.

4.7 References

1. DANINO, A.M., BASMACIOGLU, P., SAITO, S., ROCHER, F., BLANCHET-BARDON, C., REVOL, M. and SERVANT, J.M. (2001). Comparison of the Capsular Response to the Biocell RTV and Mentor 1600 Siltex Breast Implant Surface Texturing: A Scanning Electron Microscopic Study. *Plast Reconstr Surg*, 108: 2047–2052.
2. MHRA Medical Device Alert MDA/2010/025, issued 31st March 2010.
3. AFSSAPS Medical Devices Evaluation Direction. Silicone based filling gel breast implants from Poly Implant Prothèse Company: update of test results, issued 14th April 2011.
4. HEDÉN. P. *et al.* (2006). Style 410 cohesive silicone breast implants; safety and effectiveness after 5–9 years of implantation; *Plast & Recons Surg*, 118, 6, 1281–1287.
5. HOLMICH, L.R., KJOLLER, K., VEJBORG, I., CONRAD, C., SLETTING, S., MCLAUGHLIN, J.K., FRYZEK, J., BREITING, V., JORGENSEN, A. and OLSEN, J.H. (2001). Prevalence of silicone breast implant rupture among Danish women. *Plast Reconstr Surg*, 108, 848–858.
6. HEDÉN, P., JERNBECK, J. and HOBER, M. (2001). Breast augmentation with anatomical cohesive gel implants. The world's largest current experience. *Clin Plast Surg*, 28, 531–552.
7. TEBBETTS, J.B. (2001). Dual plane breast augmentation: optimizing implant-soft-tissue relationships in a wide range of breast types. *Plast Reconstr Surg*, 107: 1255–1272.
8. TEBBETS, J.B. (2006). Achieving a zero percent reoperation rate at 3 years in a 50-consecutive-case augmentation mammaplasty premarket approval study. *Plast Reconstr Surg*, 118, 1453–1457.
9. HALL-FINDLAY, E.J. (2011). Breast implant complications review: double capsules and late seromas, *Plast Reconstr Surg*, 128, 56–66.
10. DANINO, A., ROCHER, F. *et al.* (2001). A scanning electron microscopy study of the surface of porous-textured breast implants and their capsules. Description of the 'velcro' effect of porous-textured breast prostheses. *Ann Chir Plast Esthet*, 46, 23–30.
11. JEWELL, M.L. and JEWELL, J.L. (2010). A comparison of outcomes involving highly cohesive, form-stable breast implants from two manufacturers in patients undergoing primary breast augmentation. *Aesthet Surg J*, 30, 51–65.

5
Polyurethane foam covered breast implants

D. FLEMING, The Cosmetic Surgery Institute of Australia, Australia

Abstract: Polyurethane foam covered silicone gel breast implants have been proven to dramatically reduce the incidence of capsular contracture in primary and secondary patients in every study published over more than four decades. Analysis of capsular contracture at the molecular level and of the difference between textured and polyurethane foam surfaces shows why polyurethane foam is effective in preventing capsular contracture and texturing is not. Concerns about the safety of polyurethane foam have been exhaustively investigated and disproved. Alleged difficulties in the use and removal of these implants are discussed and revealed to be unfounded. There is no logical reason not to use polyurethane foam covered implants as first choice in all patients.

Key words: polyurethane foam, capsular contracture, displacement, rotation, 2,4 toluenediamine (2,4 TDA).

5.1 Introduction

Following the introduction of the first silicone gel filled breast implants by Cronin and Gerow in 1963,[1] it soon became evident that significant numbers of patients would notice a variable degree of hardening of their implants over time. Initially this was mild but in some patients it became worse, causing discomfort and a change in shape of the breast. In the worst cases the breast was rock hard, distorted and painful. It was apparent that this was due to contraction of the fibrous capsule around the implant, the formation of which is the body's response to the presence of a foreign body. Since that time, surgeons and patients have sought to reduce the incidence of this capsular contracture. A myriad of strategies have been employed. Postoperative massage and specific manipulative exercises[2] of the implant have sought to enlarge the pocket, so that if a small amount of contracture occurs it will not compress the implant. Other attempts focused on operative technique to try to reduce contracture. The creation of a mega-pocket at the time of surgery was the operative sister of the massage and manipulation exercises, again seeking to avoid any contracture impinging on the implant. The use of a plethora of different antibiotic regimens,[3] sometimes including steroids, have been advocated both systemically, in the pocket and, in the case of saline filled, or double lumen implants, intra-lumenally. The routine use of drains and sub-muscular placement of the implants have been proposed.[4] The literature has been contradictory when reporting the efficacy or otherwise of all of these modalities[5] and certainly none has been accepted as making such a difference to contracture rates that it has become universally accepted. Attention has also been given to the implant surface.[4,6–9] The surface, because it is the implant's interface with the capsule, inevitably must mediate the interaction between the implant and the capsule. This chapter will explore how covering the implant in a layer of polyurethane foam dramatically reduces the risks of capsular contraction and how merely mechanically texturing the surface of the implant does not.

5.1.1 History of polyurethane foam covered breast implants

The first report of the use of a silicone filled breast implant covered with a layer of polyurethane foam was made by Ashley in 1969 to the 48th Meeting of the American Association of Plastic Surgeons in San Francisco. This formed the basis for an article published in *Plastic and Reconstructive Surgery* the next year, some 18 months after Ashley had first performed the operation.[10] Ashley described a thin silicone envelope implant filled with a low viscosity gel. The implant differed from other implants of the day because not only was it covered in a 1 mm layer of polyurethane foam, but also it had an internal Y shaped septum to maintain form stability of the implant by preventing the gel from shifting. Additionally, the implant was not round and had a different width, height and projection, so it can be said that Ashley had introduced the first anatomical, form stable breast implant as well as the first polyurethane foam covered implant. Ashley reported the results in 60 patients with up to 18 months follow-up. There were no cases of capsular contraction and only one patient had required revision due to a necrosed skin flap. The absence of contraction and minimal complication rate, in both primary augmentation and reconstructive patients, was confirmed by Ashley in his update article in 1972.[11] In this article he also described the ease of removal of the implant (now called the 'Natural Y implant') in two patients in whom they were removed for non-medical reasons.

Over the next two decades, the use of polyurethane foam covered breast implants became widespread in the United States, Europe, South America and Australia. Numerous peer reviewed papers were published, all of which demonstrated reduced contracture rates compared with smooth and latterly mechanically textured implants.[12–17] In fact, mechanically textured surfaced implants were not introduced until 1984, some 16 years after Ashley's first use of polyurethane foam. It is significant that many of the patent applications for the various methods of texturizing the smooth surface of the silicone envelope of breast implants claim to simulate an open-cell foam for promoting in-growth of tissue and for preventing capsular contracture.[18,19] Indeed, one of the major manufacturers of breast implants, Mentor (Mentor Corporation, Santa Barbara, California), used a method for texturing implants involving pushing the as yet uncured, and therefore still tacky, implant shell into a mold of polyurethane foam. The result is a negative imprint of the foam on the implant surface.[20]

As their use increased, reports of difficulties with foam covered implants started to emerge. These included delamination of the foam from the implant surface,[21] late breast pain,[22] difficulty of removal[23] and infections.[24] In 1991 it was suggested that the gradual breakdown of polyurethane foam in vivo might release potentially carcinogenic metabolites.[25,26] This coincided with the growing concern about silicone breast implants in general, which ultimately led to the United States Food and Drug Administration (FDA) moratorium on their use in 1992. The manufacturer of foam implants in the United States at that time was Surgitek (now defunct), a division of Bristol Myers Squibb (New York, USA). Surgitek voluntarily decided to cease manufacturing in 1991 prior to the silicone moratorium and foam covered implants have not been available in the United States since. Silimed (Rio de Janeiro, Brazil) has manufactured polyurethane foam covered silicone gel breast implants continuously from 1989. The Silimed manufacturing process involved vulcanizing the foam to the silicone shell, whereas previously it had been glued. This has eliminated the possibility of delamination of the foam layer. More recently in 2008 Polytech (Polytech Health and Aesthetics GmbH, Dieberg, Germany) has commenced manufacture of its own polyurethane foam covered implants. Prior to 2008, Polytech sold Silimed's implants in Europe under the 'Polytech Silimed' brand.

Polyurethane foam covered silicone gel implants continue to be used in all regions outside of North America for both primary and secondary breast augmentation patients and reconstructive patients. Saline implants have never been manufactured with a polyurethane foam covering. With the evidence of the long-term FDA supervised core studies of smooth and textured silicone gel implants showing very high contracture rates,[27,28] polyurethane foam covered implants are enjoying a renaissance. At the time of writing (May 2012), no application for approval for use of polyurethane foam covered implants in the US or Canada has yet been made. Thus the only region where they are not currently available is North America, where they were invented more than 40 years ago.

5.2 Capsular contracture and the role of polyurethane foam in its prevention

To appreciate the role of polyurethane foam in the prevention of capsular contracture it is necessary to understand the process by which capsules are

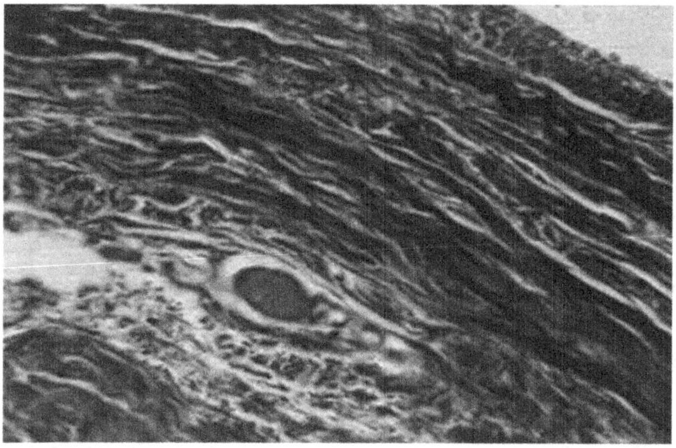

5.1 Histology of capsule of a smooth surfaced breast implant. Note parallel orientation of collagen fibers (dark grey) and relative paucity of blood vessels and cells.

formed and may subsequently contract. When foreign material is implanted into humans, the body reacts by trying to reject the foreign material or by encapsulating it in a fibrous membrane. Following implantation with a foreign body, there is an initial reactive inflammatory phase of healing which lasts 3 to 4 weeks.[21] This is characterized histologically by an infiltration of macrophages and multi-nucleate giant cells which display abundant lysosomes indicating active phagocytotic activity. There are relatively few fibroblasts present at this stage and therefore little collagen is produced. The intention is to break down the foreign material and excrete it. Over the ensuing weeks, if the implanted material is not readily biodegradable, the lysosomes diminish as the macrophages turn away from phagocytosis and instead secrete substances which induce fibroblast proliferation and the subsequent production of collagen. By 6 months this collagen has coalesced to form bundles of fibers arranged end on end and parallel to one another to surround the implant (Fig. 5.1). A complete capsule is formed around the implant and it is effectively sealed off from the patient's native tissue.

Over time the host's continuing response to the presence of a foreign body is to minimize the surface area of that foreign body. The collagen fibers therefore shorten and the foreign body is compressed within the capsule possibly mediated by the action of myofibroblasts.[29] If the implant is malleable, as is the case with breast implants, the volume of the implant will be compressed into a smaller space, the pressure within it will increase and the implant will become firmer. If the contractile force is sufficient, the implant will also change shape, causing the symptomatic complication called

Table 5.1 The Baker classification for capsular contracture

Grade 1	The breast is normally soft and appears natural in size and shape
Grade 2	The breast is a little firm, but appears normal
Grade 3	The breast is firm and appears abnormal
Grade 4	The breast is hard, painful to the touch, and appears abnormal

capsular contracture. This progressive development of capsular contracture is recognized in the universally used Baker scale classification of breast implant capsules (Table 5.1).

Published reports of capsular contracture rates vary enormously and an examination of the Baker scale classification together with an understanding of the mechanism of capsular contracture helps to explain this. By convention, only Baker grades 3 and 4 are considered to be contractures. Grade 2 capsules are not counted as contractures for the purposes of reporting contracture rates. However, a grade 2 capsule is in fact a clinical manifestation of a small degree of contraction of the capsule around the implant when compared to a grade 1, where there is no contraction and no compression of the implant. Additionally, as contracture is a progressive process, all grade 3 contractures were previously a grade 2. It is necessarily a subjective judgment, made by the examiner in each patient, whether the capsule has reached the criteria for a grade 3 and is therefore reported as a contracture, or if it is still a grade 2 and thus the patient is contracture-free. The implications for observer bias, especially when assessing one's own patients or those of an employer, are obvious. These difficulties are further magnified when the form stability of different implants is taken into consideration. Solid implants, cheek implants for example, form capsules but when these contract the implant is not deformed. Very firm silicone implants like gluteal implants are rarely compromised by symptomatic capsular contracture. The very high rates of capsular contracture of the early silicone gel implants occurred at least in part because these implants contained an easily deformed, almost liquid, gel in an under-filled envelope. Modern silicone implants are available in more form stable or less form stable gels and have a higher percentage fill. The more form stable the gel, and the more percentage fill, the firmer it feels and the more resistant it is to a compressive change of shape. The same contractile force may change the shape of a less form stable, softer implant and therefore reach the diagnostic criteria for a Baker grade 3. This is then counted as a contracture, but the same force may not change the shape of a firmer implant, which will then not reach the criteria for a grade 3 and will not be counted. This is the likely explanation for the reported reduced capsular contracture rates of highly cohesive (and therefore firmer) implants.[30] The fact that there is less deformity if the patient develops a capsular contracture, has been recognized by Spear and Hedén in their expert review of Allergan's (Santa Barbara, California) silicone gel breast implants.[31] This also explains Hall-Findlay's finding of less capsular contracture with Allergan's (now discontinued) CUI and CMH microtextured silicone implants which contain the same highly cohesive gel.[32] The disadvantage for the patient is that her implants will feel firmer even in the absence of any contracture. Manufacturers of such implants have recognized this and developed softer versions with less form stable gels. It is to be expected that the contracture rates for these softer implants will be higher than for the firmer ones.

Another often unrecognized factor contributing to the variability of reported contracture rate is the size of the patient's native breast and thickness of her adipose tissue. Visible shape change is necessary to diagnose a grade 3 capsule and therefore contracture. If an implant is covered by substantial adipose and breast tissue, lesser degrees of shape change will be camouflaged and hardening of the implant within a contracted capsule may be missed. Even if obvious firmness is detected on deep palpation, the lack of a visible change in shape of the breast will lead to the capsule being labeled as a grade 2 and thus not a contracture. Conversely, in a thin patient, a small degree of shape change will be readily seen and smaller degrees of hardening more obvious. Thus a lesser degree of contractile force may reach the diagnostic criteria for a grade 3 capsule in a thin patient with small breasts, but a greater degree of contracture in a more corpulent patient with larger breasts may not.

These factors mean the Baker classification has serious limitations. Although it is a useful method for classifying the severity of capsular contracture, it is less useful, and may even be a hindrance, in diagnosing the presence or absence of contracture. These deficiencies as a diagnostic instrument as opposed to a rating scale mean the Baker scale is far less useful for measuring the effectiveness or otherwise of interventions, such as polyurethane foam coating, designed to prevent contracture from occurring. If a method prevents contracture, it will prevent grade 2 capsules from developing, not just grades 3 and 4, and this will be missed by the Baker scale classification as it is conventionally used. In the absence of accurate and practical objective tonometry instruments, it is suggested a better, though still subjective, method for diagnosing the presence or absence of capsular contracture would be to ask the patient, 'Since your augmentation surgery have your breasts at any time been softer than they are now?' If the answer to this simple question is 'yes', then in the absence of seroma, hematoma, active infection or temporary conditions such as pregnancy or being premenstrual, capsular contracture is present.

A further factor complicating the range of reported contracture rates is the length of follow-up of many studies is short, often no more than 2 or 3 years. Capsular contracture is a progressive phenomenon as Handel has observed.[33] New cases occur many years after the original implantation and these are missed by the short follow-up studies. Meta-analyses, such as the often cited review by Barnsley,[4] which showed less capsular contracture for textured surfaced implants compared to smooth but only in the sub-glandular plane, are necessarily dependent on the limitations of the original studies they are analyzing. There has been a need for a rigorous, prospective, long-term study of both smooth and textured surfaced breast implants to provide solid data on what really happens to breast implants over time. Commenting in *Plastic and Reconstructive Surgery*, Spear has observed, 'The information that plastic surgeons will be most interested in would be that regarding single-lumen textured and smooth silicone gel implants. The very best data regarding those devices are available from the core clinical studies that were submitted to the Food and Drug Administration over the last year as part of the Premarket Approval process by both Inamed (now Allergan) and Mentor.'[34]

Commenced in 2000, these are 10 year, prospective, multi-centered studies in the United States of smooth and textured silicone gel implants. The FDA required these studies as a pre-condition for the 2006 re-approval of silicone gel implants in the United States. The FDA also required that Mentor and Allergan make available to patients the results of the core studies.

Allergan's data show a re-operation rate of 30% at 7 years for 455 primary augmentation patients operated on by multiple surgeons. Forty percent of the re-operations were for one of two reasons: capsular contracture or malposition/displacement.[35] The grade 3 and 4 contracture rate at 10 years was 19.1%[27] with no difference between textured and smooth surfaced implants.[28] Mentor's data are published for 8 years of follow-up and they have a contracture rate of 10.9%.[27] The progressive nature of capsular contracture seen in the results of the core studies have confirmed Handel *et al.*'s findings and have implications when considering the causes of contracture and therefore strategies for avoiding it. Handel observed the progressive nature of the incidence of capsular contracture '... contradicts the widely held belief that if patients remain contracture-free for a year or two they probably will not develop significant contracture. This finding may also have some relevance in understanding the cause of capsular contracture. If the risk of contracture persists for many years after implantation (as it appears to), it seems less likely that it is related to acute events such as bacterial contamination, surgical technique, drains, antibiotics, or other ancillary measures that have a short-term impact and more likely related to some chronic effect of implants on adjacent tissue.'[33]

Indeed there is no one cause of capsular contracture. Certainly there have been factors identified which increase its incidence. These include hema-

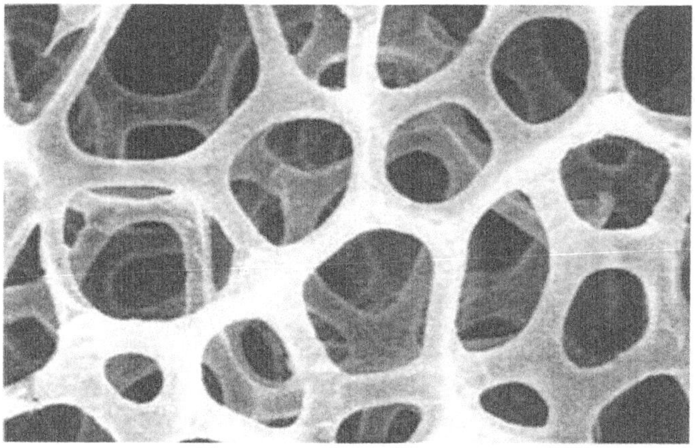

5.2 Electron microscopy of unused polyurethane foam.

toma, clinical infection, radiotherapy and evidence of the otherwise asymptomatic presence of *Staphylococcus epidermidis*.[36] The common denominator seems to be an increased inflammatory reaction exacerbating, or accelerating the body's natural response to minimize the surface area of the foreign material.

When an implant is covered in polyurethane foam, the fibroblasts encounter an up to 2.3 mm deep, three-dimensional sponge-like matrix of polyurethane struts with a very large surface area of 10 m^2/g (Fig. 5.2). Each strut is a triangular prism which has sharp borders. The intersection of the struts is irregular and multilayered. The spaces between the struts measure 200 μm–500 μm. Since both macrophages and fibroblasts have a diameter of upwards of 20 μm they are able to enter this deep matrix and recognize each individual strut as foreign material. Brand[21] has shown the histological response to the polyurethane foam is different, both spatially and chemotactically, to the response to smooth surfaced foreign material described above. After the initial invasion by macrophages and giant cells, these cells remain in phagocytotic mode and do not send out the signal for fibroblast stimulation. Thus, the production of collagen and the development of fibrosis is delayed. When it does occur, it is modified by the architecture of the foam matrix. Each individual strut becomes encapsulated by a layer of collagen and a network of micro-capsules is formed running in multiple, random vectors in three dimensions (Fig. 5.3). This process creates a spongy fibrosis with a Velcro-like attachment of the implant surface to the capsule and therefore the breast tissue.

There are two reasons why this 'stable marriage' between the implant and the patient's tissues is important. Firstly it dramatically reduces the risk of the capsule contracting around the implant.[37] The foam becomes

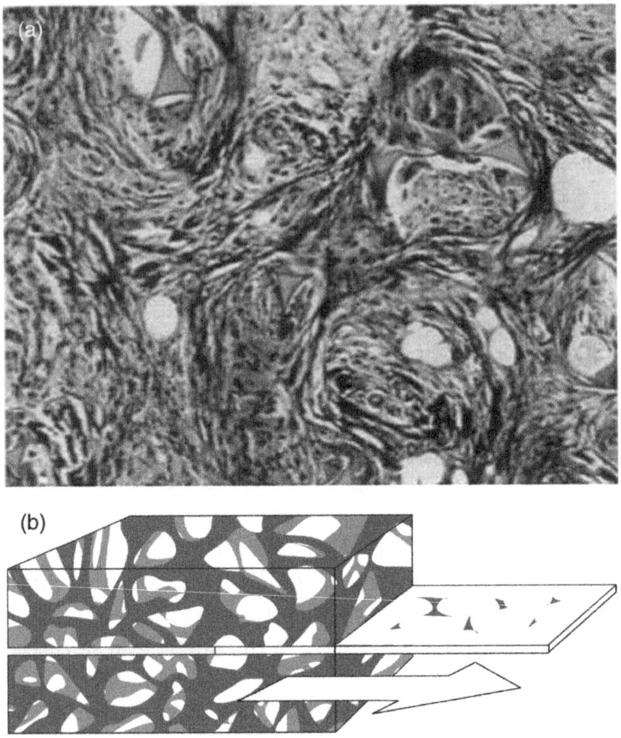

5.3 (a) Histology of a capsule of a polyurethane foam covered implant. Note prominent vascularity, increased cellular response and how the collagen fibers are disjoined as they form microcapsules around the foam struts. (b) Diagram showing how slide in panel (a) was prepared.

integrated into the full thickness of the capsule. The collagenized microcapsules around each foam strut form a three-dimensional matrix. Any contractile force compresses each strut and because these are disjoined and in multiple vectors, the forces neutralize each other. A concentric shrinkage of the capsule compressing the implant is thus avoided. Multiple papers published over the last 40 years[10–17] have universally shown reduced contracture rates with polyurethane foam covered implants when compared to smooth and textured surfaced implants. No paper has been published showing the opposite. The longest follow-up of a series of polyurethane foam implants was in a study by Vazquez and Pellon of 300 randomized patients for 18 years in a population of 1,257 patients, all of whom received polyurethane foam covered implants in a sub-glandular plane.[38] The capsular contracture rate at 15 years was 1%. Grade 2 capsules are not considered contractures and figures on their incidence are not typically reported. However, a grade 1 capsule where the implant is indistinguishable from the natural breast is the optimal outcome and a better outcome than a grade 2 capsule. For the same reasons foam covered implants have many fewer grade 3 or grade 4 capsules compared to smooth and textured implants, they also have many fewer grade 2 and more grade 1 capsules.

The second benefit of the stable marriage of the foam covered implant to the capsule and native tissue is a reduction in the risk of displacement or rotation of the implant. Polyurethane foam covered implants always adhere to the capsule as the foam becomes integrated into the full thickness of it. The only exceptions to this are in the presence of a hematoma or a seroma, or in cases of delamination of the foam layer from the implant surface, which only occurred in foam implants with the glued foam layers manufactured before 1992. Spontaneous, late loss of adherence of the implant to the capsule can occur but is rare. The Velcro-like adhesion prevents rotation or displacement of the implant, common causes of re-operations.[35,39,40] Additionally, the polyurethane foam covering has a high friction coefficient so immediately after insertion the implants are resistant to rotation and displacement even before the capsule has formed. This fact has implications for the meticulous intra-operative correct placement of these implants which will be discussed below.

5.3 Comparison of polyurethane foam covered implants with smooth and textured surfaced implants

We have seen how the polyurethane foam becomes integrated into the capsular architecture and how this neutralizes contractile forces preventing concentric shrinkage of the capsule around the implant. The architecture of the capsules formed around smooth and textured surfaced implants is very different. In both smooth and textured implant capsules the collagen fibers line up, parallel and end on end throughout the full wall of the capsule (Figs 5.1 and 5.4). If a stimulus to contract occurs (whatever it may be), the fibers can shorten over one another concentrically around the implant causing a shrink-wrap effect compressing the implant. Effectively there is one capsule around one large foreign body, the implant. This contrasts with the structure seen in a polyurethane foam covered implant capsule with its many microcapsules, running in random vectors throughout the full thickness depth of the capsule, around the multiple individual foam struts, each of which is recognized as a foreign body.

With textured surface implants, the intention is that the collagen fibers will weave into the irregular surface of the implant and a Velcro-like attachment, similar to that seen with polyurethane foam, will occur. However, even aggressively textured implants such as Allergan's Biocell® range only have a depth of texturing of about 200 μm. This contrasts with depth of the

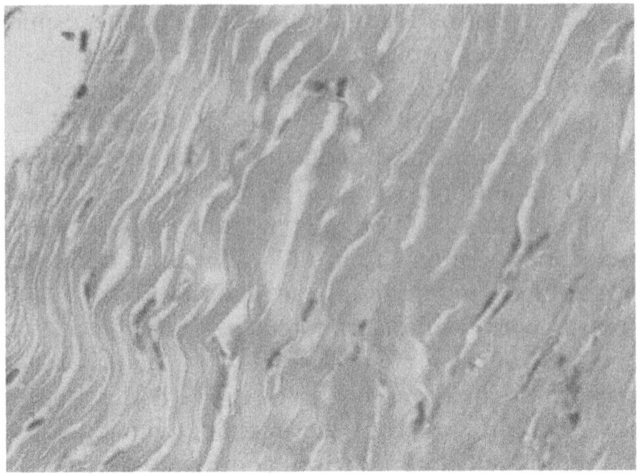

5.4 Histology of a capsule from a Biocell® textured surface implant. Note similarity of architecture with the smooth implant capsule (Fig. 5.1) with parallel orientation of collagen fibers.

polyurethane implant covering of at least 1000 μm[41] and up to 2300 μm (Fig. 5.5).[42] Inevitably therefore, the differences in the surface area of the mechanical surface texturing and the foam covering are much larger. The importance of this is revealed by the histology of textured implant capsules. This shows the texturing is unable to significantly change the capsular architecture compared with smooth surfaced implants. In fact, in most cases mechanical texturing does not create any attachment at all. When audiences of surgeons are asked, 'Of all the textured implants you have removed what percentage have had a Velcro-like attachment to the capsule?' the answer is invariably very few. Hall-Findlay has come to the same conclusion.[32]

An unpublished study by the author of 25 consecutive cases of textured implants removed for a variety of reasons including contracture, displacement, size change, rotation and leakage showed that more than 80% were not adherent to the capsule and were moving freely within it as a smooth implant would. In all patients where a unilateral complication was the indication for removal and the uncomplicated side was removed for implant replacement, there was no difference in adhesion rates between the two sides. Interestingly, in all of the patients where adherence had occurred, the implants were being removed for capsular contracture. This raises the possibility that the adherence in these cases was secondary rather than primary with the capsule contracting onto the implant surface. A similar effect occurs in reverse when textured saline tissue expanders are used. Here attachment is more likely as there is an expansile force pushing the textured surface into the enlarging capsule. This force is absent when the implant is of a fixed volume.

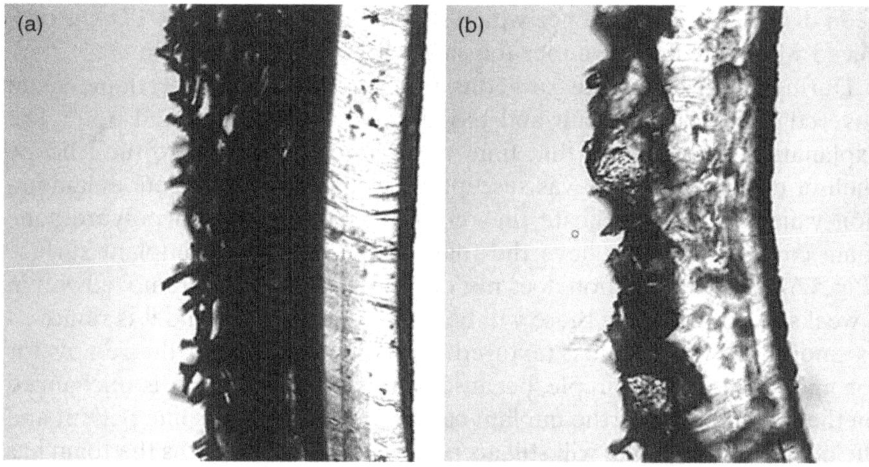

5.5 Surfaces of unused breast implants, ×40 magnification. Note the surface of the polyurethane foam implant (Silimed) (a) is not only deeper but also denser compared with the mechanically textured implant surface (Allergan Biocell®) (b). This results in a much greater surface area being exposed to the mediators of tissue in-growth.

In the case of smooth surfaced implants, the implant is not fixed to the capsule and is free to move within it. Since there is typically no attachment with textured implants, they usually behave in the same way. The core studies, the 'very best data' we have ever had according to Spear,[34] not only have shown very high contracture rates, they have also shown there is no difference between smooth and textured surfaced silicone gel implants.[28] The lack of attachment of textured implants to their capsules is also consistent with the observed high rates of rotation with textured anatomical implants and the high rates of re-operation for implant displacement in the core studies. Perhaps this explains why many surgeons advise their patients to massage their textured implants, an apparently contradictory recommendation.

Various objections have been proposed against the use of polyurethane foam implants. These have included suggestions that the implants were too difficult to remove, that there may be an increased risk of seroma or infection, that there would be a late spike in the rate of contractures as the polyurethane underwent slow biodegradation and allegations that this type of implant, with its strong attachment to the capsule, would be more likely to exhibit visible rippling. Of most concern were claims that the degradation products of the polyurethane foam included 2,4 toluenediamine (2,4 TDA), a known carcinogen in rodents in high doses.[25,26] All of these criticisms have been disproved. The evidence which showed no significant 2,4 TDA is produced will be dealt with under the safety section below (Section 5.4).

During the 1980s some surgeons found removing polyurethane foam covered implants a difficult and bloody procedure. Others did not.[43] The explanation for this is at that time the foam was glued onto the silicone shell of the implants and was susceptible to partial or complete delamination which could complicate the removal process. Modern polyurethane foam covered implants have the foam vulcanized to the implant surface (Fig. 5.6) and delamination does not occur. If the implant is removed within 3 weeks of implantation there will be no tissue in-growth and it is removed as smooth, or indeed most textured, implants would be. If the removal is for malposition for example, because at this point the foam is unchanged on the implant surface, the implant can be replaced in the same patient and the benefits of the foam will still accrue. After about 6 months the foam has fully integrated into the capsule. Because of the strong Velcro effect, the implant must be detached from the capsule prior to removal. This is easily done using blunt finger dissection with or without needle point diathermy. A typical example of such a removal by the author can be viewed on the internet.[44] The explant will now be devoid of foam (Fig. 5.7). However, it is important to recognize the foam has not disappeared. It remains in the capsule having been forcibly separated during the removal process from its otherwise enduring in vivo connection to the implant surface. Note the surface of the explant retains an imprint of the foam and is similar in appearance to the Mentor Corporation's textured implants which were manufactured by creating a negative imprint of polyurethane foam as previously described.

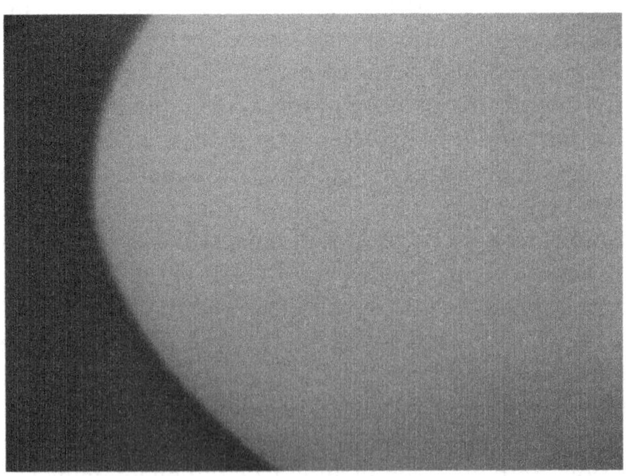

5.6 Surface of unused polyurethane foam covered implant.

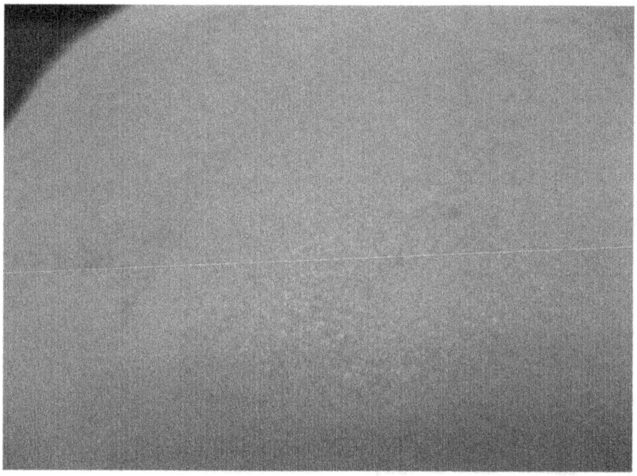

5.7 Surface of explanted polyurethane foam covered implant. Note foam remains in the capsule leaving only an imprint of its previous presence on the surface of the implant, similar to Mentor's Siltex® texturing. See text for explanation.

Between 3 weeks and 6 months the foam is becoming part of the capsule and removal at this time will result in some of the foam remaining on the implant surface and some residing in capsule. Thus if the benefits of the foam are to be retained with a removal and replacement after about 3 weeks, a new implant with an intact foam surface should be used.

There has been no evidence of a spike in capsular contracture rates as vulcanized foam implants age. Vasquez and Pellon showed only a marginal increase in contractures in their series between publishing the 10 year and 18 year follow-up data.[38,45] Handel compared the long-term outcomes, complications and patient satisfaction of smooth, textured and polyurethane foam covered breast implant patients in 2006.[33,37] He found no increase in seromas, infections, ruptures or visible rippling in polyurethane foam covered implants compared to smooth or textured surfaced implants. He confirmed a 'dramatic' reduction in capsular contracture rates in the polyurethane foam group, even though his long-term contracture rate for foam was higher than that of Vazquez and Pellon. The likely explanation for this is that Handel was using earlier models of the foam implant which had the foam layer glued to the silicone shell. Vazquez and Pellon were using more recent implants which used vulcanization to attach the foam layer. Brand, commenting on the few cases of contracture he saw in polyurethane foam covered implants manufactured using the glue technique, noted, 'Gross examination revealed in every case that the PU coating had partially or completely separated from the underlying silicone membrane, thus

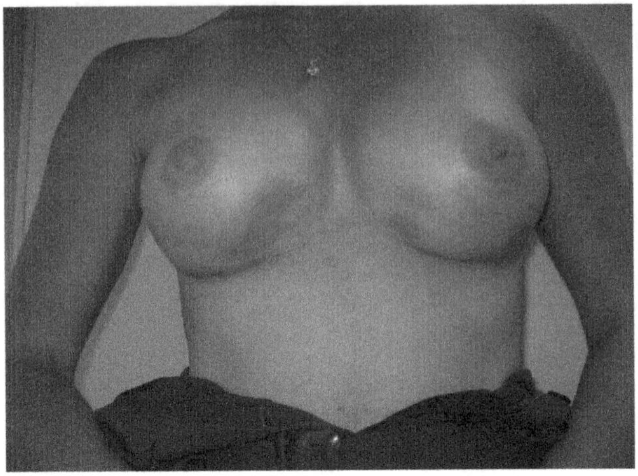

5.8 Polyurethane specific rash 2 weeks after implantation.

exposing the smooth surface. Scar-like contracted patches of fibrosis had formed in exactly those denuded areas.[21] Histological examination confirmed the gross findings.

The only complication specific to the foam implants was a temporary rash in 1–3% of patients. This rash (Fig. 5.8) appears on or around the breasts typically in the second week after implantation. It can be unilateral or bilateral. It is easily distinguished from the erythema of infection because the patient is always well and the rash almost always itchy. It is treated symptomatically with antihistamines and/or topical steroids and, in extreme cases, with a short course of oral steroids. The natural history of the rash is for it to worsen for a few days, then remain for about a week before spontaneously resolving, never to recur. The cause is not known but is presumed to be an idiopathic sensitivity. There have been reports that the rash is more common in very thin patients or reconstructive patients who have undergone mastectomy and in whom the implant is lying closer to the skin.[46]

5.4 Safety when using polyurethane foam breast implants

The polyurethane foam in the capsule does degrade very slowly over time under the influence of inflammatory cell esterases (Fig. 5.9).[47,46] Nevertheless, the protective effect of the foam against capsular contracture is enduring. Both the Handel and Vazquez and Pellon data have confirmed the long-term efficacy and safety of polyurethane foam covered breast implants.

The foam is a polyester polyurethane formed by a polymerization process using a mixture of 2,4 and 2,6 diisocyanate and there have been concerns

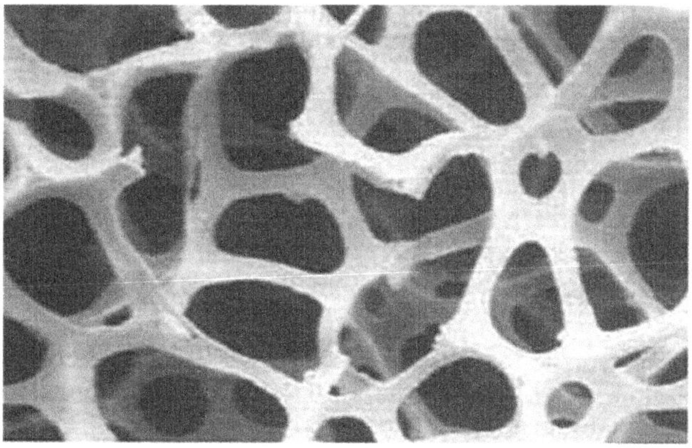

5.9 Electron micrograph of the foam after enzymatic degradation of 6-year-old capsule. Note that the foam struts are thinner but the matrix remains largely intact compared with the unused foam in Fig. 5.2. The biodegradation of the foam in vivo is very gradual and its protective effect against capsular contracture long lasting (see text).

that either the foam itself, or its potential breakdown products, might be carcinogenic. Concerns were heightened when case reports were published by Chan[25,26] showing measurable levels of 2,4 TDA in the urine of two patients who had polyurethane foam implants. Interestingly and, as it subsequently emerged, significantly, it was not found in their blood. The Health Board of Canada commissioned research by an Expert Panel on the Safety of Polyurethane-covered Breast Implants.[49] The panel could find no evidence of a significant risk but called for further investigation. This was done by Hester *et al.*[50] under FDA supervision. In their carefully designed, controlled and blinded study, they also found no free 2,4 TDA in the patients' blood. This was because it was never in the blood. Chan's method of preparing the urine samples prior to detecting 2,4 TDA is relevant. The urine was treated with six times normal hydrochloric acid and then boiled for an hour at 105°C. The elevated urinary 2,4 TDA subsequently detected was present as an artefact caused by in vitro acid hydrolysis. This had cleaved 2,4 TDA off from the harmless oligomers that are produced as part of the slow metabolism of polyurethane foam by inflammatory cell esterases.

It is also important to realize that 2,4 TDA has never been shown to be carcinogenic in humans at any concentration, and two occupational studies of workers exposed to it over long periods did not show any increase in cancers of any type.[51,52]

Significantly, 2,4 TDA was also detected intermittently in the urine of control subjects with no implants, indicating low-level environmental contamination with 2,4 TDA is unavoidable in humans. Hester *et al.* concluded the miniscule amounts of free 2,4 TDA found in the non-hydrolyzed urine of implanted patients posed no significant risk, a conclusion shared by the Health Board of Canada and Australia's Therapeutic Goods Administration and the FDA.[53] Even if it was assumed that 2,4 TDA was equally as carcinogenic in humans as it is in rodents, the levels found in the urine would equate to a lifetime risk of developing breast cancer increased by less than one in a million, a risk defined by the WHO as unmeasurable and described by the editors of 'Safety of Silicone Breast Implants' published by the National Academy of Sciences as 'the equivalent of developing cancer having smoked one cigarette.'[54] It is pertinent to compare this theoretical risk with the known real risk of death from a general anesthetic given to a healthy patient undergoing a capsulectomy, or surgery for an implant displacement, which she would not have needed if she had foam implants – about one in 80,000.[55] It should also be mentioned that polyurethane foam itself has no association with an increased risk of any cancer in any species and is used in other human prosthetic devices, such as pacemakers and prosthetic heart valves. The well intentioned but scientifically questionable, and ultimately erroneous, extrapolation of the results of experiments about the degradation products of polyurethane foam in vitro to the clinical setting in humans has had serious consequences. It is perhaps not an exaggeration to say that more than any other event in the history of breast augmentation, this has caused and continues to cause avoidable harm, condemning generations of patients to the miseries of capsular contracture and re-operations which might otherwise be avoided.

5.5 Use in secondary procedures

Polyurethane foam covered breast implants have measurable advantages over other types of implant in primary augmentation and reconstruction patients. These benefits are enhanced when patients have already developed complications with smooth or textured surfaced implants. The FDA instigated core studies have shown that patients who undergo a secondary breast augmentation procedure have an increased risk of needing another within 7 years compared with primary augmentation patients. Also capsular contracture occurred in 19.1% of the primary patients and 27.5 % of the revision augmentation patients by 10 years after their respective operations.[27] Therefore there is an increasing risk of complications requiring further surgery once a patient has had revisional surgery, and polyurethane foam covered implants can delay the need for the first revision by reducing the major causes of it.

In patients with capsular contracture who have a replacement with a polyurethane foam covered breast implant, the recurrence rate at up to 6 years is only 2% provided a new implant to tissue interface is created.[56]

This means either plane change, or the creation of a neo-pocket or total capsulectomy. If only capsulotomy is performed and the polyurethane foam covered implants are placed into an enlarged, previously contracted pocket, the recurrence rate for contracture by 6 years is at least 45%. To obtain the full benefits of replacement with a polyurethane foam covered implant, a new capsule with the foam fully integrated must be formed. This requires a virgin tissue–implant interface, not simply a polyurethane foam implant being placed into an old capsule.

There is no data published on whether the other advantages of the foam, namely the increased initial friction and long-term adherence to the capsule, also require a virgin tissue interface. These benefits are helpful in cases of implant displacement, rotation of anatomical implants, and in the treatment of symmastia. Once the inter-mammary space has been recreated with sutures in symmastia cases, or a capsulorrhaphy performed in inferiorly displaced implants, polyurethane foam implants, because of their high friction coefficient, will not exert the same force on the sutures as other types of implant. Thus the repair is less likely to break down with a recurrence of the symmastia or displacement. In the absence of definitive data it is logical to assume that if a virgin tissue interface with the foam implant is created these benefits will be maximized, particularly in the long term. However, this must be balanced against the risk of creating that virgin tissue interface. The risks of capsulectomy including tissue loss are well known. Plane change may be inappropriate in a particular patient because of the risks of creating visible rippling or the pseudo ptosis known as the 'Snoopy' deformity. The creation of a neo-pocket may be difficult. The author has had the experience of replacing inferiorly displaced textured silicone implants with polyurethane foam covered implants. Bilateral capsulorrhaphy was performed and the foam implants placed in the existing pocket. The displacement did not recur but 2 years later the patient suffered a blunt trauma injury to the left implant resulting in an intra-capsular rupture. The patient decided that as she needed surgery anyway, she would have both implants replaced with larger ones. At explant the unruptured implant was adherent to the capsule and a Velcro-like attachment was present, albeit a less strong attachment than is seen in implants placed into a pocket with a virgin tissue interface. Significantly, the explant was denuded of foam which had become integrated into the old capsule. This demonstrated that the capsule of a textured implant (and most likely of smooth implants as well), are not static but dynamic entities, capable of incorporating polyurethane foam into them.

The gold standard must remain creating a virgin tissue interface when replacing smooth or textured implants with polyurethane foam covered ones. However, unless capsular contracture is present it is not mandatory. In each case the reduced benefits of placing the foam implants in a pre-existing capsule must be weighed against the risks of creating the virgin tissue interface.

5.6 Disadvantages of polyurethane foam breast implants

The main disadvantage of polyurethane foam covered breast implants is that surgeons unfamiliar with their use need to make slight modifications to their operative technique when commencing using them. There is a learning curve but it is not difficult, provided appropriate instruction has been given and received. The choice of operative plan is no different for these implants. The incision site, implant plane, size, profile and shape are the same as for other implants. It has been suggested that a larger incision is necessary because of the high friction of the foam surface. This is not the case. Both manufacturers of foam implants include a sterile plastic sleeve, open at both ends, through which the implant can be inserted. The technique for doing this can be viewed on the internet.[57] Alternatively the implant can be liberally smeared in a film of sterile aqueous gel prior to insertion. This renders the implant slippery during insertion which can then occur without the sleeve. Because the aqueous gel is absorbed by the body within minutes, the friction of the foam covering is rapidly regained once the implant has been inserted.

The most important modification surgeons need to make if they have previously been using smooth and textured implants is to position foam covered implants at the final desired height. Although this may seem obvious, a common mistake made by surgeons switching to foam covered implants is positioning the implants too high. Because smooth and textured implants do not have the high friction coefficient of foam, postoperatively they will 'settle' into the inferior extent of the pocket. Thus if a patient returns a week after augmentation with smooth or textured implants complaining that her implants are slightly high, they are typically advised, correctly, to wait, because by 6 weeks the implants will have 'dropped' or 'settled' into the pocket. Polyurethane foam covered implants do not do this. They stay where they are put. If the implant is too high the day or the week after the surgery it will remain so. This is managed preferably by early operative repositioning during the first 3 weeks using the same implant, or waiting until the capsule is fully formed at 6 months and then replacing with a new implant for the reasons explained earlier. The author has considerable experience in teaching the use of polyurethane foam covered implants, and has observed that many surgeons initially find it difficult to force themselves to position the implants lower than they would using smooth or textured implants, even when they are aware of and understand the need to do this. To avoid placing the implants too high, and thus minimize this aspect of the learning curve, it is suggested patients are sat up intra-operatively prior to closure of the wounds. The implants should then be adjusted so the inferior margin of the implant is at the desired postoperative height. This helps to avoid malposition caused by artefactual upper pole appearances due to swelling or muscle spasm.

The second disadvantage of polyurethane foam covered breast implants is that if the pocket is insufficiently dissected, and a buckle or fold is present in the implant, this will not go away postoperatively. It is necessary therefore to ensure a generous pocket is made. Because the capsule integrates with the foam the pocket will always exactly conform to the exact shape of the implant. Thus, if there is a fold in the implant surface the capsule will conform to this fold and it will remain. In the case of smooth implants, which never adhere to the capsule and in textured implants, which usually do not adhere, the pocket is larger than the implant so the implant is free to move within it. In the absence of contracture, folds and buckles can therefore self correct.

Surgeons should not be fearful of making the pocket larger than the implant even when using anatomical polyurethane implants. The friction of the foam surface will keep the implant in position until the foam becomes attached to the forming capsule. No special bandaging or strapping is required and rotation with polyurethane foam covered implants has not been described. In summary the learning curve has three simple points.

1. Familiarize yourself with the insertion techniques.
2. Make a generous pocket to ensure no buckling.
3. Ensure the implants are positioned at the final desired height.

It has been shown that polyurethane foam covered breast implants are no more likely to become infected than smooth or textured implants.[21,37,46] Some surgeons have theorized that if infection does occur, then total capsulectomy will be needed to remove all foreign material because the foam is integrated into the capsule. This is rarely necessary. Superficial infections without implant exposure will usually settle with antibiotic therapy alone. If an infection involving the implant cavity occurs within 3 weeks of the augmentation, the foam will not be incorporated in the capsule and implant removal and delayed replacement can be performed in the usual way. If infection with implant exposure occurs later, management depends on whether it is localized to the wound or generalized involving the entire peri-prosthetic pocket. If localized, the capsule will be adherent to the implant at the margins of the exposure. In such cases, local and systemic antibiotics will usually allow healing by secondary intention with the implant left in situ. Suturing can also be used to accelerate healing if the tissues are viable and the infection resolving. If the infection involves the cavity beyond the exposed area, the capsule will not be adherent to the implant and it must be removed. Usually this will allow antibiotic therapy to clear the infection as any residual foam is in the well-vascularized capsule. Very deep-seated, long-standing infections may require a total capsulectomy. This situation is rare and occurs typically when treatment has been inadequate or delayed, or a resistant organism is the cause. Polyurethane foam capsulectomy can be performed in the usual way, with careful piecemeal diathermy excision of the capsule. 'Mutilating surgery with removal of significant amounts of surrounding soft tissue is never necessary.'[46]

The specific polyurethane rash previously described occurs in about 1%–3% of patients and is a temporary disadvantage. A further temporary disadvantage is that polyurethane foam covered implants take longer to start softening than smooth or textured implants. This is because of the prolonged inflammatory reaction also previously described. This causes micro-edema, stiffening the tissues around the implant during the post-operative phase. Thus the breasts of a patient with polyurethane foam covered implants will typically feel firmer than those of a patient with smooth or textured implants for the first few months after augmentation. The foam implant patient's breasts start to become softer at 5–6 weeks after the operation, and then continue to become gradually softer and softer over the ensuing months as the micro-edema resolves and the spongy capsule develops. The softening process is usually complete by 9 months. Because of the protective effect against even minor degrees of capsular contracture, they are more likely to remain soft compared with those of patients with textured or smooth surfaced implants.

5.7 Conclusions

Polyurethane foam covered breast implants have the lowest rates of capsular contracture, the commonest complication of breast augmentation and the commonest reason for re-operation. They also reduce the second commonest reason for reoperation, implant displacement. The low rates of these complications are known to be sustained for at least 15 years post implantation. There is no evidence that the advantages of polyurethane foam covered implants over smooth and mechanically textured implants diminishes in the long term. Polyurethane foam covered implants have been proven to be safe over more than four decades of use in humans. Theoretical concerns about possible carcinogenicity have been exhaustively investigated and disproved.

Textured implants were developed as an attempt to mimic the proven efficacy of polyurethane foam covered implants before the safety of foam had been established beyond doubt. Textured implants have failed to deliver the benefits of foam.

Foam covered implants are not difficult to use but they are different to use. The learning curve for surgeons wishing to give their patients the reduced risks of polyurethane foam is simple once understood.

Surgeons often start using foam implants in secondary cases where the patient already has contracture, rotation or displacement. Other than a fear of making a mistake in a primary patient, there is no logical reason for this and patients are better served with primary use of foam covered implants to reduce their risk of becoming a secondary patient. Other authors agree.

> There is nothing ... to suggest that polyurethane foam, or its in vivo breakdown products, pose a threat to the health or safety of patients. Polyurethane implants have measurable advantages over smooth and mechanically textured gel-filled prostheses and do not appear to be associated with an increased risk of complications or morbidity. (Handel[37])

> Currently, given our wide experience with the use of polyurethane-coated silicone gel implants, we may state they are the best option for augmentation mammoplasty, and have the lowest incidence of fibrous contracture. (Vázquez and Pellón[38])

> During the span of this author's practice, he has never been able to match the number and quality of superior results exemplified by these patients when using other devices. (Hester *et al.*[48])

> I think the evidence in favour of preferable use of PU covered implants is overwhelming compared to smooth or textured implants and it is clinically negligent to not put these facts to the patient. (J. Frame, Professor of Aesthetic Plastic Surgery, Anglia Ruskin University, UK, personal communication, 2011)

Frame's view is based on more than 40 years of accumulated evidence of the safety and efficacy of polyurethane foam as a covering for breast implants and the undeniable results of the core studies, showing the much higher rate of complications with both smooth and textured implants. Unless the patient is in one of the few countries where polyurethane foam implants are not available, it is unethical, and is increasingly likely to be found to be negligent, not to inform patients seeking breast augmentation of the fact that using polyurethane foam covered implants reduces the risk of the surgery. In the United States, which gave the world polyurethane foam covered implants in 1968, they remain unavailable. Because of the FDA's policy of requiring US based trials prior to approval of a specific breast implant, no matter what the duration and weight of evidence from other countries, patients will be denied access to the safest type of breast implants for many years yet. Ironically senior surgeons in the United States already know this. Dr Leroy Young commented following his presentation updating delegates about polyurethane foam covered implants at the 2009 American Association of Aesthetic Plastic Surgeons' annual breast meeting in Santa Fe, '... there were a number of surgeons who had used the devices when they were available in the US who uniformly said they were the best implants they ever used' (L. Young, Plastic Surgeon, St Louis, personal communication, 2009).

5.8 References

1. CRONIN TD, GEROW F. Augmentation mammaplasty. A new natural-feel prosthesis. Transactions of the Third International Congress of Plastic Surgery, 1963, Amsterdam, Excerpta Medica Foundation, 1963; p. 41.
2. CAMIRAND A, DOUCET J, HARRIS J. Breast augmentation: Compression. A very important factor in preventing capsular contracture. *Plast Reconstr Surg* 1999; 104: 529.
3. ADAMS WP JR, RIOS JL, SMITH SJ. Enhancing patient outcomes in aesthetic and reconstructive breast surgery using triple antibiotic breast irrigation: six-year prospective clinical study. *Plast Reconstr Surg* 2006 Jan; 117: 30–36.
4. BARNSLEY GP, SIGURDSON LJ, BARNSLEY SE. Textured surface breast implants in the prevention of capsular contracture among breast augmentation patients: A meta-analysis of randomized controlled trials. *Plast Reconstr Surg* 2007; 117: 2182–2190.
5. ARACO A, CARUSO R, ARACO F, OVERTON J, GRAVANTE G. Capsular contractures: a systematic review. *Plast Reconstr Surg* 2009; 124: 1808–1819.
6. HAKELIUS L, OHLSÉN L. Tendency to capsular contracture around smooth and textured gel-filled silicone mammary implants: a five-year follow-up. *Plast Reconstr Surg* 1997; 100: 1566–1569.
7. WONG CH, SAMUEL M, TAN BK, SONG C. Capsular contracture in subglandular breast augmentation with textured versus smooth breast implants: a systematic review. *Plast Reconstr Surg* 2006; 118: 1224–1236.
8. ASPLUND O, GYLBERT L, JURELL G, WARD C. Textured or smooth implants for submuscular breast augmentation: a controlled study. *Plast Reconstr Surg* 1996; 97: 1200–1206.
9. TARPILA E, GHASSEMIFAR R, FAGRELL D, BERGGREN A. Capsular contracture with textured versus smooth saline-filled implants for breast augmentation: a prospective clinical study. *Plast Reconstr Surg* 1997; 99: 1934–1939.
10. ASHLEY FL. A new type of breast prosthesis; preliminary report. *Plast Reconstr Surg* 1970; 45: 421–424.
11. ASHLEY FL. Further studies on the Natural Y breast prosthesis. *Plast Reconstr Surg* 1972; 49: 414–419.
12. GASPERONI C, SALGARELLO M, GARGANI G. Polyurethane covered mammary implants: a 12-year experience. *Ann Plast Surg* 1992; 29: 303–308.
13. PENNISI VR. Polyurethane-covered silicone gel mammary prosthesis for successful breast reconstruction. *Aesthetic Plast Surg* 1985; 9: 73–77.
14. COHNEY BC, COHNEY TB, HEARNE VA. Augmentation mammaplasty–a further review of 20 years using the polyurethane-covered prosthesis. *J Long Term Eft Med Implants* 1992; 1: 269–279.
15. CAPOZZI A, PENNISI VR, SPIRA M. Clinical experience with polyurethane-covered gel-filled mammary prostheses. *Plast Reconstr Surg* 1981; 68: 512–520.
16. HESTER TR. The Polyurethane-covered mammary prosthesis: Facts and fiction. *Perspectives in Plastic Surgery* 1988; 2, 1: 135–169.

17. PITANGUY I, BRENTANO J, DE CASTRO RAMALHO M, JOAO PORTO M. Implante de silicone gel comrevestimento de poliuretano. *Rev Bras Cir* 1990; 80: 119–130.
18. QUAID J. Method for making open-cell, silicone-elastomer medical implant. US patent 4889744. 1989.
19. YAN J, PURKAIT B. Method of making textured surface prosthesis implants. US patent 5022942, 1991.
20. BARR S, BAYAT A. Breast implant surface development: Perspectives on development and manufacture. *Aesth Surg J* 2011; 31: 56–67.
21. BRAND K. Foam-covered mammary implants. *Clin Plast Surg* 1988; 15: 533–539.
22. JABALAEY M, DAS S. Late breast pain following reconstruction with polyurethane-covered implants. *Plast Reconstr Surg* 1986; 78: 390–395.
23. PRADO A, ANDRADES P, BENITEZ S. A word of caution on the explantation of polyurethane breast implants. *Plast Reconstr Surg* 2006; 117: 1655–1657.
24. OKUNSKI M, CHOWDARY R. Infected Meme implants: Salvage reconstruction with latissimus dorsi myocutaneous flaps and silicone implants. *Aesth Plast Surg* 1987; 11: 49–51.
25. CHAN SC, BIRDSELL DC, GRADEEN CY. Detection of toluenediamines in the urine of a patient with polyurethane-covered breast implants. *Clin Chem* 1991; 37: 756.
26. CHAN SC, BIRDSELL DC, GRADEEN CY. Urinary excretion of free toluenediamines in a patient with polyurethane-covered breast implants. *Clin Chem* 1991; 37: 2143.
27. http://www.fda.gov/downloads/MedicalDevices/ProductsandMedicalProcedures/ImplantsandProsthetics/BreastImplants/UCM260090.pdf.
28. Surface texturing. http://www.allergan.com/assets/pdf/M1209–02_Silicone_Aug_Label.pdf p. 44.
29. BAKER J, CHANDLER M, LEVIER R. Occurrence and activity of myofibroblasts in human capsular tissue surrounding mammary implants. *Plast Reconstr Surg* 1981; 68: 905.
30. HEDÉN P. *et al.* Long-term safety and effectiveness of style 410 highly cohesive silicone breast implants. *Aesthetic Plast Surg* 2009; 33: 430–436.
31. SPEAR S, HEDÉN P. *Expert Rev Med Devices* 2007; 4: 699–708.
32. HALL-FINDLAY E. Breast implant complication review: Double capsules and late seromas. *Plast Reconstr Surg* 2011; 127: 56–66.
33. HANDEL N, CORDRAY T, GUTIERREZ J, JENSEN JA. A long-term study of outcomes, complications, and patient satisfaction with breast implants. *Plast Reconstr Surg* 2006; 117: 3.
34. HANDEL N, CORDRAY T, GUTIERREZ J, JENSEN JA. A long-term study of outcomes, complications, and patient satisfaction with breast implants. *Plast Reconstr Surg* 2006; 117: 3, discussion 768–770.
35. What are the main reasons for reoperation? http://www.allergan.com/assets/pdf/M1209-02_Silicone_Aug_Label.pdf p.36.
36. SHAH Z, LEHMAN J, TAN J. Does infection play a role in breast capsular contracture? *Plast Reconstr Surg* 1981; 68: 34–38.
37. HANDEL N. Long-term safety and efficacy of polyurethane foam-covered breast implants. *Aesthetic Surg J* 2006; 26: 265–274.
38. VÁZQUEZ G, PELLÓN A. Polyurethane-coasted silicone gel breast implants used for 18 years. *Aesthetic Plast Surg* 2007; 31: 330–336.
39. SCHOTS J, FECHNER M, HOOGBERGEN M, VAN TITS H. Malrotation of the McGhan Style 510 prosthesis. *Plast Reconstr Surg* 2010; 126: 261–265.

40. BAEKE J. Breast deformity caused by anatomical or teardrop implant rotation. *Plast Reconstr Surg* 2002; 109: 2555–2564.
41. BARR S, HILL E, BAYAT A. Current implant surface technology: An examination of their nanostructure and their influence on fibroblast alignment and biocompatibility. *ePlasty* 2009; 9: e22.
42. Data on file Silimed, Rio de Janeiro, Brazil.
43. HOEFFLIN S. Extensive experience with polyurethane breast implants. *Plast Reconstr Surg* 1990; 86: 1.
44. FLEMING D. Removal of pu foam breast implant.mov (http://www.youtube.com/watch?v=Z3uMZY5qsxo).
45. VAZQUEZ G. A ten year experience using polyurethane-covered breast implants. *Aesth Plast Surg* 1999; 23: 189–196.
46. HESTER TR. Diagnosis and treatment of complications occurring with polyurethane-covered breast implants. *Perspect Plast Surg* 1990; 4: 105–121.
47. SINCLAIR T, KERRIGAN C, BUNTIC R. Biodegradation of the polyurethane covering of breast implants. *Plast Reconstr Surg* 1993; 92: 1003.
48. HESTER TR, TEBBETTS J, MAXWELL GP. The Polyurethane-covered mammary prosthesis: Facts and fiction (II). A look back and a 'peek' ahead. *Clinics Plast Surg* 2001; 28: 579–585.
49. Expert Panel on the Safety of Polyurethane-covered Breast Implants. *Can Med Assoc J* 1991; 145: 1125.
50. HESTER TR, FORD NF *et al.* Measurement of 2,4-toluenediamine in urine and serum samples from women with Même or Replicon breast implants. *Plast Reconstr Surg* 1997; 100: 1291–1298.
51. SORAHAN T, POPE D. Mortality and cancer morbidity of production workers in the UK flexible polyurethane foam industry. *Br J Indus Med* 1993; 50: 528.
52. HAGMAR L, WELINDER H, MIKOCZY Z. Cancer incidence and mortality in the Swedish polyurethane foam manufacturing industry. *Br J Indus Med* 1993; 50: 537.
53. MDDI Reports: The Gray Sheet: Polyurethane foam-covered breast implant cancer risk is negligible. 1995, July 3.
54. BONDURANT S, ERNSTER VL, HERDMAN R. *Safety of Silicone Breast Implants*. Committee on the Safety of Silicone Breast Implants, Institute of Medicine. Washington, DC: National Academies Press; 1999.
55. LIENHART A *et al.* Survey of anesthesia-related mortality in France. *Anesthesiology* 2006; 105: 1087–1097.
56. HESTER TR, MAXWELL GP, TEBBETTS JB. Capsular contracture following augmentation mammoplasty: Long-term follow up of treatment with polyurethane-covered prostheses. Unpublished.
57. FLEMING D. Insertion technique for polyurethane foam covered breast implants.mov (http://www.youtube.com/watch?v=RYlsJBus1s8).

6
The safety of breast implants: epidemiologic studies

L. LIPWORTH and J. K. McLAUGHLIN,
International Epidemiology Institute, USA and
Vanderbilt University Medical Center, USA

Abstract: The safety of silicone gel-filled breast implants has been studied more rigorously and extensively than any other medical device in the medical literature. This chapter summarizes the epidemiologic evidence regarding the safety of silicone gel-filled breast implants. The chapter emphasizes results drawn from the most recent epidemiologic investigations and from studies with long-term follow-up, often longer than three decades, as well as those that address some of the historically widespread adverse outcome claims regarding cosmetic breast implants, including connective tissue disease, local complications, offspring health effects, implant rupture, cancer, and psychologic outcomes including suicide.

Key words: epidemiology, connective tissue disease, cancer, local complication, rupture, suicide.

6.1 Introduction

Few implantable medical devices have been studied more rigorously or extensively for more adverse outcomes than silicone gel-filled breast implants. Although their design has been altered over the years, including changes to the cohesiveness of the silicone gel filler and texturing of the shell, the basic device design remains a silicone elastomer shell surrounding a viscous cross-linked silicone gel. Following a de facto ban on silicone breast implants by the United States (US) Food and Drug Administration (FDA) in 1992, the Institute of Medicine (IOM), which was established by the National Academy of Sciences to examine policy matters pertaining to the health of the public, published a review in 1999 of the safety of silicone breast implants (Bondurant *et al.*, 1999). The IOM specifically examined the safety concerns that had been raised about implants beginning in the 1980s, including connective tissue or rheumatic disease, neurological disease, effects on pregnancy, lactation, and offspring, risk of reoperations, specific local and perioperative complications, and cancer and effects on breast imaging. The IOM report did much to clarify the extent of knowledge and to identify gaps in information as of 1998 about the safety of silicone gel-filled breast implants.

This chapter summarizes the epidemiologic evidence regarding the safety of silicone gel-filled breast implants, emphasizing extensive additional data published in the years following the release of the IOM report. Much of the evidence reviewed herein derives in the main from large, nationwide, long-term investigations performed in Scandinavia, where unique population-based databases and well-established data linking possibilities exist. Many of these studies had, on average, at least 10 years of follow-up, including over three decades of surveillance for the longest-term implant recipients. Rather than reviewing every study we have cited, many of which have been summarized in detail in previous comprehensive reviews, we emphasize results drawn from the most recent epidemiologic investigations and from studies with long-term follow-up, as well as those that address some of the historically widespread adverse outcome claims regarding cosmetic breast implants. Many of the specific safety issues addressed in this review were initially raised by self-declared implant safety advocates, product liability lawyers and the actions of the FDA, largely based on letters and anecdotal reports published in medical journals in the early 1990s and sensationalized stories in the media during that entire decade.

6.2 Connective tissue disease

Initially, the primary concern regarding breast implants was the occurrence of systemic sclerosis and other connective tissue diseases (CTDs), including systemic lupus erythematosus (SLE), rheumatoid arthritis, Sjögren's syndrome, and fibromyalgia. It had also been hypothesized that women with breast implants experience symptoms of apparent connective tissue, rheumatic, or autoimmune origin that bear some resemblance to fibromyalgia but do not fulfill established diagnostic criteria for any known CTD, including cognitive dysfunction, severe joint and muscle pain, incapacitating fatigue, and skin abnormalities (Kallenberg, 1994; Wolfe, 1999). Although unsubstantiated claims still appear from time to time regarding an association between silicone breast implants and known or atypical CTDs, these have been unequivocally refuted by the reassuringly consistent epidemiologic evidence from published large-scale cohort (Breiting *et al.*, 2004; Brinton *et al.*, 2004; Brown *et al.*, 2001; Edworthy *et al.*, 1998; Englert *et al.*, 2001; Friis *et al.*, 1997; Fryzek *et al.*, 2007; Gabriel *et al.*, 1994; Giltay *et al.*, 1994; Hennekens *et al.*, 1996; Holmich *et al.*, 2003b; Kjoller *et al.*, 2001; Lee *et al.*, 2010; Nyren *et al.*, 1998a; Park *et al.*, 1998a; Sanchez-Guerrero *et al.*, 1995; Schusterman *et al.*, 1993; Wells *et al.*, 1994) and case-control (Burns *et al.*, 1996; Dugowson *et al.*, 1992; Englert *et al.*, 1996; Goldman *et al.*, 1995; Hochberg *et al.*, 1996; Lai *et al.*, 2000; Laing *et al.*, 1996, 2001; Strom *et al.*,

1994; Williams *et al.*, 1997; Wolfe and Anderson, 1999) studies, as well as numerous meta-analyses and critical qualitative reviews (Bondurant *et al.*, 1999; Blackburn and Everson, 1997; Hochberg and Perlmutter, 1996; Independent Review Group, 1998; Janowsky *et al.*, 2000; Lamm, 1998; Lewin and Miller, 1997; Lipworth *et al.*, 2004a,2004b,2010; McLaughlin *et al.*, 2007; Silman and Hochberg, 2001; Silverman *et al.*, 1996; Tugwell *et al.*, 2001). Among these qualitative reviews is the US Federal court-appointed National Science Panel Report in 2001 (Tugwell *et al.*, 2001), as well as other more recent reviews (Lipworth *et al.*, 2004a, 2004b, 2010; McLaughlin *et al.*, 2007) of findings from epidemiologic studies published after the National Science Panel's review, all of which have concluded that there is no credible evidence of an association between breast implants and any of the traditional CTDs evaluated individually or in combination, or atypical CTD.

6.2.1 Established connective tissue disease

In an early, large, well-designed epidemiologic cohort study of US female health professionals, evidence initially suggestive of a relation between well-defined CTDs and breast implants was reported (Hennekens *et al.*, 1996; Lee *et al.*, 2010). In the first analysis, there was a small but significant overall increased risk of self-reported (not validated) CTDs among women with breast implants (Hennekens *et al.*, 1996). Due to the self-reported nature of the CTD result, a subsequent medical record validation of these data was performed by the same investigators, showing clear evidence of over-reporting of CTD by the participants, as only 22.7% of self-reported cases of definite CTD could be confirmed by a review of patient records (Karlson *et al.*, 1999). In the latest update from the same study population (Lee *et al.*, 2010), initially statistically significantly elevated relative risks (RR) of 1.6–1.8 for self-reported CTDs or for CTDs ascertained using a specialized CTD screening questionnaire (CSQ) were again found to be greatly attenuated and no longer significant when the analysis was restricted to CTD cases confirmed by medical records. Among women with implants, CTD diagnoses were confirmed for only 27% of women who screened positive for CTD on the CSQ, and for 18% of women who self-reported a CTD. The most informative result of this study, therefore, is the high level of CTD over-reporting by women with implants, particularly among US women with implants when there was nationwide litigation, sensational media reports, and a government de facto ban of the use of silicone-filled cosmetic breast implants. For most other industrialized countries, this was not the environment.

Over-reporting was similarly evident in a US cohort study (Brinton *et al.*, 2004) of 7234 women with breast implants, in which only a small minority of self-reports of rheumatoid arthritis, scleroderma and Sjögren's syndrome were considered 'likely' (i.e., likely to be real) after medical record review by a panel of expert rheumatologists. For the remainder, the diagnoses were not supported, either because records were incomplete or because clinical criteria were not met. Based on these 'likely' diagnoses, RRs among women with implants were non-significantly elevated for the three disorders combined (RR = 2.5; 95% CI 0.8–7.8) or for rheumatoid arthritis alone (RR = 1.9; 95% CI 0.6–6.2). The US study also found that women with breast implants were not more likely to have fibromyalgia than women with other types of plastic surgery, based on self-reports (RR = 1.3; 95% CI 0.9–1.7).

In a study of Danish women (Breiting *et al.*, 2004) with long-term follow-up, up to 35 years after implantation, no significant association for all CTDs combined was reported among 190 women with cosmetic silicone breast implants when compared with either 186 breast reduction controls (RR = 0.8) or 149 women in the general population (RR = 1.4). This study was able to identify women who had received their implants on average almost two decades earlier, but due to the relatively small sample size had limited statistical power to observe associations with rare outcomes such as individual CTDs.

Fryzek *et al.* (2007) reported on the occurrence of CTD in an extended follow-up of an earlier study of 2761 Danish women with breast implants and 8807 comparison women who underwent breast reduction surgery (Kjoller *et al.*, 2001). The women with implants were followed with virtually complete follow-up for an average of 13.4 years, and all CTD outcomes were based on hospital records and were medically verified through medical chart review to evaluate possible misclassification of these diseases at discharge in the study cohorts. Over 85% of CTDs diagnosed in hospital records were confirmed through medical chart review for women with breast implants. Compared with either general population rates or with women with breast reduction, women in the implant cohort had no significant increase in the incidence of combined CTDs or of any specific CTD, including rheumatoid arthritis, dermato- and polymyositis, systemic sclerosis, SLE, and Sjögren's syndrome. Direct comparison of the implant and comparison cohorts showed no relation for breast implants with confirmed fibromyalgia. Nyren *et al.* (1998a) conducted a large Swedish cohort study that included 3500 women with cosmetic breast implants, followed for a mean of 10.3 years, and 3353 women with breast reduction followed for a mean of 9.9 years. This study relied on a medical record data review to correct for all misclassified and pre-existing (prevalent) CTD diagnoses in both cohorts. In a direct comparison with women who had undergone breast reduction, the RR for hospitalization for total CTDs was 0.8, and no significant increases were found among women with breast implants for any specific CTD, including rheumatoid arthritis, SLE, Sjögren's, or scleroderma. The RR for fibromyalgia among women with breast implants was 1.0 (95% CI 0.3–3.0) compared with women who had undergone breast reduction.

Englert *et al.* (2001) conducted a retrospective cohort study in Australia of 458 women who received cosmetic breast implants between 1979 and 1983, and 687 women with other types of plastic surgery. Diagnoses of CTDs subsequent to implantation or other plastic surgery were self-reported and then validated through medical record review. There was no statistically significant difference between women with breast implants and controls in the reporting of any CTD or of systemic sclerosis, SLE, or rheumatoid arthritis.

With respect to fibromyalgia, a case-control study by Wolfe and Anderson (1999) found no association between silicone breast implants and the subsequent development of fibromyalgia. Utilizing a longitudinal clinical databank of patients seen at a rheumatic disease clinic from 1991 through 1994, history of breast implantation (including date of implantation) was ascertained among 508 women with fibromyalgia, as well as among 464 women with rheumatoid arthritis and 261 rheumatic disease controls with osteoarthritis. The fibromyalgia patients were the least likely to have had breast implantation prior to their diagnosis. When women with fibromyalgia were compared with women with osteoarthritis, who were selected by the investigators to serve as the relevant disease control group, the odds ratio (OR) for fibromyalgia diagnosed after implantation was 0.77 (95% CI 0.13–4.65), highlighting the importance of determining, in studies of breast implants, whether self-reported CTDs or symptoms occurred before or after breast augmentation surgery.

Similarly, Lai *et al.* (2000) conducted a case-control study of women seen at a rheumatology practice in Atlanta from 1986 through 1992 to ascertain prior history of breast implantation and fibromyalgia. Medical records were reviewed for 2500 women, of whom 131 had a history of breast implantation and 484 met the American College of Rheumatology criteria for fibromyalgia. There was no association between breast implantation and fibromyalgia. In addition to the studies reported above, a number of earlier cohort studies, most with shorter follow-up and fewer study subjects, also found no increased risk of definite CTDs among women with cosmetic breast implants when compared with either women who had undergone breast reduction or women in the general population, although the relatively small numbers of rare outcomes such as specific CTDs reported in these studies often precluded meaningful comparisons. Included among these early studies are the 'Mayo Clinic Study' of 749 women in Minnesota, who received silicone breast implants between 1964 and 1991 and were followed for an average of 7.8 years (Gabriel *et al.*, 1994); a study of 1183 women with breast implants identified from the Harvard Nurses' Health

Study cohort (Sanchez-Guerrero *et al.*, 1995); and a nationwide Danish Hospital Discharge Register study (Friis *et al.*, 1997) of 1135 women with cosmetic breast implants.

6.2.2 'Atypical' connective tissue disease

Studies that evaluated undifferentiated or atypical CTD as an outcome, defined as having a case definition distinct from the other established CTDs and substantive symptoms (Williams *et al.*, 1997), have consistently reported no credible evidence of an association with silicone breast implants or of a rheumatic symptom profile unique to these women and/or indicative of a specific atypical CTD (Bondurant *et al.*, 1999; Breiting *et al.*, 2004; Brinton *et al.*, 2004; Fryzek *et al.*, 2001a, 2007; Jensen *et al.*, 2001a, 2001b; Kjoller *et al.*, 2001; Laing *et al.*, 2001; Lipworth *et al.*, 2004b, 2010; Tugwell *et al.*, 2001).

In the Danish follow-up study (Fryzek *et al.*, 2007), unspecified rheumatism (which included fibromyalgia and myalgia) was statistically significantly elevated in both the implant cohort (standardized incidence ratio (SIR) = 1.9; 95% CI 1.6–2.2) and in the comparison cohort of 8807 women who underwent breast reduction surgery (SIR = 1.5; 95% CI 1.4–1.7) cohorts, when compared with the general population. A validation of the diagnosis 'unspecified rheumatism' (Jensen *et al.*, 2001b) did not reveal a rheumatic symptom profile unique to women with silicone breast implants or suggestive of atypical CTD. Jensen *et al.* (2001a) examined rheumatic diagnoses and related symptoms among women with implants with and without a prior diagnosis of muscular rheumatism, and observed that the frequency of fibromyalgia and the number of tender points were markedly increased among women with earlier muscular rheumatism, compared with women without a prior diagnosis of muscular rheumatism. These results, again, indicate the importance of taking prior rheumatic complaints and diseases into consideration when evaluating current rheumatic diseases among women with breast implants. In the US study of CTDs by Brinton *et al.* (2004), the authors included a category of self-reported conditions termed 'other disorders'. The RR for these self-reported disorders among women with implants compared with other plastic surgery controls was 1.4 (95% CI 0.8–2.6) for the period before 1992 and 3.6 (95% CI 1.9–7.0) for the period after 1992, during which breast implant litigation and media reports were widespread in the United States, suggesting strong reporting bias inherent in these self-reports of CTDs during a period of widespread litigation and publicity. Moreover, the authors indicate that most of these 'other CTDs' were 'vaguely defined or should not have been considered CTDs.'

In the largest study to date to examine symptom reporting for a pattern unique among breast implant recipients (Fryzek *et al.*, 2001a), 1546 Swedish implant patients and 2496 breast reduction controls completed a questionnaire regarding rheumatologic and other symptoms. Women with breast implants reported a multitude of symptoms, but with a clear lack of specificity. Thus, after extensive cluster analysis, there was no identifiable cluster of symptoms indicative of a specific 'atypical' CTD, nor was there a unique pattern of inflammatory rheumatic disorders or soft-tissue complaints among women with breast implants.

6.3 Offspring effects

There have been isolated case reports of children born to or breastfed by women with silicone breast implants who developed swallowing difficulties, irritability, nonspecific skin rashes, fatigue, and other symptoms (Gedalia *et al.*, 1995; Levine and Ilowite, 1994; Levine *et al.*, 1996a, 1996b, 1996c; Teuber and Gershwin, 1994). Besides the lack of a control group in these case series or small clinical studies, selection bias is a major concern due to the referral of children to a gastroenterology clinic because of a concern about breast implants, including those whose mothers were involved in implant litigation (Bartel, 1994; Cook, 1994; Epstein, 1994; Placik, 1994). In addition, some of the children were born to families with a history of scleroderma and esophageal dysmobility, so genetic or familial factors cannot be ruled out, and sedation of the children during testing may have affected esophageal pressures.

Four population-based retrospective cohort studies have examined health outcomes among children born to mothers with silicone breast implants, and none has found evidence of such a relationship. Kjoller *et al.* (1998) examined the occurrence of esophageal disorders, CTD, and congenital malformations among 399 Danish children of mothers who received breast implants at public hospitals between 1977 and 1992, compared with 3906 children of mothers who had undergone breast reduction. After a mean follow-up of 5.5 years (range up to 15.7 years), higher than expected rates of esophageal disorders were found among children born to mothers with implants, compared with the general population; however, similar excesses were observed among the control group of offspring born to mothers with breast reduction surgery, and excesses were also observed among children born prior to the mother's implant surgery. The observation of an increased occurrence of esophageal disorders among the offspring of women with implants both before and after implant surgery, and women with breast reduction suggests confounding by some characteristics of women who undergo cosmetic breast operations in general as a likely explanation for the observed excesses. There were no significant increases in CTD or congenital malformations in either the breast implant or breast reduction cohorts. Kjoller *et al.* (2002a) reported on an additional cohort of children of Danish women who received implants at private plastic surgery clinics between 1973 and 1995, and updated the follow-up of the earlier public hospital implant and reduction cohorts (Kjoller *et al.*, 1998). The mean follow-up after breast implantation for the private clinic and public hospital cohorts combined was 6.0 years (range up to 19 years). Esophageal disorders, rheumatic disease, and congenital malformations were examined among 2854 children born to Danish women with implants and 5805 children born to women who underwent breast reduction or other plastic surgery. Significantly higher than expected rates of esophageal disorders were observed for children born before (SIR = 2.0; 95% CI 1.3–2.8) but not after (SIR = 1.3; 95% CI 0.5–2.9) maternal implant surgery; similar excesses were observed among children born before (SIR = 2.1; 95% CI 1.5–2.8) and after (SIR = 1.6; 95% CI 1.1–2.3) maternal breast reduction surgery. Risks of rheumatic disease were not significantly elevated and were similar among children born before and after maternal breast implant surgery. A borderline significant excess of congenital malformations of the digestive organs was observed among children born after maternal implant surgery (SIR = 1.8; 95% CI 1.0–3.1), but a similar excess was observed among children born to women in the breast reduction cohort after their surgeries (SIR = 1.9; 95% CI 1.4–2.4). The risk of malformations overall was not statistically significantly higher than expected among children born after cosmetic breast surgery. Any observed elevated risks of adverse health outcomes appear unrelated to breast implants per se, because similar findings were observed among children born both before and after the mother's implant surgery, as well as among children born to control mothers in the breast reduction cohort.

Similarly, a retrospective cohort study conducted in Sweden found no evidence of increased risk of adverse health outcomes among children born to women with breast implants, after a mean follow-up of 8.9 years (range up to 24 years) (Signorello *et al.*, 2001). The investigators evaluated hospitalization rates for rheumatic and esophageal disorders, incidence rates for cancer, and prevalence rates for congenital malformations among 5874 children born to women with cosmetic breast implants compared with 13274 children born to women who had undergone breast reduction surgery. Compared with children of women who had undergone breast reduction, children of women with cosmetic breast implants were not at increased risk for rheumatic disease (RR = 1.1; 95% CI 0.2–5.3), esophageal disorders (RR = 1.0; 95% CI 0.7–1.6), congenital malformations overall (RR = 1.0; 95% CI 0.6–1.5), congenital malformations specifically involving the digestive organs (RR = 0.5; 95% CI 0.2–1.3), cancer (RR = 0.3; 95% CI 0.0–2.5) or perinatal death (RR = 0.9; 95% CI 0.5–1.8).

A fourth study, conducted in Finland (Hemminki *et al.*, 2004), attempted to evaluate perinatal health outcomes among infants born to women with silicone breast implants, as well as pregnancy and birth patterns among these women. In general, this study suffered from numerous methodological shortcomings, including biased control selection and uncontrolled confounding. As a result of these flaws the null results are uninterpretable.

6.4 Neurological disease

Flawed case reports have described neurologic disorders, including a multiple sclerosis-like syndrome and motor and peripheral neuropathies, among women with cosmetic breast implants. To date, three large, nationwide, population-based cohort studies, with average follow-up of approximately 10 years and with some subjects being followed for up to 20 years, have been conducted to evaluate risk for neurologic disease among women with cosmetic breast implants (Nyren *et al.*, 1998b; Winther *et al.*, 1998, 2001), and no associations have emerged.

Prior to the publication of these large epidemiologic studies on neurologic disease among women with breast implants, the American Academy of Neurology (Ferguson, 1997) published a report which concluded that the existing case reports concerning allegations of neurologic symptoms were insufficient to establish a causal association with silicone, given the methodologically unsound nature of the reports. In 1998, in an editorial (Ferguson, 1998) accompanying the Swedish (Nyren *et al.*, 1998b) and Danish (Winther *et al.*, 1998) studies published in *Neurology*, Ferguson, the editor-in-chief, concluded that these studies 'offer the best epidemiologic data to date of the lack of association between breast implants and neurologic disease.'

6.5 Implant rupture

In 1999, the IOM defined silicone breast implant rupture as a breach of any size in the implant shell and reported that all silicone gel implants were susceptible to silicone bleed through the implant shell (Bondurant *et al.*, 1999). However, because the larger weight molecules of the silicone gel cannot diffuse through the shell, gel does not appear outside the implant unless the shell has ruptured. Rupture has been suspected to occur as a result of biochemical degradation of silicone, physical trauma to the elastomer at the time of implantation, 'fold-flaw' failures, or as a result of mechanical injury, e.g., during mammograms, closed capsulotomies, or accidents (Cook *et al.*, 2002).

Intracapsular rupture, which is most commonly identified via MRI, represents a loss of integrity of the implant shell and is diagnosed when silicone gel is present outside the implant but within the intact fibrous capsule. Intracapsular rupture can go unrecognized as there may be no accompanying change in the configuration of the breast, no patient complaints, and no physical diagnostic finding. Leakage of gel outside the fibrous capsule surrounding an implant, or extracapsular rupture, is typically identified by MRI or at explantation surgery.

6.5.1 Rupture incidence

The IOM concluded that quantitative data on rupture incidence over time were lacking for all breast implant types, including third generation implants (Bondurant *et al.*, 1999). Only one study has employed a valid study design to detect true rupture incidence (Holmich *et al.*, 2003a). The study design included examination of the incidence rate of breast implant rupture via an initial MRI in 1999 followed 2 years later by a second MRI. The study was comprised of 271 Danish women (533 implants) with cosmetic breast implants. At baseline, 141 (26%) of implants in 97 (36%) women were ruptured, with a median implantation time of 12 years at first MRI (Holmich *et al.*, 2001). Of the ruptures, 31 (22%) were extracapsular, affecting 23 women (8%) in the study group. Extracapsular rupture was significantly associated with a prior closed capsulotomy. A true rupture incidence analysis was performed based on 317 implants (in 186 women) that were intact at the baseline MRI (n = 280) or were intact at baseline but removed before the second MRI (n = 37) (Holmich *et al.*, 2003a). The authors observed an overall rupture incidence rate for definite ruptures of 5.3% per year. The rupture rate increased significantly with implant age. For third generation implants (barrier-coated, low bleed implants available since 1988), the rupture-free survival was estimated as 98% at 5 years and 83%–85% at 10 years.

6.5.2 Rupture prevalence

Estimates of breast implant rupture prevalence range widely, in part because the methods of estimating rupture prevalence rates differ among studies (Bondurant *et al.*, 1999; Brown *et al.*, 2000; Handel *et al.*, 2006; Heden *et al.*, 2006a, 2006b; Marotta *et al.*, 1999, 2002; Robinson *et al.*, 1995; Slavin and Goldwyn, 1995). Determination of the frequency of gel migration outside the fibrous capsule is more difficult than ascertainment of rupture prevalence, unless there is implant retrieval (which is usually done in symptomatic women) and examination of explant and tissue. Marotta *et al.* (1999) conducted a retrospective failure analysis for explanted silicone gel-filled breast implants (8000 explants from 35 studies) and found a statistically significant correlation between implant duration and elastomer shell failure

(25% within 3.9 years and 71.6% at 18.9 years). An update of that analysis (9774 explanted implants from 42 studies) revealed 26% failure at 3.9 years, 47% at 10.3 years, and 69% at 17.8 years (Marotta *et al.*, 2002). These percentages were arrived at by studying only women who elected to undergo explantation. Because women with severe enough complaints to undergo explantation likely have much higher rupture rates than asymptomatic women, the reported rupture prevalence rates overestimate the rupture prevalence for all women with implants, as asymptomatic women are usually not part of the studies. Marotta *et al.* found a general reduction in tensile strength, tear strength, and elongation of explanted silicone elastomer shells and concluded that their explant rupture data are representative of the implant aging properties and rupture characteristics of the general population of silicone gel-filled breast implants that remain implanted. The fact that prevalence of rupture increases over time is not surprising since prevalence is a cumulative measure at a given moment in time. This, however, does not mean that the *probability* of rupture during a specified time period (incidence) increases with increasing implant age, a conclusion that cannot be drawn from the highly selected cross-sectional data analyzed by Marotta and co-workers. Finally, damage to implants during explantation can also lead to an overestimation of in vivo failure prevalence (Slavin and Goldwyn, 1995). Brown *et al.* (2000) determined the prevalence of rupture diagnosed by MRI in the selected group of 344 women (687 implants) with breast implants from two plastic surgery clinics. Overall, 265 (77%) of the women had at least one breast implant that was rated by radiologists as being ruptured or indeterminate (55% of implants were ruptured, affecting 69% of women). The median implant age at rupture was estimated to be 10.8 years, and over 90% of the implants included in the study were the less durable second generation implants. Extracapsular migration of gel was seen in 85 (12.4%) breasts in 73 (21.2%) of the women.

Handel *et al.* (2006) conducted a study of 1529 consecutive women who received 3494 implants (1137 saline-filled, 778 double lumen, 1537 silicone gel-filled, 38 other) for augmentation, reconstruction or revision at a clinical practice between 1979 and 2004. Rupture diagnosis was based on clinical confirmation at the time of explantation and not on the basis of mammography, ultrasound or MRI findings. After a mean follow-up of 37.4 months (range, 0–23.3 years), silicone implant ruptures occurred in 14 of 1123 smooth implants, six of 618 textured implants, and eight of 568 polyurethane foam-covered implants, yielding crude prevalence rates of 1.2%, 1.0% and 1.4%, respectively.

Finally, MRI rupture screening of 144 Swedish women with 286 fourth generation cohesive silicone breast implants yielded a rupture prevalence of 0.3–1.0% at an average of 6 years post-implantation (Heden *et al.*, 2006a). In a recent multi-center European study, MRI examination of rupture in women with 199 third generation silicone gel-filled breast implants with a median implantation time of almost 11 years revealed a rupture prevalence rate of 8% (Heden *et al.*, 2006b).

It is difficult to compare the results of cross-sectional rupture prevalence studies, for several reasons. Studies often include women with different generations of implants (often not the third or fourth generation single-lumen silicone gel-filled implants currently in use), saline and silicone implants, and implants made by different manufacturers. Studies of rupture prevalence are also likely to be biased in favor of higher rupture prevalence, since many publications present rupture data for implants that had already been explanted because rupture was suspected. Moreover, studies present data on women with different follow-up periods, and determination of rupture has been based on different detection methods (e.g., explantation, ultrasound, mammography, MRI, clinical survey results in patient cohorts), all with varying sensitivity and specificity. As a result, findings cannot be generalized for all women with breast implants. Implant age has been commonly noted in the literature as a determinant of rupture, with risk of implant rupture increasing with implant age (De Camara *et al.*, 1993; Feng and Amini, 1999; Holmich *et al.*, 2003a; Rohrich *et al.*, 1998). Holmich *et al.* (2001) found that age of implant was significantly associated with rupture prevalence among second and third generation implants. However, the prevalence of rupture among first generation implants, which had thick shells and highly viscous gel, was substantially lower than thin-shelled second generation implants, despite the longer implantation time, although this observation suffered from the small number of first generation implants.

To date, only one prospective study has addressed the possible health implications of ruptured, *in situ* silicone breast implants. In this unique study, Holmich and colleagues (2004) examined the possible health implications, including changes over time in MRI findings, serological markers, or self-reported breast symptoms, of untreated silicone breast implant ruptures. Sixty-four women with implant rupture diagnosed by MRI were followed for 2 years, and a second MRI was performed. A control group of women with no evidence of rupture on either MRI was used for comparison. The majority of women had no visible MRI changes of their ruptured implants. Progression of silicone leakage (either herniation of silicone within the fibrous capsule, migration from the intracapsular space into the surrounding tissue, or progression of extracapsular silicone) was observed in 11 implants (11%) in ten women; in most cases the changes were small. There was no increase in autoantibody levels, and no increase in reported breast hardness among these women. They did report a significant increase in non-specific breast changes compared with women in the control group. The authors concluded that, for most women, rupture is a harmless condition which does not appear to progress or to produce significant clinical symptoms. Based on their findings, they argue against routine explantation in asymptomatic women with ruptures; instead, they recommend that such women be followed regularly by clinical examination (Holmich *et al.*, 2004).

6.5.3 Connective tissue disease and implant rupture

It has been hypothesized that women with ruptured implants may experience increased exposure to silicone, which in turn could induce an immunological reaction leading to a higher risk of specific symptoms or systemic diseases (Press *et al.*, 1992; Melmed, 1998; Solomon, 1994). As previously reviewed by Holmich *et al.* (2007), only two studies of either CTDs or related symptoms evaluated by implant rupture status were based on patients not thought to be selected by the clinical course or symptoms.

In a magnetic resonance imaging (MRI) study by Brown *et al.* (2001), 236 (68.6%) of 344 women from two volunteer plastic surgery clinics had at least one ruptured implant; 73 of these 236 women had an extracapsular rupture. Women with breast implant rupture (overall or extracapsular rupture) were no more likely than women with intact implants to self-report a diagnosis of any of the definite CTDs studied, including fibromyalgia, or symptoms including joint symptoms, skin rash, cognitive disorder, fatigue, or hair loss. When women with extracapsular silicone were compared with a combined group of women with intracapsular rupture and women with intact implants, excesses were found for self-reported Raynaud's syndrome (OR = 4.2; 95% CI 1.1–16.0) and fibromyalgia (OR = 2.8; 95% CI 1.2–6.3). However, there is no biologic or scientific rationale for comparing women with extracapsular rupture with a combined group of women with intracapsular rupture and women with intact implants, since women with intracapsular rupture had fibromyalgia rates substantially lower (8%) than women with intact implants (14.8%). If the analyses had been conducted appropriately, based on three separate categories of implant status (intact, intracapsular rupture, extracapsular rupture), the fibromyalgia OR for extracapsular rupture compared with intact implants would be 1.9 (95% CI 0.8–4.3), substantially lower than the 2.8 reported by the authors (Lipworth *et al.*, 2004a). Moreover, the study had considerable potential for selection bias due to recruitment procedures and low response rates, and could not determine whether self-reported conditions occurred before or after breast augmentation (Lipworth *et al.*, 2004a).

In a sample of women from the Danish implant cohort who were randomly selected to undergo MRI to detect rupture, Holmich *et al.* (2003b) evaluated risk of CTD by rupture status among 238 women with cosmetic silicone breast implants. Ninety-two (39%) of the women had MRI-diagnosed ruptures, of which 69 were intracapsular and 23 were extracapsular, and 146 had intact implants. One year prior to the MRI, information was obtained on self-reported CTDs and symptoms with onset after breast augmentation. Two women in the ruptured group (both with extracapsular ruptured implants) and three women with intact implants self-reported a diagnosis of definite CTD, yielding ORs of 0.9 (95% CI 0.1–6.7) for women with ruptured implants overall and 3.8 (95% CI 0.4–35.1) for women with extracapsular ruptures compared with women with intact implants. For undefined CTD or other chronic inflammatory conditions, including fibromyalgia, the corresponding ORs were 1.0 (95% CI 0.3–3.0) and 0.8 (95% CI 0.1–4.5), respectively. Two cases of fibromyalgia were reported, one in the group with intact implants (0.7%) and one in the group with intracapsular rupture (1.4%). None of the women with extracapsular rupture reported fibromyalgia. These rates of fibromyalgia are consistent with the estimated prevalence rate of 3.4% for US women (Wolfe *et al.*, 1995), as opposed to the much higher rates of fibromyalgia reported among women with intact implants or intracapsular ruptures in the study by Brown *et al.* (2001), again suggesting biased selection of women in that study.

6.6 Local complications

Women with silicone gel-filled breast implants sometimes develop local and perioperative complications including serious infections, severe or chronic breast pain, hematoma and the need for additional surgery. Many of these postoperative complications are not unique to breast implantation but occur following various types of surgery in general. The reported frequency of local complications among silicone breast implant recipients generally ranges between 17% and 36% (Spear *et al.*, 2007; Cunningham, 2007; Hvilsom *et al.*, 2009; Kjoller *et al.*, 2002b; Henriksen *et al.*, 2003, 2005; Fryzek *et al.*, 2001b; Kulmala *et al.*, 2004). This variability among studies reflects differences in patients' physical conditions and co-morbidities, implant design, and timing of occurrence of complications. Studies including newer generations of implants and textured implants generally report lower complication frequencies compared with studies of earlier generations of implants. Typically, the most frequent local complication is capsular contracture, with frequencies ranging from 1.9% to 23% in recent reports, while complications such as pain, hematoma, and wound infection are substantially less common and occur during the acute postoperative period, with frequencies generally less than 2%. Additional surgery after primary implantation has been reported as a result of complications in 10% to 30% of implantations. Capsular contracture is the most frequent reason for additional surgery in women with breast implants.

Reports of complications following implantation with the newer generations of implants were published recently by two large implant manufacturers. Spear *et al.* (2007) reported results for 455 women (with 908 Inamed/Allergan implants). During 6 years of follow-up, the most common local complication was severe capsular contracture (Baker III/IV) which occurred in 15% of the women and was the primary indication for approximately 30% of reoperations. Other complications reported after primary augmentation were implant malposition and asymmetry occurring in 5.2% and 3.0% of the women, respectively. Twenty-eight percent of the women underwent a reoperation within 6 years, seven of whom had more than one reoperation. Cunningham *et al.* (2007) reported results for 551 patients with Mentor implants and 3 years of follow-up. Severe capsular contracture (Baker III/IV) was the most common complication observed in 8.1% of the women. Fifteen percent of the women underwent a reoperation within 3 years, of which 36.7% were due to capsular contracture, 11% to hematoma and 4.6% to asymmetry.

Cohort studies conducted in Denmark (Hvilsom *et al.*, 2009; Kjoller *et al.*, 2002b; Henriksen *et al.*, 2003, 2005), Sweden (Fryzek *et al.*, 2001b) and Finland (Kulmala *et al.*, 2004) have investigated local complications among women with cosmetic breast implants. Hvilsom *et al.* (2009) reported the most recent, long-term prospectively acquired data on local complications from the population-based Danish Registry for Plastic Surgery of the Breast. The incidence and severity of short-term complications was examined in 5373 women (10 640 implants) who underwent primary cosmetic breast implantation between 1999 and 2007, with a mean follow-up of 3.8 years (range up to 8.7 years). The frequencies of complications among women in this study were generally lower than those reported in other studies, likely to be due to some underestimation of complications attributable to passive long-term surveillance used by the Registry, as opposed to regular and frequent examination according to protocol in some clinical studies. During the entire follow-up period, 16.7% of women developed at least one adverse effect and 4.8% developed a complication requiring surgery. Within 30 days of implantation, the most common adverse events were infection (1.1%) and hematoma (1.2%), while change of tactile sense (8.7%), asymmetry/displacement of the implant (5.2%) and mild capsular contracture (4.2%) were most common within five years. The frequency of severe capsular contracture (Baker Grade III–IV) was 1.3% within 3 years and 1.7% within 5 years after implantation. Displacement or asymmetry (39.9%) and capsular contracture (17.3%) were the most frequent clinical indications for reoperation.

In their recent clinical practice-based study, Handel *et al.* (2006) reported that the rate of capsular contracture grade III or IV was 1.99 per 1000 patient-months after augmentation and 4.36 per 1000 patient-months after implant revision surgery. The frequency of hematoma and infection ranged between 1.5% and 2.1% following augmentation or revision surgery. For breast augmentation, 248 of 1601 (15.5%) implants required subsequent reoperation, while 21.9% of implants used for revision surgery required subsequent reoperation. The most common reason for reoperation was capsular contracture (56% of patients requiring additional surgery).

6.7 Incidence of cancer

More than a dozen epidemiologic studies, many of which have been large and able to assess long-term risks, have been conducted in North America and Europe to evaluate the potential association between cosmetic breast implants and the incidence of breast and other cancers (Breiting *et al.*, 2004; Gabriel *et al.*, 1994; Brinton *et al.*, 1996, 2000a, 2001a; Bryant and Brasher, 1995; Deapen *et al.*, 1997; Kern *et al.*, 1997; Malone *et al.*, 1992; Park *et al.*, 1998b; McLaughlin *et al.*, 1998, 2006; Mellemkjaer *et al.*, 2000; Pukkala *et al.*, 2002; Friis *et al.*, 2006; Brisson *et al.*, 2006; Lipworth *et al.*, 2008). The primary concern among breast implant patients, the medical community, and regulatory agencies was breast cancer risk because of the location of the implants, their use for reconstruction following breast cancer, and the hypothesis that they may interfere with mammographic detection of breast cancer. Some early reports also raised concern that women with silicone gel-filled breast implants may be at increased risk of developing other cancers, including lung cancer, cancers of the cervix and vulva, leukemia, and multiple myeloma. However, epidemiologic studies have been remarkably consistent in finding no evidence of increased breast cancer risk among women with breast implants, and the weight of the epidemiologic evidence is consistent with there being no causal association between breast implants and any other type of cancer. Accordingly, independent scientific reviews have unanimously concluded that there is no demonstrated excess of cancer of any type among women with silicone breast implants (Bondurant *et al.*, 1999; McLaughlin *et al.*, 2007; EQUAM, 2000; International Agency for Research on Cancer, 1999; National Institutes of Health, 2005). Indeed, in 1999, the International Agency for Research on Cancer (IARC) took the unusual step of concluding that there was evidence of a lack of breast carcinogenicity in women with silicone breast implants, and this conclusion was supported by that of the independent report of the IOM Committee on the Safety of Silicone Breast Implants (Bondurant *et al.*, 1999).

Numerous epidemiologic studies have continued to evaluate risk of breast and other cancers in women with silicone gel-filled breast implants. In a pooled analysis of the two large Scandinavian, nationwide cohort studies with virtually complete follow-up and cancer ascertainment

(Lipworth *et al.*, 2008), 3486 Swedish women (McLaughlin *et al.*, 2006) and 2736 Danish women (Friis *et al.*, 2006) who received cosmetic implants between 1965 and 1993 were followed for up to 37 years, with more than half followed for 15 years or more. There was no statistically significant increase in cancer incidence overall, compared with the general population of age-matched women. Similarly, Pukkala *et al.* (2002) conducted a cohort study of 2171 Finnish women with cosmetic breast implants, with a mean length of follow-up of 8.3 years. Cancer incidence overall was similar to that expected in the general population. Brinton *et al.* (1996, 2000a) conducted a retrospective cohort study of the incidence and mortality of cancers of various types among 13488 women with silicone breast implants compared with 3936 women who had other types of plastic surgery, as well as with women in the general population. There was a slight excess of cancer incidence overall among women with implants (SIR = 1.2; 95% CI 1.1–1.4) when compared with women in the general population, but not when compared with other plastic surgery patients (Brinton *et al.*, 2000a). In the large Canadian cohort study, the incidence rate for cancer at all sites combined was significantly reduced among 24558 women with implants compared with the general population (SIR = 0.75; 95% CI 0.70–0.81) and was similar to that among other plastic surgery patients (Brisson *et al.*, 2006). The incidence of breast cancer was below expectation in virtually all the large-scale epidemiologic studies, with risk ratios suggesting a reduction of 10%–50%. Few statistically significantly increased or decreased SIRs were observed for other types of cancers in any of the studies. A significant increase in lung cancer (SIR = 2.2; 95% CI 1.3–3.4) was observed among women with implants in the Swedish study (McLaughlin *et al.*, 2006). An earlier survey based on a randomly selected subset of these Swedish women with breast implants found that they were 2.8 times more likely to be current smokers than the general population of Swedish women (Fryzek *et al.*, 2000). This difference in smoking habits is likely to explain the increase in lung cancer risk among women in this study, as well as the excess of lung cancer mortality among women with breast implants in the Swedish mortality study (Lipworth *et al.*, 2007). The slight excess of total cancer in the study by Brinton *et al.* (2000a) was due primarily to statistically significant increased risks of cervical, vulvar, and brain cancer, and leukemia compared with the general population. Substantial differences in demographic, lifestyle, and/or reproductive characteristics between women with implants and both women with other types of cosmetic surgery and women in the general population have been reported in several epidemiologic studies (Fryzek *et al.*, 2000; Kjoller *et al.*, 2003; Cook *et al.*, 1997; Brinton *et al.*, 2000b) and are likely to account for these sporadic excesses of cancer, in particular vulvar, cervical and lung cancer.

Brain cancer has been studied quite extensively in several large-scale incidence studies (Pukkala *et al.*, 2002; Friis *et al.*, 2006; McLaughlin *et al.*, 2006; Brisson *et al.*, 2006; McLaughlin and Lipworth, 2004), as well as in five mortality studies (Lipworth *et al.*, 2007; Jacobsen *et al.*, 2004; Brinton *et al.*, 2001b, 2006; Pukkala *et al.*, 2003; Villeneuve *et al.*, 2006), all of which consistently failed to demonstrate any significant excess among women with cosmetic breast implants. Only one study to date has reported a significant excess of brain cancer among women with breast implants (Brinton *et al.*, 2001b), but upon further follow-up no additional deaths from brain cancer were observed (Brinton *et al.*, 2006), yielding a non-significant standardized mortality ratio (SMR) of 1.4 (95% CI 0.8–2.5) after an average of 20 years of follow-up.

6.7.1 Anaplastic large-cell lymphoma

Concerns about non-Hodgkin lymphoma (NHL) among women with breast implants have been raised by anecdotal reports of lymphomas in or near the breast among women with breast implants (Brody *et al.*, 2010; Newman *et al.*, 2006; Gaudet *et al.*, 2002; Sahoo *et al.*, 2003; Keech and Creech, 1997; Duvic *et al.*, 1995). A pooled analysis of NHL incidence in five long-term cohort studies with virtually complete follow-up of 43537 women with cosmetic breast implants in Denmark and Sweden, the US, Canada, and Finland yielded an SIR of 0.89 (95% CI 0.67–1.18), based on 48 observed NHL cases (Lipworth *et al.*, 2009). None of the studies reported a primary lymphoma of the breast. Thus, the epidemiologic evidence, based on large surveillance studies with long-term follow-up, does not provide evidence of an increased risk of NHL of any site among women with cosmetic breast implants. In the only published cancer incidence study to include women followed for at least 25 years after implantation (Lipworth *et al.*, 2008), including 3336 women followed for 15 years or more and 827 followed for at least 25 years, no significant excess of NHL was observed overall and not one primary lymphoma of the breast was observed. Moreover, the largest study to date (Brisson *et al.*, 2006), with cancer surveillance as long as 24 years, actually reported a reduced incidence of NHL among almost 25000 Canadian women with cosmetic breast implants.

Recently, a report of a case-control study from the Netherlands suggested an association of breast implants with anaplastic large cell lymphoma (ALCL) (De Jong *et al.*, 2008), although the latency period between placement of the implants and ALCL diagnosis was remarkably short (<5 years) for three of the five ALCLs diagnosed in implant women, weakening the plausibility that any observed association with implants is causal in nature. The cases in this study were reported to be all patients with ALCL of the breast identified in the Netherlands between 1990 and 2006, while all of the controls had lymphomas of the breast but of cell types other than ALCL diagnosed during the same time period. Thus, the elevated odds ratio presented in the paper does not demonstrate an increased risk of ALCL of the breast among augmented women per se. In fact, no valid conclusion at all can be drawn regarding whether there is an excess of lymphoma overall, or of ALCL in particular, among women with breast implants compared with women without implants, since control patient selection purposefully comprised only patients with breast lymphomas other than ALCL. Of interest, all five of the women with ALCL and breast implants had bilateral 'saline-filled' implants, which are used infrequently in Northern Europe, where silicone breast implants have not been taken off the market as they were in North America. Thus, the only valid conclusion that can be drawn from this study is that among women with breast lymphomas in the Netherlands, those whose pathology is of the anaplastic, large cell type variety may be more likely to have received saline implants (Lipworth *et al.*, 2009).

Lymphomas of the breast are rare, comprising 0.04–0.5% of all breast cancers (Kim *et al.*, 2011a, 2011b), and the vast majority are of B-cell origin. Anaplastic large cell lymphoma is a rare type of lymphoma, or cancer of the immune system, characterized by abnormal growth of T-lymphocytes, that occurs in several parts of the body, including lymph nodes, skin (cutaneous ALCL), breast, bones or soft tissue. ALCL is not cancer of the breast tissue; rather, implant-associated ALCL falls within a broad spectrum of lymphoproliferative disorders with a variety of clinical behaviors, raising questions about a diagnosis of malignancy in many instances (Jewell *et al.*, 2011). According to the United States National Cancer Institute, approximately 1 in 500 000 women is diagnosed with ALCL in the United States each year, with ALCL in the breast even less common, diagnosed in 3 in 100 million women per year (US FDA, 2011). In 2011, an FDA summary of the literature through May 2010 identified at least 34 unique cases of ALCL among women with breast implants, and concluded that women with breast implants may have a very small but increased risk of developing ALCL in the scar capsule adjacent to the implant (US FDA, 2011). Of the 34 cases, the median time from breast implantation to ALCL diagnosis was 8 years (range 1–23 years), and ALCL in women with breast implants is generally located in the region immediately surrounding the breast implant (seroma or fibrous capsule) but without invasion of the breast parenchyma. Most ALCL patients were diagnosed at the time of medical treatment for complications such as persistent seromas, capsular contracture or peri-implant masses. The evidence on implant characteristics, in particular implant surface, is too limited to evaluate whether implants with textured or smooth outer shell are associated with ALCL. As stated by the FDA, 'the totality of the evidence continues to support a reasonable assurance that FDA-approved breast implants are safe and effective when used as labeled.'

Several independent reviews of the literature pertaining to ALCLs among women with breast implants have been published (Kim *et al.*, 2011b; Jewell *et al.*, 2011; Brody *et al.*, 2010). In a review of 36 clinical cases of NHLs involving the breast among women with implants, 29 were ALCLs (Kim *et al.*, 2011b). However, 12 of the 29 women with ALCLs had a prior history of cancer other than T-cell lymphoma and two had a prior history of T-cell lymphoma. Similarly, Brody *et al.* (2010) identified 34 cases of T-cell ALCL among women with breast implants, all presenting as late peri-implant seromas, capsular contracture or peri-capsular tumor masses. The authors obtained preliminary data on brand and style of implant for 25 of the cases, and reported that 23 of them had a specific textured surface created by the lost salt method. Most if not all of these cases likely overlap with those reviewed by the FDA.

In summary, a potential association between ALCL and breast implants in general, or implants with particular characteristics such as a textured shell in particular, has been suggested by anecdotal reports of small numbers of women. A causal link between breast implants has not been established, nor has an association been evaluated in a large, well-designed epidemiologic study to date.

6.7.2 Breast cancer detection

The IOM (Bondurant *et al.*, 1999) suggested that implants may make screening mammography more challenging by obscuring a variable part of breast tissue. Based on the findings of a few case series (Fajardo *et al.*, 1995; Silverstein *et al.*, 1988,1990,1992), many originating from the same clinic, a hypothesis was generated that opaque breast implants may interfere with physical breast examination or mammographic visualization of breast tumors, leading to delays in breast cancer diagnosis and worse prognosis among women receiving implants. However, the interpretation of these clinical case series is hampered by potential referral or ascertainment bias, small sample size and absence of a control group. Furthermore, many of the women included in these case series underwent their mammograms prior to the implementation of Eklund's implant displacement technique which improved the accuracy of mammograms for women with breast implants (Eklund *et al.*, 1988), although a portion of the breast may still not be adequately visualized.

Numerous epidemiologic studies have evaluated whether implants delay the detection of breast cancer by comparing the stage distribution among women with implants at breast cancer diagnosis with an appropriate comparison group. Virtually all of these studies indicate that, although the sensitivity of mammography may be reduced somewhat in women with breast implants, these women do not in fact present with more advanced stages of breast cancer or suffer from reduced survival after breast cancer diagnosis (Friis *et al.*, 2006; McLaughlin *et al.*, 2006; Deapen *et al.*, 2000; Hoshaw *et al.*, 2001; Miglioretti *et al.*, 2004; Holmich *et al.*, 2003c). Most recently, Xie *et al.* (2010) reported on stage distribution and prognosis among 182 and 202 incident cases of breast cancer identified in the large Canadian cohorts of women with breast implants and women with other plastic surgery procedures. Women with breast implants were more likely to be diagnosed with a more advanced stage of breast cancer compared with other plastic surgery patients; however, there were no differences in tumor size and breast cancer-specific survival was similar in both groups. Moreover, none of the mortality studies to date has demonstrated an increased risk for death from breast cancer among women with implants compared with women in the general population (Lipworth *et al.*, 2007; Jacobsen *et al.*, 2004; Brinton *et al.*, 2006; Villeneuve *et al.*, 2006).

6.8 Occurrence of suicide

Five large epidemiologic mortality studies, conducted in various populations during the past decade, have reported with remarkable consistency that women with cosmetic breast implants have a two- to three-fold higher rate of suicide than similar-aged women in the general population (Lipworth *et al.*, 2007; Jacobsen *et al.*, 2004; Brinton *et al.*, 2001b, 2006; Pukkala *et al.*, 2003; Villeneuve *et al.*, 2006). To our knowledge, prior to these mortality studies, there were no case reports or case series in the literature to suggest a suicide excess among women with cosmetic breast implants.

Three nationwide cohort studies have been conducted in Scandinavia to evaluate cause-specific mortality among women with breast implants. In the Swedish cohort of 3521 women who had breast implants and were followed for an average of 18.7 years (up to 38 years) after implantation, a statistically significant threefold excess rate of suicide compared with the general population was observed based on 24 deaths (SMR = 3.0; 95% CI, 1.9–4.5). The excess rate of suicide in this study became apparent 10 years after implantation and continued to increase with extended follow-up to an SMR of 4.5 (95% CI, 2.6–7.7) among women 10 to 19 years after implantation and 6.0 (95% CI, 2.7–13.4) among women 20 or more years after implantation (Lipworth *et al.*, 2007).

Jacobsen *et al.* (2004) reported an increased risk of suicide (SMR = 3.1; 95% CI 1.7–5.2), based on 14 observed suicides compared to an expected 4.5 in the Danish implant cohort of 2788 women with implants, with a mean follow-up of 11.5 years (range, 4–26 years). No clear pattern emerged in the

SMRs for suicide according to length of follow-up, with substantial excesses observed in all time periods. This was the first and to date only mortality study to explore pre-implant psychopathology among women undergoing cosmetic breast implant surgery, by examining their preoperative history of hospitalization for psychiatric illness. The results of this study indicate that the Danish women who underwent breast implantation had a higher prevalence of psychiatric admissions prior to cosmetic surgery (8.0%; 95% CI 7.0%–9.0%) than women who underwent breast reduction (4.7%; 95% CI 4/2%–5.2%) or other types of cosmetic surgery (5.5%; 95% CI 4.5%–6.7%). When compared with all control groups, the risk ratio for prior psychiatric admission was 1.7 (95% CI 1.4–2.0). In fact, seven of 14 women with breast implants who committed suicide in the study had a history of preoperative psychiatric hospitalization. The study did not, however, provide information on history of specific psychiatric diagnoses or treatments prior to breast implantation.

Brinton and co-workers (2006), in their mortality analysis for the US cohort of 12 144 women who received cosmetic breast implants, reported an increased risk of suicide among implanted women when compared with the general population (SMR = 1.6; 95% CI 1.1–2.3, based on 29 observed suicides) or when compared with other cosmetic surgery patients (RR = 2.6; 95% CI 0.9–7.8). The risk of death from suicide was not elevated during the first 10 years of follow-up but was increased in all subsequent time periods.

In the mortality analysis of the large Canadian cohorts (Villeneuve *et al.*, 2006), significantly higher rates of suicide were observed in both the implant (SMR = 1.7; 95% CI 1.3–2.2) and other plastic surgery groups (SMR = 1.6; 95% CI 1.1–2.2) compared with the general population, based on 58 and 33 observed suicides, respectively. In the Finnish cohort of 2166 women who had cosmetic breast implantation and were followed for a mean of 10.3 years (Pukkala *et al.*, 2003), a statistically significantly increased SMR for suicide was observed among implanted women compared with the general Finnish female population (SMR = 3.2; 95% CI 1.53–5.86, based on ten suicides compared to an expected 3.1).

In addition to the increased risk of suicide among women with cosmetic breast implants, excesses of other external causes of deaths due to drug and alcohol abuse and dependence, atypical motor vehicle accidents, and other self-harm causes were also reported in the five published mortality studies (Lipworth and McLaughlin, 2010). The consistently higher rate of suicide, as well as the observed excesses of other drug- and alcohol-related external causes of death, among women with cosmetic breast implants is unlikely to represent a causal association, but rather reflects an increased prevalence of preexisting underlying psychiatric problems and other important risk factors for suicide among a subset of these women prior to their implantation. However, direct empirical research on these women prior to surgery for cosmetic implants is limited.

Women with cosmetic breast implants have been shown to have a higher prevalence of cigarette smoking and alcohol use, younger age at first pregnancy, history of induced abortions, and lower-than-average body weight (Fryzek *et al.*, 2000; Kjoller *et al.*, 2003; Cook *et al.*, 1997; Brinton *et al.*, 2000b; Didie and Sarwer, 2003), perhaps reflecting an increased prevalence of eating disorders among a subset of these women. Moreover, there is some evidence that women who seek cosmetic breast implantation experience preoperative psychological symptoms indicative of depressive disorders or report a history of psychiatric treatment substantially more frequently than women undergoing other cosmetic surgery (Didie and Sarwer, 2003; Sarwer *et al.*, 2000, 2003; Young *et al.*, 1994). These and other characteristics may influence rates of suicide and related causes of death. The prevalence and severity of pre- and post-implant psychiatric disorders or other factors needs to be further investigated to identify whether some women who undergo cosmetic breast implantation are at high risk of suicide.

6.9 Conclusion

In summary, the safety of silicone gel-filled breast implants has been studied far more extensively than any other medical device in the scientific literature, with much of the evidence drawn from large cohort studies with long-term follow-up, often longer than three decades. Paradoxically, the unexpected finding of an excess of suicide is the only consistently observed serious adverse outcome reported among women with cosmetic implants, despite initial claims of implants causing a large number of serious systemic illnesses, such as cancer and various connective tissue diseases. The results of the most recent investigations are remarkably consistent with earlier epidemiologic evidence in demonstrating that cosmetic breast implants are not associated with a subsequent increased occurrence of individual CTDs or all CTDs combined, including fibromyalgia. Moreover, there is no credible evidence for the conjectured excess of 'atypical' CTD among women with cosmetic breast implants. The epidemiologic evidence indicates that offspring of women with breast implants are not at increased risk for esophageal disorders, rheumatic diseases, or congenital malformations, and large, nationwide cohort studies with long-term follow-up have found no evidence of a causal association between silicone breast implants and neurological disease. The epidemiologic evidence consistently demonstrates that the incidence of short- and long-term local complications following breast implantation is relatively low and does not typically require additional surgery. Surgical intervention occurs most frequently as a result of capsular contracture. Large-scale incidence studies have consistently found no credible evidence of a causal association between breast implants and any type of cancer.

6.10 Acknowledgments

Dr McLaughlin has served as a consultant to the Inamed Corporation. The International Epidemiology Institute has received research funding for projects from Dow Corning Corporation, 3M Company and the Plastic Surgery Educational Fund of the American Society of Plastic Surgeons. Neither of the authors was compensated for this chapter.

6.11 References

BARTEL D R (1994), Re: Sclerodermalike esophageal disease in children of mothers with silicone breast implants (letter), *JAMA*, 272, 767.

BLACKBURN W D JR and EVERSON M P (1997), Silicone-associated rheumatic disease: an unsupported myth, *Plast Reconstr Surg*, 99, 1362–1367.

BONDURANT S, ERNSTER V and HERDMAN R (1999), *Safety of Silicone Breast Implants, Report of the Committee on the Safety of Silicone Breast Implants (IOM)*, Washington, D.C., National Academy Press.

BREITING V B, HOLMICH L R, BRANDT B, FRYZEK J P, WOLTHERS M S, KJOLLER K, MCLAUGHLIN J K, WIIK A and FRIIS S (2004), Long-term health status of Danish women with silicone breast implants, *Plast Reconstr Surg*, 114, 217–226.

BRINTON L A, MALONE K E, COATES R J, SCHOENBERG J B, SWANSON C B, DALING J R and STANFORD J L (1996), Breast enlargement and reduction: results from a breast cancer case-control study, *Plast Reconstr Surg*, 97, 269–275.

BRINTON L A, LUBIN J H, BURICH M C, COLTON T, BROWN S L and HOOVER R N (2000a), Breast cancer following augmentation mammoplasty, *Cancer Causes Control*, 11, 819–827.

BRINTON L A, BROWN S L, COLTON T, BURICH M C and LUBIN J (2000b), Characteristics of a population of women with breast implants compared with women seeking other types of plastic surgery, *Plast Reconstr Surg*, 105, 919–927.

BRINTON L A, LUBIN J H, BURICH M C, COLTON T, BROWN S L and HOOVER R N (2001a), Cancer risk at sites other than the breast following augmentation mammoplasty, *Ann Epidemiol*, 11, 248–256.

BRINTON L A, LUBIN J H, BURICH M C, COLTON T and HOOVER R N (2001b), Mortality among augmentation mammoplasty patients, *Epidemiology*, 12, 321–326.

BRINTON L A, BUCKLEY L M, DVORKINA O, LUBIN J H, COLTON T, MURRAY M C and HOOVER R (2004), Risk of connective tissue disorders among breast implant patients. *Am J Epidemiol*, 160, 619–627.

BRINTON L A, LUBIN J H, MURRAY M C, COLTON T and HOOVER R N (2006), Mortality rates among augmentation mammoplasty patients: an update, *Epidemiology*, 17, 162–169.

BRISSON J, HOLOWATY EJ, VILLENEUVE P J, XIE L, UGNAT A M, LATULIPPE L and MAO Y (2006), Cancer incidence in a cohort of Ontario and Quebec women having bilateral breast augmentation, *Int J Cancer*, 118, 2854–2862.

BRODY G, DEAPEN D and GILL P (2010), T-cell non Hodgkin's anaplastic lymphoma associated with one style of breast implants, In: *89th Annual Meeting, American Association of Plastic Surgeons*, San Antonio, TX.

BROWN S L, MIDDLETON M S, BERG W A, SOO M S and PENNELLO D (2000), Prevalence of rupture of silicone gel breast implants revealed on MR imaging in a population of women in Birmingham, Alabama, *AJR Am J Roentgenol*, 175, 1057–1064.

BROWN S L, PENNELLO G, BERG W A, SOO M S and MIDDLETON M S (2001), Silicone gel breast implant rupture, extracapsular silicone, and health status in a population of women, *J Rheumatol*, 28, 996–1003.

BRYANT H and BRASHER P (1995), Breast implants and breast cancer – reanalysis of a linkage study, *N Engl J Med*, 332, 1535–1539.

BURNS C J, LAING T J, GILLESPIE B W, HEERINGA S G, ALCSER K H, MAYES M D, WASKO M C M, COOPER B C, GARABRANT D H and SCHOTTENFELD D (1996), The epidemiology of scleroderma among women: Assessment of risk from exposure to silicone and silica, *J Rheumatol*, 23, 1904–1911.

COOK L S, DALING J R, VOIGT L F, DEHART M P, MALONE K E, STANFORD J L, WEISS N S, BRINTON L A, GAMMON M D and BROGAN D (1997), Characteristics of women with and without breast augmentation, *JAMA*, 277, 1612–1617.

COOK R R (1994), Re: Sclerodermalike esophageal disease in children of mothers with silicone breast implants (letter), *JAMA*, 272, 767–768.

COOK R R, BOWLIN S J, CURTIS J M, HOSHAW S J, KLEIN P J, PERKINS L L and AUSTAD E D (2002), Silicone gel breast implant rupture rates: research issues, *Ann Plast Surg*, 48, 92–101.

CUNNINGHAM B (2007), The Mentor core study on silicone MemoryGel breast implants, *Plast Reconstr Surg*, 120, 19S–29S.

DE CAMARA D L, SHERIDAN J M and KAMMER BA (1993), Rupture and aging of silicone gel breast implants, *Plast Reconstr Surg*, 91, 828–834.

DE JONG D, VASMEL W L E, DE BOER J P, VERHAVE G, BARBE E, CASPARIE M K and VAN LEEUWEN F E (2008), Anaplastic large-cell lymphoma in women with breast implants, *JAMA*, 300, 2030–2035.

DEAPEN D M, BERNSTEIN L and BRODY G S (1997), Are breast implants anticarcinogenic? A 14-year follow-up of the Los Angeles study, *Plast Reconstr Surg*, 99, 1346–1353.

DEAPEN D, HAMILTON A, BERNSTEIN L and BRODY G S (2000), Breast cancer stage at diagnosis and survival among patients with prior breast implants, *Plast Reconstr Surg*, 105, 535–540.

DIDIE E R and SARWER D B (2003), Factors that influence the decision to undergo cosmetic breast augmentation surgery, *J Womens Health*, 12, 241–253.

DUGOWSON C E, DALING J, KOEPSELL T D, VOIGT L and NELSON J L (1992), Silicone breast implants and risk for rheumatoid arthritis. 56th Annual Meeting. American College Rheumatology, *Arthr Rheum*, 35(Suppl), S66.

DUVIC M, MOORE D, MENTER A and VONDERHEID E C (1995), Cutaneous T-cell lymphoma in association with silicone breast implants, *J Am Acad Dermatol*, 32, 939–942.

EDWORTHY S M, MARTIN L, BARR S G, BIRDSELL D C, BRANT R F and FRITZLER M J (1998), A clinical study of the relationship between silicone breast implants and connective tissue disease, *J Rheumatol*, 25, 254–260.

EKLUND G W, BUSBY R C, MILLER S H and JOB J S (1988), Improved imaging of the augmented breast, *AJR Am J Roentgenol*, 151, 469–473.

ENGLERT H, MORRIS D and MARCH L (1996), Scleroderma and silicone gel breast prostheses–the Sydney study revisited, *Aust N Z J Med*, 26, 349–55.

ENGLERT H, JOYNER E, MCGILL N, CHAMBERS P, HORNER D, HUNT C, MAKAROFF J, O'CONNOR H, RUSSEL N and MARCH L (2001), Women's health after plastic surgery, *Intern Med J*, 31, 77–89.

EPSTEIN, W A (1994), Re: Sclerodermalike esophageal disease in children of mothers with silicone breast implants (letter), *JAMA*, 272, 768.

EUROPEAN COMMITTEE ON QUALITY ASSURANCE and MEDICAL DEVICES IN PLASTIC SURGERY (EQUAM) (2000), *Consensus declaration on breast implants, 23–6-2000: 4th Consensus Declaration*, Israel, European Committee on Quality Assurance.

FAJARDO L L, HARVEY J A, MCALEESE K A, ROBERTS C C and GRANSTROM P (1995), Breast cancer diagnosis in women with subglandular silicone gel-filled augmentation implants, *Radiology*, 194, 859–862.

FENG L J and AMINI S B (1999), Analysis of risk factors associated with rupture of silicone gel breast implants, *Plast Reconstr Surg*, 104, 955–963.

FERGUSON J H (1997), Silicone breast implants and neurologic disorders. Report of the Practice Committee of the American Academy of Neurology, *Neurol*, 48, 1504–1507.

FERGUSON J H (1998), Breast implants redux: this time with data, *Neurol*, 50, 849–852.

FRIIS S, MELLEMKJAER L, MCLAUGHLIN J K, BREITING V, KJAER S K, BLOT W and OLSEN J H (1997), Connective tissue disease and other rheumatic conditions following breast implants in Denmark, *Ann Plast Surg*, 39, 1–8.

FRIIS S, HOLMICH L R, MCLAUGHLIN J K, MELLEMKJAER L, KJOLLER K, FRYZEK J P, HENRIKSEN T and OLSEN J H (2006), Cancer risk among Danish women with cosmetic breast implants, *Int J Cancer*, 118, 998–1003.

FRYZEK J P, WEIDERPASS E, SIGNORELLO L B, HAKELIUS L, LIPWORTH L, BLOT W J, MCLAUGHLIN J K and NYREN O (2000), Characteristics of women with cosmetic breast augmentation surgery compared with breast reduction surgery patients and women in the general population of Sweden, *Ann Plast Surg*, 45, 349–356.

FRYZEK J P, SIGNORELLO L B, HAKELIUS L, FELTELIUS N, RINGBERG A, BLOT W J, MCLAUGHLIN J K and NYREN O (2001a), Self-reported symptoms among women after cosmetic breast implant and breast reduction surgery, *Plast Reconstr Surg*, 107, 206–213.

FRYZEK J P, SIGNORELLO L B, HAKELIUS L, LIPWORTH L, MCLAUGHLIN J K, BLOT W J and NYREN O (2001b), Local complications and subsequent symptom reporting among women with cosmetic breast implants, *Plast Reconstr Surg*, 107, 214–221.

FRYZEK J P, HOLMICH L, MCLAUGHLIN J K, LIPWORTH L, TARONE R E, HENRIKSEN R, KJOLLER K and FRIIS S (2007), A nationwide study of connective tissue disease and other rheumatic conditions among Danish women with long term cosmetic breast implantation, *Ann Epidemiol*, 17, 374–379.

GABRIEL S E, O'FALLON W M, KURLAND L T, BEARD C M, WOODS J E and MELTON LJ III (1994), Risk of connective-tissue diseases and other disorders after breast implantation, *N Engl J* Med, 330, 1697–1702.

GAUDET G, FRIEDBERG J W, WENG A, PINKUS G S and FREEDMAN A S (2002), Breast lymphoma associated with breast implants: two case reports and a review of the literature, *Leuk Lymphoma*, 43, 115–119.

GEDALIA A, CUELLAR M L and ESPINOZA L R (1995), Skin rash and anti-Ro/SS-A antibodies in an infant from a mother with silicone breast implants, *Clin Exp Rheumatol*, 13, 521–523.

GILTAY E J, BERNELOT MOENS H J, RILEY A H and TAN R G (1994), Silicone breast prostheses and rheumatic symptoms: A retrospective follow up study, *Ann Rheum Dis*, 53, 194–196.

GOLDMAN J A, GREENBLATT J, JOINES R, WHITE L, AYLWARD B and LAMM S H (1995), Breast implants, rheumatoid arthritis, and connective tissue diseases in clinical practice, *J Clin Epidemiol*, 48, 571–582.

HANDEL N, CORDRAY T, GUTIERREZ J and JENSEN J A (2006), A long-term study of outcomes, complications, and patient satisfaction with breast implants, *Plast Reconstr Surg*, 117, 757–767.

HEDÉN P, BONÉ B, MURPHY D K, SLICTON A and WALKER P S (2006a), Style 410 cohesive silicone breast implants, safety and effectiveness at 5 to 9 years after implantation, *Plast Reconstr Surg*, 118, 1281–1287.

HEDÉN P, NAVA M B, VAN TETERING J P, MAGALON G, FOURIE LE R, BRENNER R J, LINDSEY L E, MURPHY D K and WALKER P S (2006b), Prevalence of rupture in Inamed silicone breast implants, *Plast Reconstr Surg*, 118, 303–308.

HEMMINKI E, HOVI S L, SEVON T, and ASKO-SELJAVAARA S (2004), Births and perinatal health of infants among women who have had silicone breast implantation in Finland, 1967–2000, *Acta Obstet Gynecol Scand*, 83, 1135–1140.

HENNEKENS C H, LEE I, COOK N R, HERBERT N R, KARLSON EW, LAMOTTE F, WHITE B and WISLEY FM (1996), Self-reported breast implants and connective tissue diseases in female health professionals. A retrospective cohort study, *JAMA*, 275, 616–621.

HENRIKSEN T F, HOLMICH L R, FRYZEK J P, FRIIS S, MCLAUGHLIN J K, HOYER A P, KJOLLER K and OLSEN J H (2003), Incidence and severity of short-term complications after breast augmentation: results from a nationwide breast implant registry, *Ann Plast Surg*, 51, 531–539.

HENRIKSEN T F, FRYZEK J P, HOLMICH L R, MCLAUGHLIN J K, KJOLLER K, HOYER A P, OLSEN J H and FRIIS S (2005), Surgical intervention and capsular contracture after breast augmentation: a prospective study of risk factors, *Ann Plast Surg*, 54, 343–351.

HOCHBERG M C and PERLMUTTER D L (1996), The association of augmentation mammoplasty with connective tissue disease, including systematic sclerosis (scleroderma): a meta-analysis, *Curr Top Microbiol Immunol*, 210, 411–417.

HOCHBERG M C, PERLMUTTER D L, MEDSGER T A JR, NGUYEN K, STEEN V, WEISMAN M H, WHITE B and WISLEY F M (1996), Lack of an association between augmentation mammoplasty and systemic sclerosis (scleroderma), *Arthr Rheum*, 7, 1125–1131.

HOLMICH L R, KJOLLER K, VEJBORG I, CONRAD C, SLETTING S, MCLAUGHLIN J K, FRYZEK J P, BREITING V, JORGENSEN A and OLSEN J H (2001), Prevalence of silicone breast implant rupture among Danish women, *Plast Reconstr Surg*, 108, 848–858.

HOLMICH L R, FRIIS S, FRYZEK J P, VEJBORG I, CONRAD C, SLETTING S, KJOLLER K, MCLAUGHLIN J K and OLSEN J (2003a), Incidence of silicone breast implant rupture, *Arch Surg*, 138, 801–806.

HOLMICH L R, KJOLLER K, FRYZEK J P, HOIER-MADSEN M, VEJBORG I, CONRAD C, SLETTING S, MCLAUGHLIN JK, BREITING V and FRIIS S (2003b), Self-reported diseases and symptoms by rupture status among unselected Danish women with cosmetic silicone breast implants, *Plast Reconstr Surg*, 111, 723–732.

HOLMICH L R, MELLEMKJAER L, GUNNARSDOTTIR K A, TANGE U, KRAG C, MELLER S and MCLAUGHLIN J K (2003c), Stage of breast cancer at diagnosis among women with cosmetic breast implants, *Br J Cancer*, 88, 832–838.

HOLMICH L R, VEJBORG I M, CONRAD C, SLETTING S, HOIER-MADSEN M, FRYZEK J P, MCLAUGHLIN J K, KJOLLER K, WIIK A and FRIIS S (2004), Untreated silicone breast implant rupture, *Plast Reconstr Surg*, 114, 204–216.

HOLMICH LR, LIPWORTH L, MCLAUGHLIN JK and FRIIS S (2007), Breast implant rupture and connective tissue disease: a review of the literature, *Plast Reconstr Surg*, 120, 62S–69S.

HOSHAW S J, KLEIN P J, CLARK B D, COOK R R and PERKINS L L (2001), Breast implants and cancer: causation, delayed detection, and survival, *Plast Reconst Surg*, 107, 1393–1407.

HVILSOM G B, HOLMICH L R, HENRIKSEN T F, LIPWORTH L, MCLAUGHLIN J K and FRIIS S (2009), Local complications after cosmetic breast augmentation: results from the Danish Registry for Plastic Surgery of the Breast, *Plast Reconstr Surg*, 124, 919–925.

INDEPENDENT REVIEW GROUP (1998), *Silicone Gel Breast Implants: the Report of the Independent Review Group*, Cambridge, England, Crown.

INTERNATIONAL AGENCY FOR RESEARCH ON CANCER (1999), *Surgical implants and other foreign bodies. IARC Monograph on the Evaluation of Carcinogenic Risks to Humans, Volume 74*, Lyon, IARC Press.

JACOBSEN P H, HÖLMICH L R, MCLAUGHLIN J K, OLSEN J, JOHANSEN C, KJOLLER K and FRIIS S (2004), Mortality and suicide among Danish women with cosmetic breast implants, *Arch Intern Med*, 164, 2450–2455.

JANOWSKY E C, KUPPER L L and HULKA B S (2000), Meta-analyses of the relation between silicone breast implants and the risk of connective tissue disease, *N Engl J Med*, 342, 781–790.

JENSEN B, BLIDDAL H, KJOLLER K, WITTRUP H, FRIIS S, HOIER-MADSEN M, ROGIND H, MCLAUGHLIN J K, LIPWORTH L, DANNESKIOLD-SAMSOE B and OLSEND J H (2001a), Rheumatic manifestations in Danish women with silicone breast implants, *Clin Rheumatol*, 20, 345–352.

JENSEN B, KJOLLER K, MCLAUGHLIN JK, DANNESKIOLD-SAMSOE B, BLIDDAL H, BLOT W J and OLSEN J H (2001b), Muscular rheumatism following breast surgery in Denmark, *Clin Exp Rheumatol*, 19, 229.

JEWELL M, SPEAR S L, LARGENT J, OEFELEIN M G and ADAMS W P JR (2011), Anaplastic large T-cell lymphoma and breast implants: a review of the literature, *Plast Reconstr Surg*, 128, 651–661.

KALLENBERG C G (1994), Overlapping syndromes, undifferentiated connective tissue disease and other fibrosing conditions, *Curr Opin Rheumatol*, 6, 650–654.

KARLSON E W, LEE I M, COOK N R, MANSON J E, BURING J E and HENNEKENS C H (1999), Comparison of self-reported diagnosis of connective tissue disease with medical records in female health professionals: the Women's Health Cohort Study, *Am J Epidemiol*, 150, 652–660.

KEECH J A JR and CREECH B J (1997), Anaplastic T-cell lymphoma in proximity to a saline-filled breast implant, *Plast Reconstr Surg*, 100, 554–555.

KERN K A, FLANNERY J T and KUEHN P G (1997), Carcinogenic potential of silicone breast implants: a Connecticut statewide study, *Plast Reconstr Surg*, 100, 737–747.

KIM B, ROTH C, YOUNG V L, CHUNG K C, VAN BUSUM K, SCHNYER C and MATTKE S (2011a), Anaplastic large cell lymphoma and breast implants: results from a structured expert consultation, *Plast Reconstr Surg*, 128, 629–639.

KIM B, ROTH C, CHUNG K C, YOUNG V L, VAN BUSUM K, SCHNYER C and MATTKE S (2011b), Anaplastic large cell lymphoma and breast implants: a systematic review. *Plast Reconstr Surg*, 127, 2141–2150.

KJOLLER K, MCLAUGHLIN J K, FRIIS S, BLOT W J, MELLEMKJAER L, HOGSTED C, WINTHER J F and OLSEN J H (1998), Health outcomes in offspring of mothers with breast implants, *Pediatrics*, 102, 1112–1115.

KJOLLER K, FRIIS S, MELLEMKJAER L, MCLAUGLIN J K, WINTHER J F, LIPWORTH L, BLOT W J, FRYZEK J and OLSEN J H (2001), Connective tissue disease and other rheumatic conditions following cosmetic breast implantation in Denmark, *Arch Intern Med*, 161, 973–979.

KJOLLER K, FRIIS S, SIGNORELLO L B, MCLAUGHLIN J K, BLOT W J, LIPWORTH L, MELLEMKJAER L, WINTHER J F and OLSEN J H (2002a), Health outcomes in offspring of Danish mothers with cosmetic breast implants, *Ann Plast Surg*, 48, 238–245.

KJOLLER K, HOLMICH L R, JACOBSEN P H, FRIIS S, FRYZEK J, MCLAUGHLIN J K, LIPWORTH L, HENRIKSEN T F, JØRGENSEN S, BITTMANN S and OLSEN J H (2002b), Epidemiological investigation of local complications after cosmetic breast implant surgery in Denmark, *Ann Plast Surg*, 48, 229–237.

KJOLLER K, HOLMICH L, FRYZEK J P, JACOBSEN P H, FRIIS S, MCLAUGHLIN J K, LIPWORTH L, HENRIKSEN T F, JORGENSEN S, BITTMANN S and OLSEN J H (2003), Characteristics of women with cosmetic breast implants compared with women with other types of cosmetic surgery and population-based controls in Denmark, *Ann Plast Surg*, 50, 6–12.

KULMALA I, MCLAUGHLIN J K, PAKKANEN M, LASSILA K, HOLMICH L R, LIPWORTH L, BOICE J D, RAITANEN J and LUOTO R (2004), Local complications after cosmetic breast implant surgery in Finland, *Ann Plast Surg*, 53, 413–419.

LAI S, GOLDMAN J A, CHILD A H, ENGEL A and LAMM S H (2000), Fibromyalgia, hypermobility, and breast implants, *Rheumatol*, 27, 2237–2241.

LAING T J, GILLEPSIE B W, LACEY J V, GARABRANT D H, COOPER B C, HEERINGA S G, ALCER K H, CHO S, MAYES M D and SCHOTTENFELD D (1996), The association between silicone exposure and undifferentiated connective tissue disease among women in Michigan and Ohio, *Arthr Rheum*, 39, S150.

LAING T J, SCHOTTENFELD D, LACEY J V, GILLESPIE B W, GARABRANT D H, COOPER B C, HEERINGA S G, ALCSER K H and MAYES M D (2001), Potential risk factors for undifferentiated connective tissue disease among women: implanted medical devices, *Am J Epidemiol* 154, 610–617.

LAMM S H (1998), Silicone breast implants, breast cancer and specific connective tissue diseases: A systematic review of the data in the epidemiological literature, *Int J Toxicol*, 17, 497–527.

LEE I M, COOK N R, SHADICK N A, PEREIRA E and BURING J E (2010), Prospective cohort study of breast implants and the risk of connective tissue diseases, *Int J Epidemiol*, 40, 230–238.

LEVINE J J and ILOWITE N T (1994), Sclerodermalike esophageal disease in children breast-fed by mothers with silicone breast implants, *JAMA*, 1994, 271, 213–216.

LEVINE J J, ILOWITE N T, PETTEI M J and TRACHTMAN H (1996a), Increased urinary NO3(-) + NO2- and neopterin excretion in children breast fed by mothers with silicone breast implants: evidence for macrophage activation, *J Rheumatol*, 23, 1083–1087.

LEVINE J J, LIN H C, ROWLEY M, COOK A, TEUBER S S and ILOWITE N T (1996b), Lack of autoantibody expression in children born to mothers with silicone breast implants, *Pediatrics*, 97, 243–245.

LEVINE J J, TRACHTMAN H, GOLD D M and PETTEI M J (1996c), Esophageal dysmobility in children breast-fed by mothers with silicone breast implants. Long-term follow-up and response to treatment, *Dig Dis Sci*, 4, 1600–1603.

LEWIN S L and MILLER T A (1997), A review of epidemiologic studies analyzing the relationship between breast implants and connective tissue diseases, *Plast Reconstr Surg*, 100, 1309–1313.

LIPWORTH L and MCLAUGHLIN J K (2010), Excess suicide risk and other external causes of death among women with cosmetic breast implants: a neglected research priority, *Curr Psychiatry Rep*, 12, 234–238.

LIPWORTH L, TARONE R E and MCLAUGHLIN J K (2004a), Breast implants and fibromyalgia: a review of the epidemiologic evidence, *Ann Plast Surg*, 52, 284–287.

LIPWORTH L, TARONE R E and MCLAUGHLIN J K (2004b), Silicone breast implants and connective tissue disease: an updated review of the epidemiologic evidence, *Ann Plast Surg*, 52, 598–601.

LIPWORTH L, NYREN O, YE W, FRYZEK J P, TARONE R E and MCLAUGHLIN J K (2007), Excess mortality from suicide and other external causes of death among women with cosmetic breast implants, *Ann Plast Surg*, 59, 119–123.

LIPWORTH L, TARONE R E, FRIIS S, YE W, OLSEN J H, NYREN O and MCLAUGHLIN J K (2008), Cancer among Scandinavian women with cosmetic breast implants: a pooled long-term follow-up study, *Int J Cancer*, 124, 490–493.

LIPWORTH L, TARONE R E and MCLAUGHLIN J K (2009), Breast implants and lymphoma risk: a review of the epidemiologic evidence through 2008, *Plast Reconstr Surg*, 123, 790–793.

LIPWORTH L, HOLMICH, L R and MCLAUGHLIN J K (2010), Silicone breast implants and connective tissue disease: no association, *Semin Immunopathol*, 33, 287–294.

MALONE K E, STANFORD J L, DALING J R and VOIGT L F (1992), Implants and breast cancer, *Lancet*, 339, 1365.

MAROTTA J S, WIDENHOUSE C W, HABAL M B and GOLDBERG E P (1999), Silicone gel breast implant failure and frequency of additional surgeries: analysis of 35 studies reporting examination of more than 8,000 explants, *J Biomed Mater Res*, 48, 354–364.

MAROTTA J S, GOLDBERG E P, HABAL M B, AMERY D B, MARTIN P J, URBANIAK D J and WIDENHOUSE C W (2002), Silicone gel breast implant failure: evaluation of properties of shells and gels for explanted prostheses and meta-analysis of literature rupture data, *Ann Plast Surg*, 49, 227–247.

MCLAUGHLIN J K and LIPWORTH L (2004), Brain cancer and cosmetic breast implants: A review of the epidemiologic evidence, *Ann Plast Surg*, 52, 115–117.

MCLAUGHLIN J K, NYREN O, BLOT W J, YIN L, JOSEFSSON S, FRAUMENI J F JR and ADAMI H O (1998), Cancer risk among women with cosmetic breast implants: a population-based cohort study in Sweden, *J Natl Cancer Inst*, 90, 156–158.

MCLAUGHLIN J K, LIPWORTH L, FRYZEK J P, YE W, TARONE R E and NYREN O (2006), Long-term cancer risk among Swedish women with cosmetic breast implants: an update of a nationwide study, *J Natl Cancer Inst*, 98, 557–560.

MCLAUGHLIN J K, LIPWORTH L, MURPHY D K and WALKER P S (2007), The safety of silicone gel-filled breast implants: a review of the epidemiologic evidence, *Ann Plast Surg*, 59, 569–580.

MELLEMKJAER L, KJOLLER K, FRIIS S, MCLAUGHLIN J K, HOGSTED C, WINTHER J F, BREITING V, KRAG C, KJAER S K, BLOT W J and OLSEN J H (2000), Cancer occurrence after cosmetic breast implantation in Denmark, *Int J Cancer*, 88, 301–306.

MELMED E P (1998), A review of explantation in 240 symptomatic women: a description of explantation and capsulectomy with reconstruction using a periareolar technique, *Plast Reconstr Surg*, 101, 1364–73.

MIGLIORETTI D L, RUTTER C M, GELLER B M, CUTTER G, BARLOW W E, ROSENBERG R, WEAVER D L, TAPLIN S H, BALLARD-BARBASH R, CARNEY P A, YANKASKAS B C and KERLIKOWSKE K, (2004), Effect of breast augmentation on the accuracy of mammography and cancer characteristics, *JAMA*, 291, 442–450.

NATIONAL INSTITUTES OF HEALTH (2005), *Breast implants: status of research at the National Institutes of Health.* Available from: http://orwh.od.nih.gov/pubs/rev305breastimplantsreport.pdf [Accessed June 20, 2011].

NEWMAN M K, ZEMMEL M J, BANDAK A Z and KAPLAN B J (2006), Primary breast lymphoma in a patient with silicone breast implants: a case report and review of the literature, *J Plast Reconstr Aesthet Surg*, 61, 822–824.

NYREN O, YIN L, JOSEFSSON S, MCLAUGHLIN J K, BLOT W J, ENGQVIST M, HAKELIUS L, BOICE J D JR and ADAMI H O (1998a), Risk of connective tissue disease and related disorders among women with breast implants: A nation-wide retrospective cohort study in Sweden, *Br Med J*, 316, 417–422.

NYREN O, MCLAUGHLIN J K, YIN L, JOSEFSSON S, ENGQVIST M, HAKELIUS L, BLOT W J and ADAMI H O (1998b), Breast implants and risk of neurologic disease: a population-based cohort study in Sweden, *Neurol*, 50, 956–961.

PARK A J, BLACK R J, SARHADI N S, CHETTY U and WATSON A C (1998a), Silicone gel-filled breast implants and connective tissue diseases, *Plast Reconstr Surg*, 101, 261–268.

PARK A J, CHETTY U and WATSON A C (1998b), Silicone breast implants and breast cancer, *Breast*, 7, 22–26.

PLACIK O J (1994), Re: Sclerodermalike esophageal disease in children of mothers with silicone breast implants (letter), *JAMA*, 272, 768–769.

PRESS R I, PEEBLES C L, KUMAGAI Y, OCHS R L and TAN E M (1992), Antinuclear autoantibodies in women with silicone breast implants, *Lancet*, 340, 1304–7.

PUKKALA E, BOICE J D JR, HOVI S L, HEMMINKI E, ASKO-SELJAVAARA S, KESKIMAKI I, MCLAUGHLIN J K, PAKKANEN M and TEPPO L (2002), Incidence of breast and other cancers among Finnish women with cosmetic breast implants, 1970–1999, *J Long Term Eff Med Implants*, 12, 271–279.

PUKKALA E, KULMALA I, HOVI S L, HEMMINKI E, KESKIMÄKI I, LIPWORTH L, BOICE J D JR and MCLAUGHLIN J K (2003), Causes of death among Finnish women with cosmetic breast implants, 1971–2001, *Ann Plast Surg*, 51, 339–342.

ROBINSON O G JR, BRADLEY E L and WILSON D S (1995), Analysis of explanted silicone implants: a report of 300 patients, *Ann Plast Surg*, 34, 1–7.

ROHRICH R J, ADAMS W P JR, BERGAN S J, RATHAKRISHNAN R, GRIFFIN J, ROBINSON J B and KENKEL J M (1998), An analysis of silicone gel-filled breast implants: diagnosis and failure rates, *Plast Reconstr Surg*, 102, 2304–2309.

SAHOO S, ROSEN P P, FEDDERSEN R M, VISWANATHA D S, CLARK D A and CHADBURN A (2003), Anaplastic large cell lymphoma arising in a silicone breast implant capsule: a case report and review of the literature, *Arch Pathol Lab Med*, 127, e115–e118.

SANCHEZ-GUERRERO J, COLDITZ G A, KARLSON E W, HUNTER D J, SPEIZER F E and LIANG M H (1995), Silicone breast implants and the risk of connective-tissue diseases and symptoms, *N Engl J Med*, 332, 1666–1670.

SARWER D B, NORDMANN J E and HERBERT J D (2000), Cosmetic breast augmentation surgery: a critical overview, *J Womens Health Gend Based Med*, 9, 843–856.

SARWER D B, LAROSSA D, BARTLETT S P, LOW D W, BUCKY L P and WHITAKER L A (2003), Body image concerns of breast augmentation patients, *Plast Reconstr Surg*, 112, 83–90.

SCHUSTERMAN M A, KROLL S S, REECE G P, MILLER M J, AINSLIE N, HALABI S and BALCH C M (1993), Incidence of autoimmune disease in patients after breast reconstruction with silicone gel implants versus autogenous tissue: A preliminary report, *Ann Plast Surg*, 31, 1–6.

SIGNORELLO L B, FRYZEK J P, BLOT W J, MCLAUGHLIN J K and NYREN O (2001), Offspring health risk after cosmetic breast implantation in Sweden, *Ann Plast Surg*, 46, 279–286.

SILMAN A J and HOCHBERG M C (2001), *Epidemiology of rheumatic diseases*. Second edition, New York, Oxford University Press.

SILVERMAN B G, BROWN S L, BRIGHT R A, KACZMAREK R G, ARROWSMITH-LOWE J B and KESSLER D A (1996), Reported complications of silicone gel breast implants: an epidemiologic review, *Ann Intern Med*, 124, 744–756.

SILVERSTEIN M J, HANDEL N, GAMAGAMI P, WAISMAN J R, GIERSON E D, ROSSER R J, STEYSKAL R and COLBURN W (1988), Breast cancer in women after augmentation mammoplasty, *Arch Surg*, 123(6), 681–685.

SILVERSTEIN M J, HANDEL N, GAMAGAMI P, GIERSON E D, FURMANSKI M, COLLINS A R, EPSTEIN M, and COHLAN B F (1992), Breast cancer diagnosis and prognosis in women following augmentation with silicone gel-filled prostheses, *Eur J Cancer*, 28, 635–640.

SILVERSTEIN M J, GIERSON E D, GAMAGAMI P, HANDEL N and WAISMAN J R (1990), Breast cancer diagnosis and prognosis in women augmented with silicone gel-filled implants. *Cancer*, 66, 97–101.

SLAVIN S A and GOLDWYN R M (1995), Silicone gel implant explantation: reasons, results, and admonitions, *Plast Reconstr Surg*, 95, 63–6.

SOLOMON G (1994), A clinical and laboratory profile of symptomatic women with silicone breast implants, *Semin Arthritis Rheum*, 24, 29–37.

SPEAR S L, MURPHY D K, SLICTON A and WALKER P S (2007), Inamed silicone breast implant core study results at 6 years, *Plast Reconstr Surg*, 120, 8S–16S.

STROM B L, REIDENBERG M M, FREUNDLICH B and SCHINNAR R (1994), Breast silicone implants and risk of systemic lupus erythematosus, *J Clin Epidemiol*, 47, 1211–1214.

TEUBER S S and GERSHWIN M E (1994), Autoantibodies and clinical rheumatic complaints in two children of women with silicone breast implants, *Int Arch Allergy Immunol*, 103, 105–108.

TUGWELL P, WELLS G, PETERSON J, WELCH V, PAGE J, DAVISON C, MCGOWAN J, RAMROTH D and SHEA B (2001), Do silicone breast implants cause rheumatologic disorders? A systematic review for a court-appointed national science panel, *Arthritis Rheum*, 44, 2477–2484.

UNITED STATES FOOD AND DRUG ADMINISTRATION (2011), Anaplastic large cell lymphoma (ALCL) in women with breast implants: preliminary FDA findings and analyses, January 2011. http://www.fda.gov/downloads/MedicalDevices/ProductsandMedicalProcedures/ImplantsandProsthetics/BreastImplants/UCM260090.pdf, accessed January 22, 2012.

VILLENEUVE P J, HOLOWATY E J, BRISSON J, XIE L, UGNAT A M, LATULIPPE L and MAO Y (2006), Mortality among Canadian women with cosmetic breast implants, *Am J Epidemiol*, 164, 334–341.

WELLS K E, CRUSE C W, BAKER J L JR, DANIELS S M, STERN R A, NEWMAN C, SELEZNICK M J, VASEY F B, BROZENA S, ALBERS S E, *et al.* (1994), The health status of women following cosmetic surgery, *Plast Reconstr Surg*, 93, 907–912.

WILLIAMS H J, WEISMANN M H and BERRY C C (1997), Breast implants in patients with differentiated and undifferentiated connective tissue disease, *Arthr Rheum*, 40, 437–440.

WINTHER J F, BACH F W, FRIIS S, BLOT W J, MELLEMKJAER L, KJOLLER K, HOGSTED C, MCLAUGHLIN J K and OLSEN J H (1998), Neurologic disease among women with breast implants, *Neurol*, 50, 951–955.

WINTHER J F, FRIIS S, BACH F W, MELLEMKJAER L, KJOLLER K, MCLAUGHLIN J K, LIPWORTH L, BLOT W J, and OLSEN J H (2001), Neurological disease among women with silicone breast implants in Denmark, *Acta Neurol Scand*, 103, 93–96.

WOLFE F (1999), 'Silicone related symptoms' are common in patients with fibromyalgia: no evidence for a new disease, *J Rheumatol*, 26, 1172–1175.

WOLFE F and ANDERSON J (1999), Silicone filled breast implants and the risk of fibromyalgia and rheumatoid arthritis, *J Rheumatol*, 26, 2025–2028.

WOLFE F, ROSS K, ANDERSON J, RUSSELL I J and HEBERT L (1995), The prevalence and characteristics of fibromyalgia in the general population, *Arth Rheum*, 38, 19–28.

XIE L, BRISSON J, HOLOWATY E J, VILLENEUVE P J and MAO Y (2010), The influence of cosmetic breast agumentation on the stage distribution and prognosis of women subsequently diagnosed with breast cancer, *Int J Cancer*, 126, 2182–2190.

YOUNG V L, NEMECEK J R and NEMECEK D A (1994), The efficacy of breast augmentation: breast size increase, patient satisfaction, and psychological effects, *Plast Reconstr Surg*, 94, 958–969.

7

Retrieval and analysis of breast implants emphasizing strength, durability, and failure mechanisms

H. J. BRANDON, K. L. JERINA and C. J. WOLF,
Washington University, USA and
V. L. YOUNG, BodyAesthetic Plastic Surgery and
Skin Care Center, USA

Abstract: The environmental durability and useful life of a breast implant is of major concern to both the patient and the plastic surgery community. The influence of complex environmental factors, both chemical and physical effects, on the basic properties of breast implants are discussed in this chapter. A large variety of physical-analytical methods were used to determine what change, if any, occurred in a variety of implants prepared by several different manufactures over several generations of implant development. Implants explanted from patients after implantation periods as long as 32 years were directly compared to available control samples. Explants and controls were investigated by a broad combination of mechanical testing, chemical analysis, and scanning electron microscopy.

Key words: breast implants, strength, failure mechanisms.

7.1 Introduction

Since the early 1990s, significant experience has been gained in testing and analyzing silicone gel breast implants, and to a lesser extent, saline-filled devices. Based on this experience, a systematic method was developed for collecting and evaluating these implants in a way that would permit different laboratories to compare their data. The developed protocol[1] offered the plastic and reconstructive surgery community a standardized method for analyzing explanted silicone gel and saline-filled breast implants. The protocol also gave surgeons a clearly defined approach for removing, handling, documenting, and shipping explanted breast implants. At the same time, biomaterials researchers could use the protocol to acquire implant data with reliable and reproducible methods. The protocol emphasizes data collection to determine the effect of implantation time on the strength and durability of breast implants. In addition, the protocol outlines the microscopy techniques for establishing modes and causes of shell failure. The

FDA guidance document[2] for breast implants recommends the protocol for a description of the type of information to consider in a retrieval study (e.g. control group of unimplanted devices, mechanical testing, chemical analyses, and scanning electron microscopy).

In this chapter, mechanical property data, chemical analyses, and failure analyses of explants that were obtained at Washington University (WU) in St. Louis using the protocol are presented along with data from other research organizations. Any investigation into the effects of implantation time on the durability of implant shells should separate the implants according to type, so that explants can be compared with the proper controls. This is necessary because the strength of implant shells can vary considerably according to the manufacturer, the implant type, and the lot-to-lot variability for the given type. For this reason, control implant data are also presented with the explant data wherever possible. The emphasis of this chapter is placed on silicone gel breast implants, since most published data are on these devices. A separate section in this chapter is devoted to saline breast implants. In addition, very limited mechanical property data have been published for recent silicone gel breast implants that are currently marketed. For this reason, most of the data presented in this chapter is for implants manufactured before the 1992 FDA moratorium on silicone gel implants. However, the failure analysis includes analyses of some recent generation implants. Additionally, the mechanical property data are primarily for single-lumen silicone gel-filled breast implants manufactured by Dow Corning (Midland, Mich.). The four major types of single-lumen silicone gel-filled breast implants manufactured by Dow Corning and their approximate production dates are as follows: Cornin seamed (1964 to 1968), Silastic 0 (1969 to 1974), Silastic I (1975 to 1986), and Silastic II (1981 to 1992). The chapter concludes with a review of data from recent clinical studies.

7.2 Silicone gel explants with longest implantation times

The various types of single-lumen silicone gel breast implants manufactured by Dow Corning that have long implantation times are listed in Table 7.1. The explants listed in Table 7.1 are the oldest known explants of their type that have been tested.[3] The Cronin seamed explants had the longest implantation times of any type of silicone implant tested to date. All of the explants were intact except for the Silastic I explant, which had a pinhole and was classified as exhibiting heavy bleeding. One of the Cronin seamed explants and one of the Silastic 0 explants were damaged during explantation procedures. The mechanical, chemical, and physical properties of the explants with long implantation times are compared with the corresponding

Table 7.1 Silicone gel explants with longest implantation times (reprinted with permission from ref. 3. Copyright 2003 Wolters Kluwer Health)

Explant	Years	Status
Cronin seamed	32	Intact*
Cronin seamed	32	Intact
Silastic 0	28	Intact*
Silastic 0	28	Intact
Silastic I	20	Pinhole
Silastic II	13	Intact
Silastic II	13	Intact

*Shell damaged during explantation procedure.

control values for as-received shells in Table 7.2 and for extracted shells in Table 7.3.

The two explants with 32 years of implantation time are the oldest known silicone gel explants that have been tested. Data for one control are also presented. Because only one control shell was tested, the assessment of in vivo aging for the explants was limited. However, a qualitative assessment of the effects of in vivo aging could be performed. The most important observation was that there was no catastrophic decrease in the ultimate properties with implantation times of up to 32 years. The maximum reduction in tensile strength for an explant, relative to its control, was 35% for a shell as received and 24% for a shell from which the non-cross-linked components had been removed (extracted). A similar comparison for elongation yielded reductions of 24% and 14% for as-received and extracted shells, respectively. These values are subject to interpretation because the effect of lot-to-lot variability is not known. The 200% and 400% modulus values for these explants were within 20% and 25% of the control values, respectively. The shell thicknesses of the two explants were within a few percentage points of the control value. The amounts extracted were 6% and 21% higher for the explants, compared with the control. The cross-link densities for the explants were 7% and 2% higher than that for the control specimen. The two Cronin seamed explants with the longest times in vivo of all silicone gel prostheses tested to date are presented, with the control, in Fig. 7.1. The explants appeared very similar to the control, even after 32 years of implantation. All of the Silastic 0 explant data except for the shell thickness and the percent extracted were within control ranges. The thicknesses of the explanted shells were above the control range, whereas the amounts extracted from the explants were approximately 10% below the control range.

Table 7.2 Properties of control and explanted shells with longest implantation times (reprinted with permission from ref. 3. Copyright 2003 Wolters Kluwer Health)

Implant	Strength (psi)	Elongation (%)	Tear resistance (P/I)	200% Modulus (psi)	400% Modulus (psi)	Thickness (inches)
Cronin seamed	428	418	40	119	394	0.02384
Cronin seamed	464	400	25	145	412	0.02253
Control	661	479	34	143	493	0.02284
Silastic 0	827	475	47	209	636	0.01475
Silastic 0	977	517	59	226	658	0.01541
Control range	356–1080	405–645	27–63	101–312	265–953	0.00885–0.0125
Silastic I	901	453	61	244	749	0.008156
Control range	356–1080	405–645	27–63	101–312	265–953	0.00885–0.0125
Silastic II	825	804	59	249	359	0.01487
Silastic II	962	907	74	255	382	0.01423
Lot-matched control	1501	1061	110	259	378	0.01500

psi, pounds per square inch; P/I, pounds per inch.

Table 7.3 Properties of extracted control and explanted shells with longest implantation times (reprinted with permission from ref. 3. Copyright 2003 Wolters Kluwer Health)

Implant	Strength (psi)	Elongation (%)	200% Modulus (psi)	400% Modulus (psi)	Percent extracted (%)	Cross-link density (mol/cm^3)
Cronin seamed	746	544	156	470	39.5	0.934×10^{-4}
Cronin seamed	854	474	224	655	34.7	0.890×10^{-4}
Control	978	553	186	581	32.6	0.870×10^{-4}
Silastic 0	1445	615	240	713	18.7	1.70×10^{-4}
Silastic 0	1511	642	228	691	18.9	1.67×10^{-4}
Control range	1216–1775	565–764	135–295	297–808	21.2–38.2	1.28×10^{-4}–2.12×10^{-4}
Silastic 1	1031	531	197	652	19.4	1.60×10^{-4}
Control range	1216–1775	565–764	135–295	297–808	21.2–38.2	1.28×10^{-4}–2.12×10^{-4}
Silastic II	1395	1017	263	377	29.3	1.22×10^{-4}
Silastic II	1890	1093	286	415	25.5	1.31×10^{-4}
Lot-matched control	1852	1138	257	377	10.7	1.20×10^{-4}

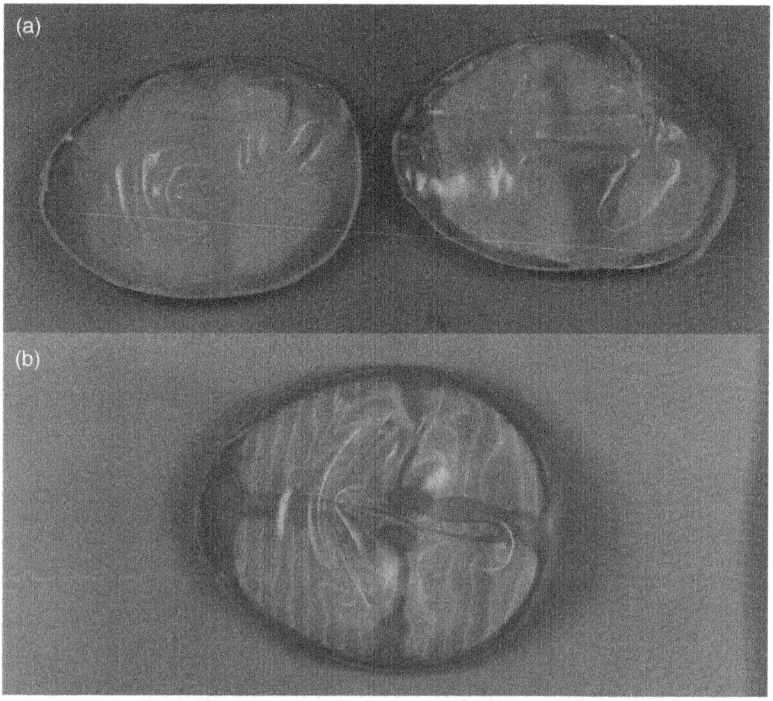

7.1 Cronin seamed explants with 32 years in vivo (a) and a control (b). Reprinted with permission from ref. 3. Copyright 2003 Wolters Kluwer Health.

The Silastic I explant data were within the control ranges except for the shell thickness, and the tensile strength and elongation values for the extracted shells. The tensile strength and elongation were approximately 15% and 6% below the control range, respectively. The shell thickness was approximately 8% below the control range.

A comparison of Silastic II explant and lot-matched control properties indicated the following for unextracted samples. The tensile strength, elongation, and tear resistance were approximately 40%, 20%, and 40% below the lot-matched control values, respectively. The explant modulus values were all within approximately 10% of the control values. The explanted shell thicknesses were less than 5% below the control values. For extracted samples, the tensile strength and elongation were 11% and 7% below the lot-matched control values, respectively. The most significant difference between explant values and control values was observed for the percent extracted from the Silastic II explants. The amounts extracted from the Silastic II explants were greater than the lot-matched control value by a factor of approximately 2.5. Figure 7.2 demonstrates that the explant with

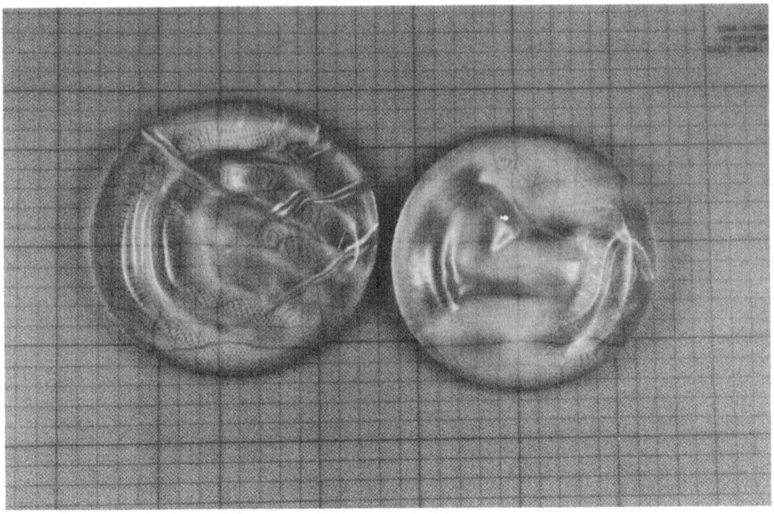

7.2 Silastic II explant with 13 years of implantation (left) and a lot-matched control (right). Reprinted with permission from ref. 3. Copyright 2003 Wolters Kluwer Health.

13 years in vivo appeared very similar to the lot-matched control, except that the explant had a slightly larger planform diameter (8%).

An interesting aspect of the data presented in Table 7.3 is the large degree of swelling for the explants, ranging from 18.7% to 39.5%. Implant failure has been attributed to degradation of the shell mechanical properties because of swelling of the elastomeric shell by the non-cross-linked silicones from the gel.[4] The results in Table 7.3 demonstrate that this is not necessarily the case. Various types of silicone gel breast implants have remained intact from 13 to 32 years in vivo, even with a large degree of swelling.

7.3 Shell properties of silicone gel implants as a function of implantation time

7.3.1 Ultimate strength properties of Silastic 0 and Silastic I implants

The ultimate strength properties of Silastic 0 and Silastic I implant shells were recently analyzed.[5] In that study, the two types of implant shells were analyzed together because the same basic process was used to prepare the elastomeric shell. The difference between these two types of implants was in the viscosity of the gel. That study included 60 explants, with implantation times ranging from 6 to 28 years, and 15 control samples. The data were obtained at five different laboratories.

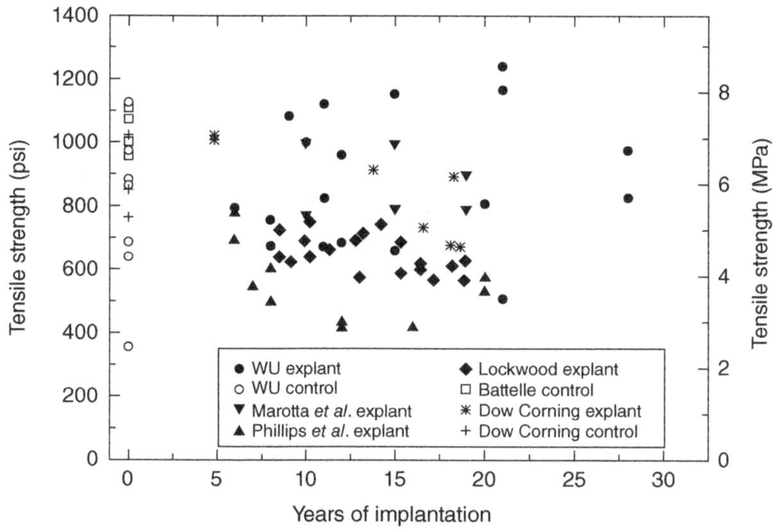

7.3 Tensile strength of Silastic 0 and Silastic I implant shells as a function of time in vivo. WU, Washington University. Reprinted with permission from ref. 5. Copyright 1999 Sage Publications.

Table 7.4 Status of explants at time of analysis (reprinted with permission from ref. 5. Copyright 1999 Sage Publications)

	Washington University	Marotta *et al.*	Phillips *et al.*	Lockwood	Dow Corning
Intact	12	2	5	6	1
Ruptured	2	4	3	10	6
Pinhole leak	4	–	2	3	–
Totals	18	6	10	19	7

Tensile stress data for Silastic 0 and Silastic I implant shells as a function of implantation time are summarized in Fig. 7.3. The control data for unimplanted shells are plotted at time zero, and the explant data correspond to implantation periods ranging from 6 to 28 years. Data are for 15 single-lumen controls and 60 single-lumen explants. The status of the explants at the time of analysis according to each of the investigators[6–10] is summarized in Table 7.4. Twenty-six of the explants were intact, 25 were ruptured, and 9 had small pinholes. The explants tested by Phillips[7] and Lockwood[8] that were listed as leaking are categorized as pinhole leaks in Table 7.4.

The large range in tensile strength of the control implants is primarily due to lot-to-lot variability among the shells.[11] The scatter in the explant data is also primarily due to lot-to-lot variability and the effect of different testing techniques used in the various studies. Nonetheless, the explant data

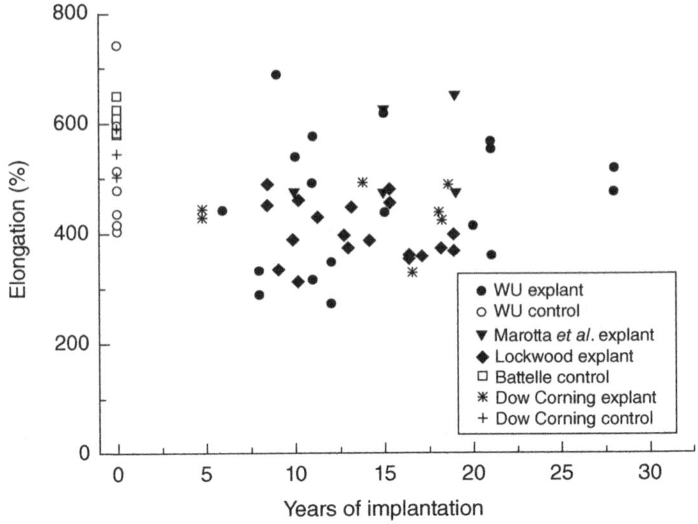

7.4 Elongation of Silastic 0 and Silastic I implant shells as a function of time in vivo. Reprinted with permission from ref. 5. Copyright 1999 Sage Publications.

from the six different studies are in general agreement; they indicate that there is no time-dependent degradation in the average shell tensile strength during 28 years of implantation. We also found no significant difference in the tensile strength of intact shells, ruptured shells, or shells containing a pinhole.

A summary of all of the published data from 15 controls and 50 explants on the elongation-to-failure of Silastic 0 and Silastic I implant shells as a function of implantation time is presented in Fig. 7.4. Elongation data were not reported by Phillips. Twenty-one of the explants were intact, 22 were ruptured, and 7 had pinholes. Again, we found no significant difference in the elongation of intact and failed implants and no significant shell degradation as a function of time in vivo. A considerable number of explants have elongations below the minimum control value of 405%. The explants with the four lowest elongation-to-failure values – three samples measured in our laboratory (273%, 288%, and 315%) and one from Lockwood (312%) – had implantation times ranging from 8 to 12 years; all of these were intact, even though their elongation-to-failure values were below the ASTM-recommended value of 350%.[12]

The tear strength data for 7 controls (plotted at implantation time zero) and 17 explants as a function of implantation time is shown in Fig. 7.5. All of the data were taken at Washington University. The tear resistance data published by Marotta and Morey[9] are not included inasmuch as those data were obtained through use of a different test protocol

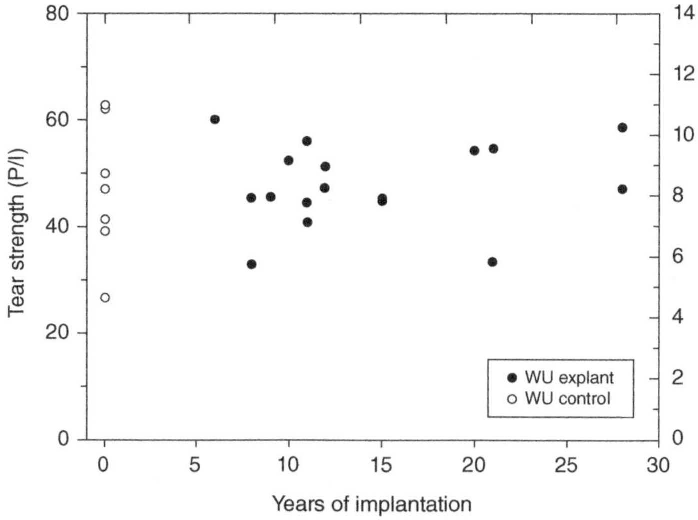

7.5 Tear strength of Silastic 0 and Silastic I implant shells as a function of time in vivo. Reprinted with permission from ref. 5. Copyright 1999 Sage Publications.

that does not allow a direct comparison with the present data. The explants have implantation times ranging from 6 to 28 years. Eleven of the explants were intact, two were ruptured, and four had pinholes. As with tensile stress and elongation, the tear data are not a function of whether the explant was intact, was ruptured, or had a pinhole. The explants with the lowest values for tear resistance were intact, unruptured implants.

The data on Silastic 0 and Silastic I implants published to date clearly indicate that the ultimate mechanical properties of the shell do not appreciably degrade in vivo. An additional study by Marotta[13] evaluated the properties of four additional standard Dow Corning gel-filled explants, with implantation times ranging from 10 to 15 years. Their tensile strength and elongation data were within the control ranges shown in Figs 7.3 and 7.4.

7.3.2 Ultimate strength properties of Silastic II implants

All published data on the ultimate properties of Silastic II implants were analyzed and reported.[14] Figure 7.6 summarizes all of the published mean tensile strength data for Silastic II implant shells as a function of implantation time. These data include lot-matched data and non-lot-matched data from WU as well as Silastic II non-lot-matched data from the literature. The control data are plotted at time zero, and the explant shell in vivo times vary from 0.3 to 13.2 years. Data are for 53 single-lumen controls and 34 single-lumen explants tested at five different laboratories and published

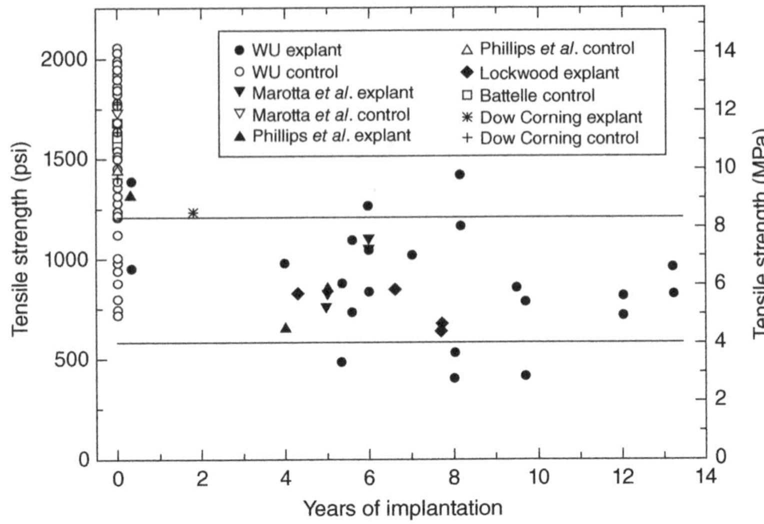

7.6 Average tensile strength of lot-matched, non-lot-matched, and literature data versus time in vivo. Reprinted with permission from ref. 14. Copyright 2000 Sage Publications.

in six different studies. The large range in tensile strength of the control implants is primarily due to shell strength variations associated with lot-to-lot variability. The scatter in the explant data is also due to lot-to-lot variability, as well as to differences in the testing techniques used in the various studies. Nonetheless, the control and explant data from the six different studies are in general agreement.

The tensile strength of the ruptured shells and the shells containing pinhole leaks fell within the scatter band of the intact shells. Hence, we found no difference in the tensile strength of intact shells, ruptured shells, and shells containing pinhole leaks. The upper and lower lines in Fig. 7.6 show the predicted tensile strength of the explants based on the strongest and weakest lots from a regression model. These predicted upper and lower strengths were determined from 16 lot-matched explants that were tested; they could have a wider range if additional lot-matched explants are tested. The predicted range of strength was based on a regression analysis of the mean measurement. However, essentially the same range was predicted through use of a regression analysis of the individual and median measurements.

Tensile strength initially decreases after the implantation process. More explant data are needed from the first few years of implantation to determine the time it takes for the tensile strength to reach its equilibrium value. However, the results of the regression analysis show that there is no difference in the ultimate strength as a function of long term implantation time

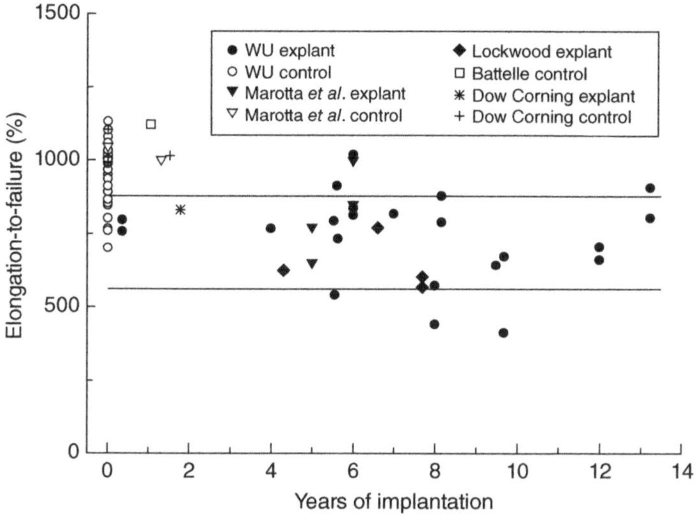

7.7 Average elongation-to-failure of lot-matched, non-lot-matched, and literature data versus time in vivo. Reprinted with permission from ref. 14. Copyright 2000 Sage Publications.

at a significance of 0.01. Regression of the means, medians, and ranked data leads to the same conclusion. Therefore, it is unlikely that the conclusions drawn from the regression analysis are influenced by scale artifacts or outliers. Data from the literature agree with the range predicted by the regression model.

A summary of all the published data on the elongation-to-failure of Silastic II implant shells as a function of implantation time is shown in Fig. 7.7, which provides data from 52 controls and 31 explants. Elongation-to-failure data were not published in the report of Phillips. Twenty-eight of the explants were intact, one was ruptured, and two had pinholes. Again, we found no differences in elongation-to-failure among intact, ruptured, and pinhole shells, indicating that the properties of the elastomers do not degrade during in vivo aging. The two explants with the lowest values of elongation-to-failure, 413% and 440%, had implantation times of 10 and 8 years, respectively, and were intact. As with tensile strength, there is an initial decrease in elongation-to-failure after implantation, but the regression analysis shows no difference in the ultimate elongation-to-failure as a function of long-term implantation at a level of significance of 0.01. Data from the literature agree with the range predicted by the regression model.

The average tear resistance data of 42 controls and 22 explants as a function of implantation time are shown in Fig. 7.8. Twenty of the explants were intact, one was ruptured, and one had a pinhole. All of the data were taken

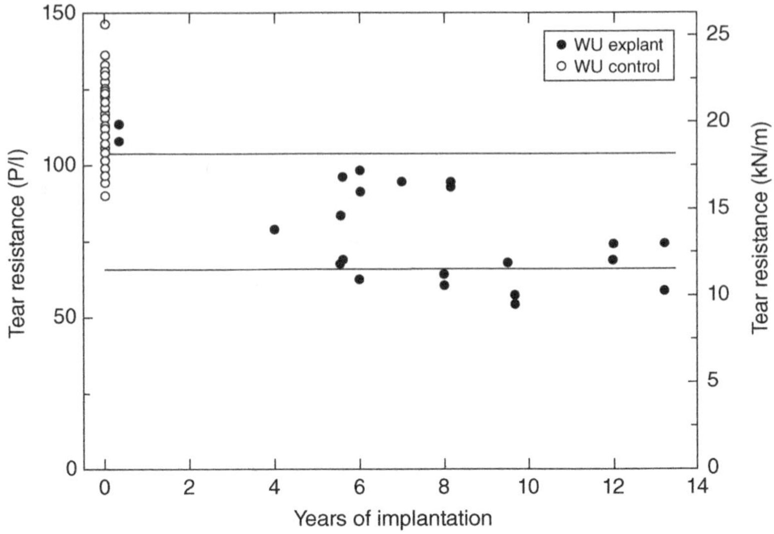

7.8 Average tear resistance of lot-matched, non-lot-matched, and literature data versus time in vivo. Reprinted with permission from ref. 14. Copyright 2000 Sage Publications.

at WU. The tear resistance results published in Marotta and Morey are not included, inasmuch as those data were obtained by a different test protocol that does not allow a direct comparison with the present data. As with tensile strength and elongation-to-failure, the tear strength data are not a function of whether the explant was intact, ruptured, or had a pinhole. The two explants with the lowest values of tear resistance after 10 years in vivo were intact. The regression coefficient of time for the median ultimate tear resistance as a function of long-term implantation was insignificant at 0.01 level. This conclusion is not as significant for the analysis of the individual measurements, the ranked data, or the means.

Silastic II implants were the newest devices to be analyzed for mechanical property data in detail in this chapter. Apparently, manufacturers have not released their data on implants being marketed currently. However, an independent study of current implants was recently reported,[15] and a discussion of that study is in order. Mechanical tests were conducted on 100 explants of current designs that were implanted from 1996 to 2006. The manufacturers were not named, and no elongation data were obtained. Implantation times varied from 0.5 to 11 years and the average was 4.9 years; 33% of the explants were ruptured. The authors reported that the absolute values of shell strength were lower than the ones in the literature. The average tensile strength for all 100 explants was 3.38 MPa which is significantly lower than the averages presented herein. However, the differences in strength before and after extraction are consistent with the outcomes from our studies. No ruptures were found when the ultimate stress was higher than 4 MPa. Unfortunately, no control implants were tested, so it is difficult to properly assess the results of that study except to state that the strength of current silicone gel implants is less than the strength of some previous designs. This result provides additional support for separating implants according to type, manufacturing lots, and manufacturers. An important future study would be a failure analysis of the current explants already mechanically tested, and a subsequent correlation of failure modes with shell strength characteristics and implantation time.

7.3.3 Moduli and cross-link density properties

The durability of breast implant shells is a function of their mechanical and chemical properties. Ultimate mechanical properties (tensile strength, elongation, and tear) can depend on material flaws and their subsequent propagation in the shell. However, modulus values are dependent on the bulk structure of the material. For this reason, modulus values tend to be more reproducible than ultimate properties. Modulus values were examined[3] to investigate the bulk material stability of explanted breast implant shells. The 200% and 400% moduli for unextracted and extracted Silastic I/Silastic 0 implant shells and the 200%, 400% and 600% moduli for unextracted and extracted Silastic II implant shells are presented in Figs 7.9 and 7.10. The controls are given at time 0. These data, which were obtained at Washington University,[3] Battelle,[9] and Dow Corning,[16] represent all known modulus data for these types of implants. Most of the explant data for unextracted and extracted Silastic I/Silastic 0 shells were within the ranges measured for the unextracted control shells (plotted at 0 years). This indicates that neither swelling nor in vivo aging affected the lower portion of the stress-strain curve. Unlike the ultimate properties, the modulus values for Silastic II explants did not decrease after the implantation process. The 200%, 400% and 600% moduli for Silastic II shells did not vary with implantation time. This demonstrates that a significant portion of the stress-strain curve is not affected by swelling or in vivo aging. The modulus properties were essentially not affected by implantation for time periods of up to 13 years for Silastic II implants and up to 28 years for Silastic I/Silastic 0 implants. The fact that the explant modulus values were essentially independent of implantation time provides evidence of long-term material stability of these breast implants. The 200% and 400% modulus properties were insensitive to long-term exposure to a biological environment.

If the silicone elastomer in an implant shell undergoes a chemical reaction during implantation, then a change in the cross-link density of the elastomer would be expected. An increase in cross-link density should be

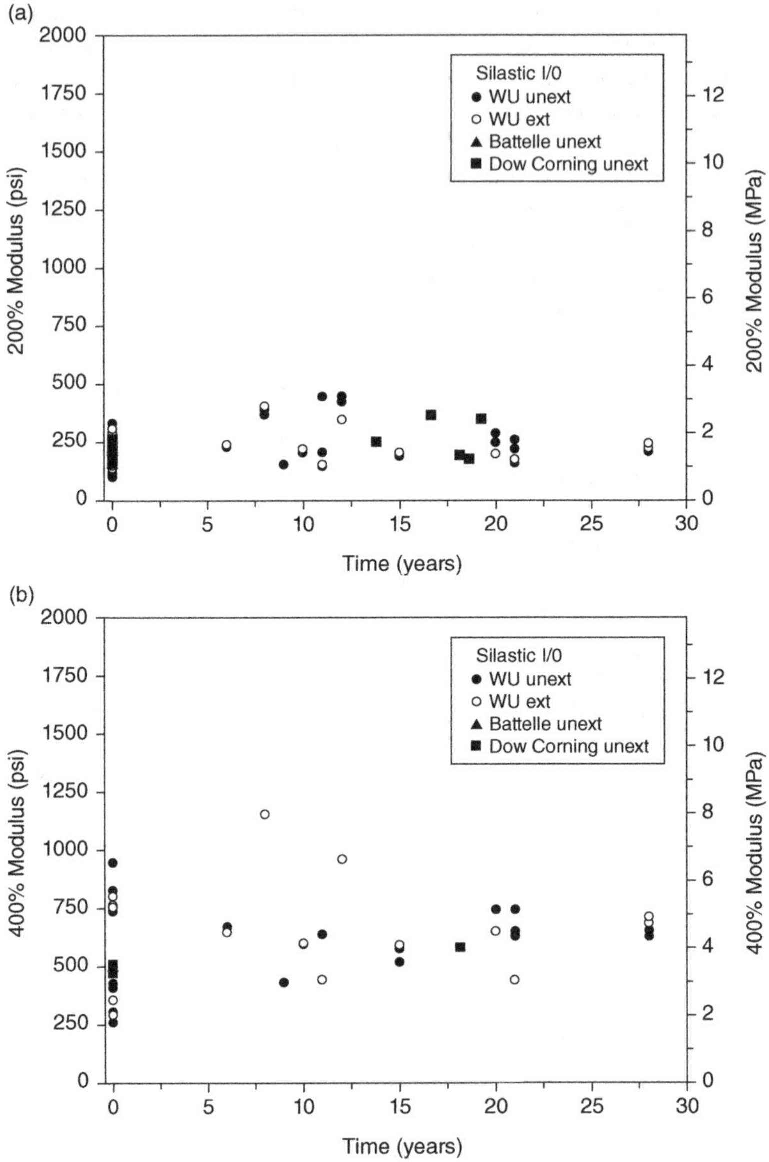

7.9 Modulus values for Silastic I implant shells as a function of time in vivo. (a) 200% modulus. (b) 400% modulus. WU, Washington University; unext, unextracted; ext, extracted; psi, pounds per square inch. Reprinted with permission from ref. 3. Copyright 2003 Wolters Kluwer Health.

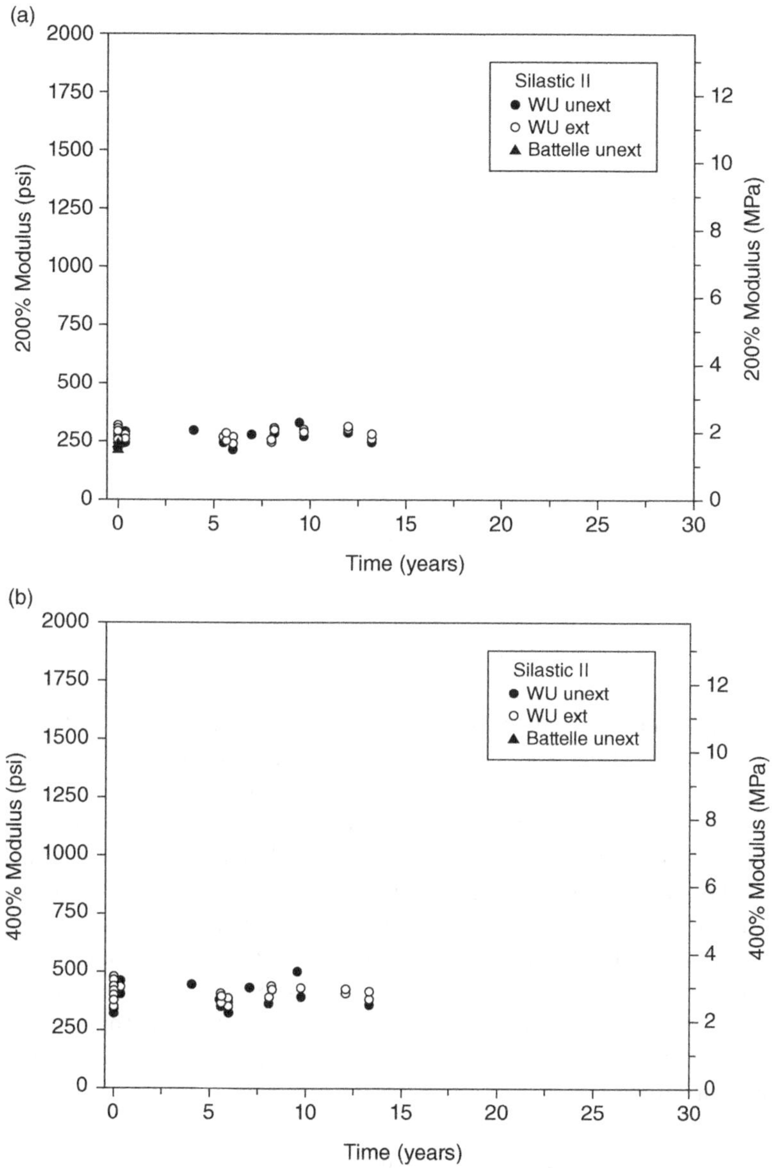

7.10 Modulus values for Silastic II implant shells as a function of time in vivo. (a) 200% modulus. (b) 400% modulus. (c) 600% modulus. WU, Washington University; unext, unextracted; ext, extracted; psi, pounds per square inch. Reprinted with permission from ref. 3. Copyright 2003 Wolters Kluwer Health.

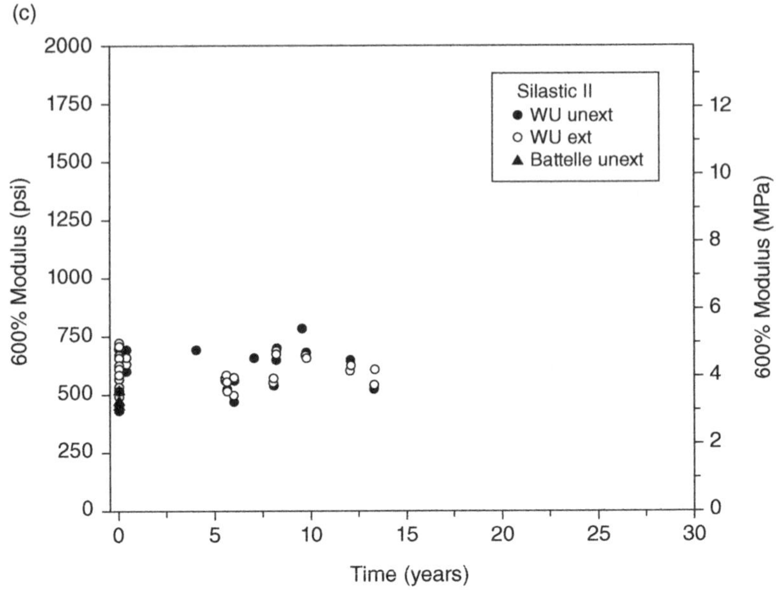

7.10 Continued.

accompanied by an increase in Young's modulus and associated embrittlement of the shell; a decrease in cross-link density suggests degradation of the elastomer and an overall loss of strength. The cross-link densities, determined from swelling measurements, as a function of implantation time for Silastic I/Silastic 0 and Silastic II implant shells are presented in Fig. 7.11. All data were obtained at Washington University.[3] All explant data were within the ranges for the control implants, indicating that the polymer does not degrade. Therefore, the cross-link densities were essentially independent of implantation time for 13 years for Silastic II implants and for 28 years for Silastic I/Silastic 0 implants. This suggests that the cross-link density of the silicone elastomer undergoes little or no change during implantation.

7.3.4 Effects of shell swelling on ultimate properties

The diffusion of non-cross-linked silicones from the gel into the shell and the associated swelling can significantly reduce the tensile strength and elongation of implant shells. This effect was observed for Silastic I/Silastic 0 and Silastic II implant shells, as depicted in Figs 7.12, 7.13 and 7.14 which present the ratios of tensile strength and elongation in unextracted to extracted (diluents removed) shells as a function of the extracted fraction for both control and explanted shells.[3,14] The strength and elongation decreased as the amount of extractable material increased. The effect of

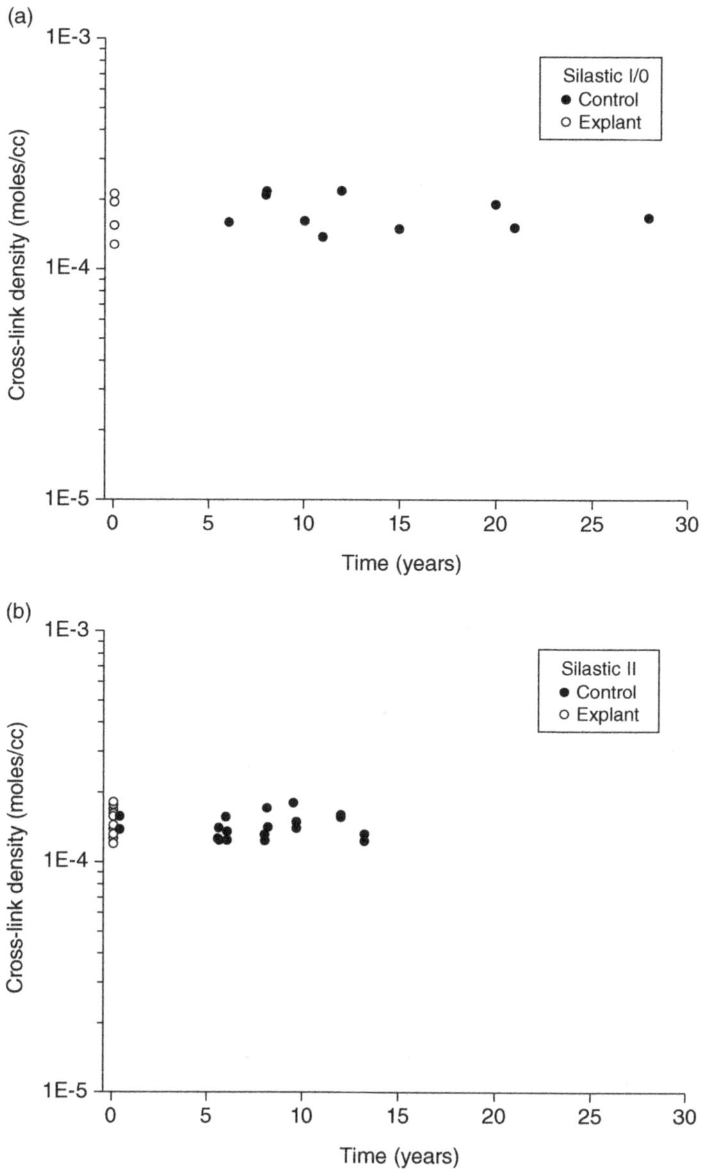

7.11 (a) Cross-link density of Silastic I implant shells as a function of time in vivo. (b) Cross-link density of Silastic II implant shells as a function of time in vivo. Reprinted with permission from ref. 3. Copyright 2003 Wolters Kluwer Health.

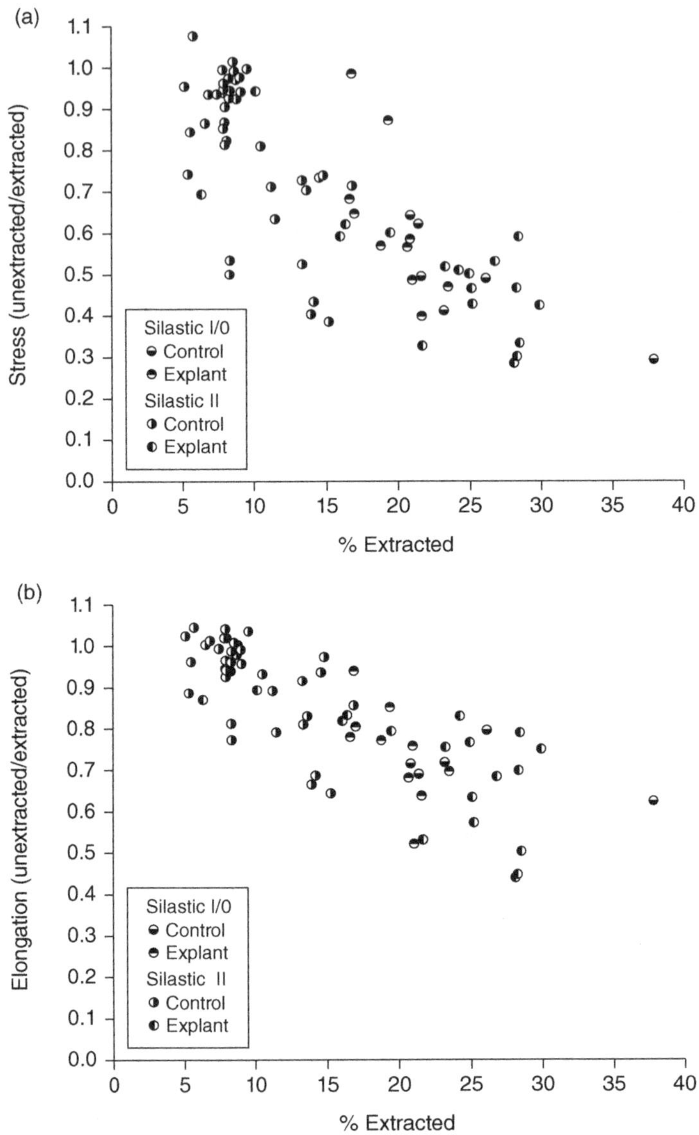

7.12 (a) Unextracted shell/extracted shell tensile stress ratio versus percent extracted. (b) Unextracted shell/extracted shell elongation ratio versus fraction extracted. Reprinted with permission from ref. 3. Copyright 2003 Wolters Kluwer Health.

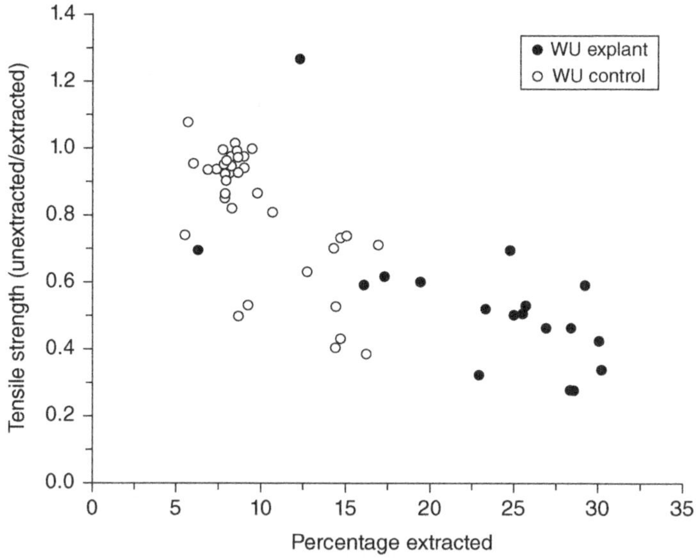

7.13 Tensile strength ratio of unextracted shell to extracted shell versus percent extracted for Silastic II implants. Reprinted with permission from ref. 14. Copyright 2000 Sage Publications.

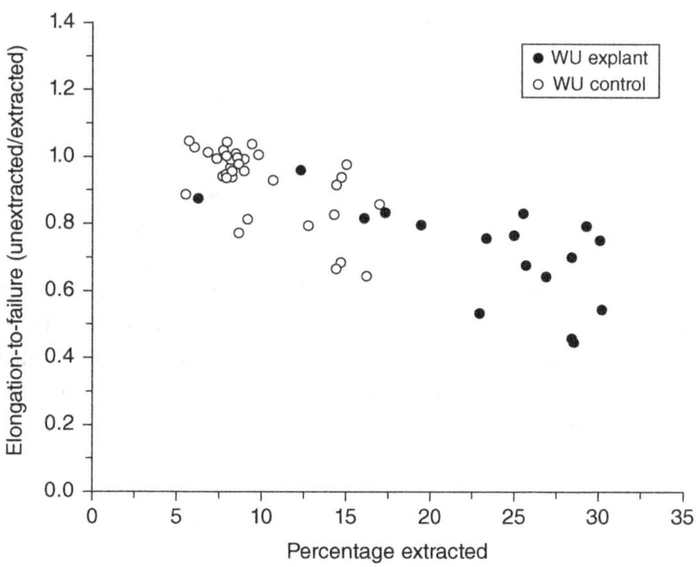

7.14 Elongation-to-failure ratio of unextracted shell to extracted shell versus percent extracted for Silastic II implants. Reprinted with permission from ref. 14. Copyright 2000 Sage Publications.

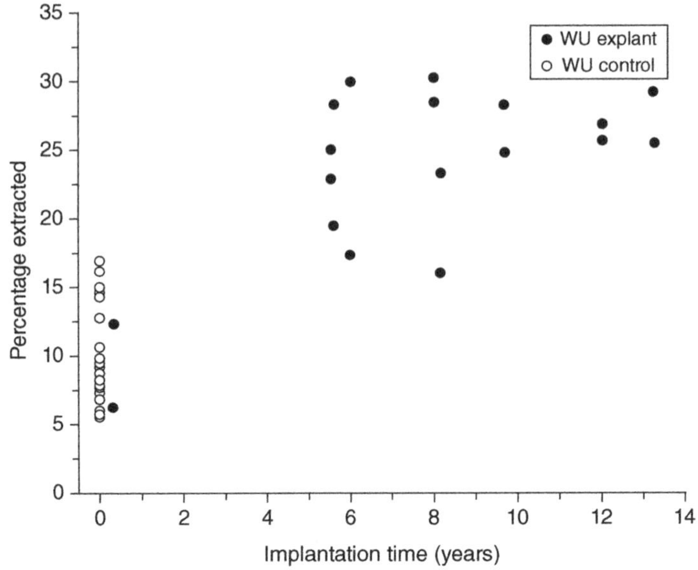

7.15 Percentage extracted as a function of time in vivo for Silastic II implants. Reprinted with permission from ref. 14. Copyright 2000 Sage Publications.

swelling on tensile strength is much greater because the stress-strain curve rises so rapidly near failure. For the shell with the largest percent extracted (38.2 weight %), the tensile strength was reduced 71% and the elongation was reduced 27%. Correlations with tear resistance data are not presented because tear data were not obtained for extracted shell specimens.

The effects of the swelling agent on the mechanical properties of the shells were investigated by extracting the swelling agent with hexane and measuring the amount extracted and the properties of the extracted elastomer. For Silastic II shells, the results[14] demonstrated that the amount extracted was initially a function of implantation time, as shown in Fig. 7.15. The increase in swelling during the initial period of implantation probably results from the enhanced diffusion of non-cross-linked silicones from the gel into the shell. After a certain length of time, the equilibrium swelling appears to be reached. The time required for the swelling equilibrium to be reached is unknown, but equilibrium seems to occur within the first few years after implantation. This phenomenon may be associated with the barrier coating. Silastic I/Silastic 0 shells do not have a barrier coating and thus may not have an extractable amount that is dependent on the time in vivo. As indicated in Fig. 7.16, analysis of the extracted fraction as a function of implantation time supports this hypothesis.[3] The data for the explants were essentially independent of time, but many of the data points were below the scatter band for the control shells. The Silastic 0 shells tended to

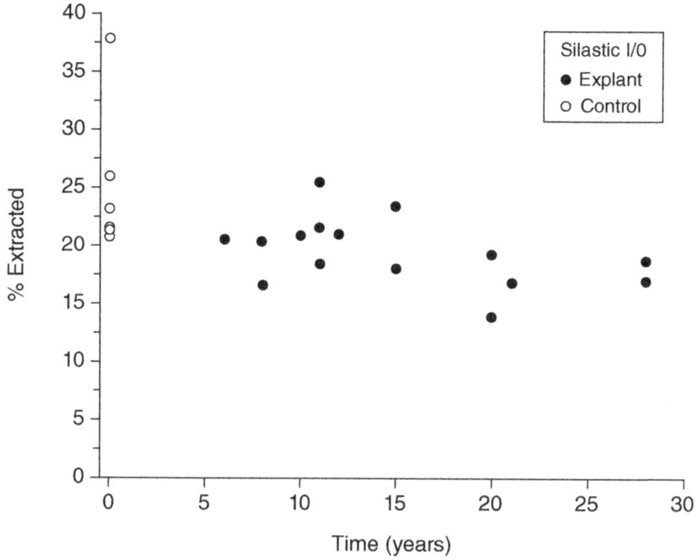

7.16 Percentage extracted as a function of time in vivo for Silastic I/0 implants. Reprinted with permission from ref. 3. Copyright 2003 Wolters Kluwer Health.

be less swollen, because the more viscous gel used in that type of implant contained fewer low-molecular-weight silicones.

There was little or no degradation of the base polydimethylsiloxane during in vivo aging in any of the implants we examined. However, the ultimate mechanical properties of the elastomeric shell can decrease because of swelling. The diluent has no long-term effect on the silicone polymer, but markedly decreases the interaction between the silicone and the silica filler. In general, more material is extraced from the explant shells than from the control shells. The total amount of extractable material varies with implantation time and can be as high as 30 wt%.

7.4 Lot-matched control study

The mechanical and chemical properties of 16 Silastic II prostheses that had been implanted for time periods ranging from 0.3 to 13 years were measured and directly compared with lot-matched controls prepared from the same batch of elastomer at the same manufacturing time.[17] The measurements include tensile strength, elongation, moduli, tear resistance, cross-link density, and percentage of extractables.

The physical properties of the two explants with 13 years in vivo are compared with the lot-matched control values in Table 7.5. The average planform diameter of the two explants with 13 years in vivo was 8% greater

Table 7.5 Physical properties of explants (13 years in vivo) and lot-matched control (reprinted with permission from ref. 17. Copyright 2002 Wolters Kluwer Health)

Implant	Years in vivo	Weight (g)	Planform diameter (in)
Explant (left)	13	272	5.57
Explant (right)	13	274	5.63
Control	–	275	5.17

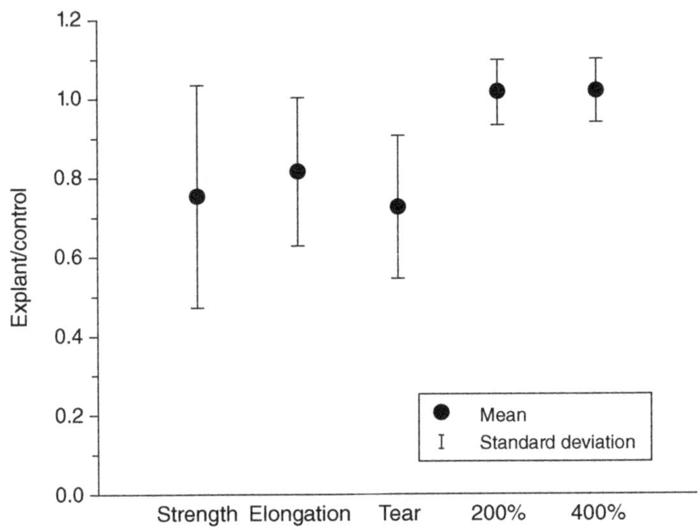

7.17 Mean ratio of properties of the explant shell to the lot-matched control shell. Data points show means ± standard deviation. Reprinted with permission from ref. 17. Copyright 2002 Wolters Kluwer Health.

than the lot-matched control planform diameter. The weights of the two explants were within 1% of the lot-matched control weight. The shell thickness increase of the two explants attributable to swelling was approximately 8% compared with 3.5% for the control.

Mechanical and chemical properties were obtained for all 16 explant shells and their lot-matched controls. For each shell property, the ratio of the explant value to the lot-matched control value was calculated for all 16 explants. The mean ratio was then computed for the 16 ratios. Figure 7.17 presents the mean ratio of the explant property to the corresponding lot-matched control property for tensile strength, elongation, tear resistance, and 200% and 400% moduli for the unextracted shells. The mean ratio for the same properties except for the tear resistance are presented for the extracted shells in Fig. 7.18, together with the cross-link density. The mean

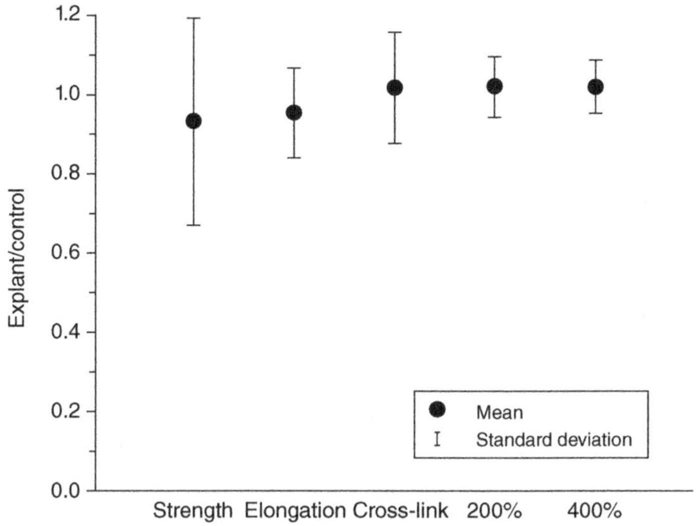

7.18 Mean ratio of properties of the extracted explant shell to the extracted lot-matched control shell. Data points show means ± standard deviation. Reprinted with permission from ref. 17. Copyright 2002 Wolters Kluwer Health.

values are given by the solid circles in these two figures. The standard deviations of the mean ratios are also shown in the two figures. A mean ratio of 1.0 for any given property indicates that on average no change occurred in that particular property during the implantation period. Hence, the ultimate explant shell properties are below the control shell properties but are only slightly below the control values for the extracted samples. There is essentially no change in either the moduli or the cross-link density because of implantation.

For the unextracted shells, the ultimate properties of tensile strength, elongation, and tear resistance of the explants were on average 18% to 27% below the lot-matched control values. The reduction in the explant ultimate property values was primarily caused by the increased swelling of the explant shells compared with the control shells. On average, the percentage extracted from an explant shell was approximately twice as great as its lot-matched control value. We previously have shown that Silastic II explant shells, including the 16 explants analyzed herein, exhibit a decrease in strength property values shortly after implantation and are essentially constant thereafter. The amount of time required for the properties to reach equilibrium is not known; however, data reported herein suggest that it occurs within the first few years of implantation. The initial reduction in the ultimate strength properties of the explants in comparison with those of the lot-matched controls probably arises from the enhanced diffusion of

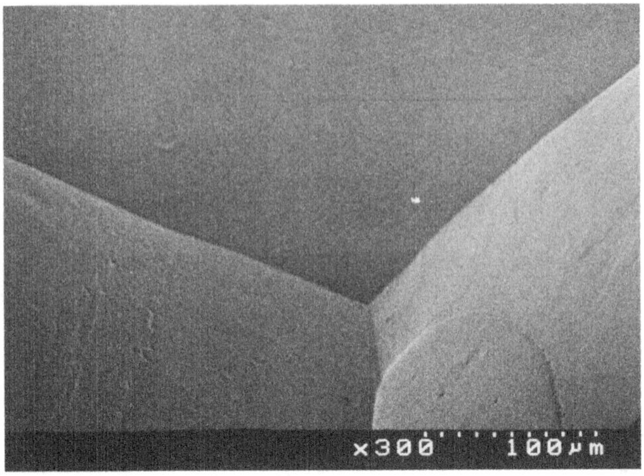

7.19 Outside surface of Silastic II explant with 10 years in vivo. Original magnification, ×300. Reprinted with permission from ref. 17. Copyright 2002 Wolters Kluwer Health.

the non-cross-linked silicones from the gel into the shell. Extracted explant shells are less affected by implantation than those of the unextracted explant shells. For the extracted shells, the tensile strength and elongation of the explants are within 5% to 7% of their original values. On average, the 200% and 400% moduli of the explanted shells are within 2% of the control values for both unextracted and extracted shells. The cross-link density of the explanted shells is also within 2% of the lot-matched control shells.

Breast implants are subjected to some degree of stress and deformation during the surgical procedure of insertion. A study discussed later in this chapter has shown that the surgical process of implanting a breast implant can have a small but statistically significant reduction in the average strength properties of the elastomer shell of the implant. Another factor that could explain some of the differences in the mechanical properties of the explants and their lot-matched controls is property variation within a lot that is not considered in the study.

In addition to comparing the physical, mechanical and chemical properties of explant and lot-matched control shells, the morphological features of the explant and control shells were also compared by using scanning electron microscopy. A typical scanning electron microscopy micrograph obtained in this study is presented in Fig. 7.19, which shows a section of a Silastic II explant shell that was explanted after 10 years in vivo. The outside surface of the shell is the large planar area in the micrograph. A 100 μm scale is shown in the lower right-hand corner. Figure 7.20 shows a similar micrograph for the explant's lot-matched control. There is essentially no

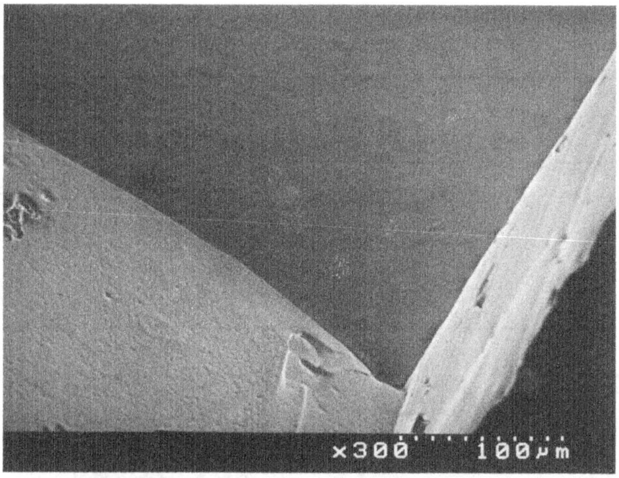

7.20 Outside surface of Silastic II lot-matched control. Original magnification, ×300. Reprinted with permission from ref. 17. Copyright 2002 Wolters Kluwer Health.

change in the outer surface of the explant shell exposed to a biological environment for 10 years compared with the unimplanted control shell manufactured at the same time and from the same lot of silicone elastomer.

7.5 Effect of implantation time on shell properties of saline implants

7.5.1 Ultimate strength properties

Most published implant properties data relate to silicone gel devices. The mechanical properties of explanted saline-filled breast implants have not received as much scientific attention. The lack of information on inflatable shells can be addressed only by testing them with methodologies such as those outlined in this chapter. For both silicone gel and saline implants, we must have sufficient experimental data to determine whether implantation degrades the elastomer, how in vivo aging affects the shell, and what processes might contribute to the failure.

We have recently applied our protocol to investigating several saline explants that were removed after varying implantation times.[1] A brief description of the five explants tested is presented in Table 7.6. To our knowledge, the Simaplast device, with 23 years in vivo, is the oldest saline implant analyzed to date. It was manufactured in France and explanted at the University of Toronto by Prof. Walter Peters. A photograph of the anterior surface of this intact explant, which is extensively calcified, is shown in

Table 7.6 Implantation time and status of five tested saline explants (reprinted with permission from ref. 1. Copyright 2003 Begell House)

Manufacturer	Years of implantation	Implant status at explantation	Shell type
Simaplast	23	Intact	Smooth
Heyer-Schulte	22	Intact	Smooth
Heyer-Schulte	21	Failed	Smooth
McGhan	5.5	Failed	Textured
McGhan	3	Failed	Textured

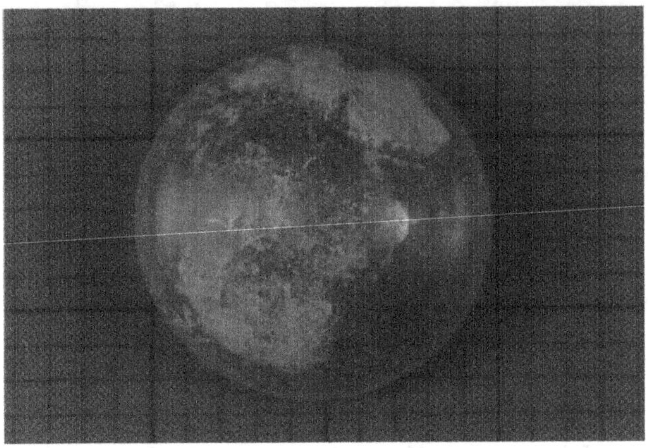

7.21 Anterior surface of intact Simaplast saline implant removed after 23 years. Extensive calcification is evident. Reprinted with permission from ref. 1. Copyright 2003 Begell House.

Fig. 7.21. We believe the intact Heyer-Schulte explant with 22 years of implantation (Fig. 7.22) is the oldest US-made saline device that has been tested. Data from a failed Heyer-Schulte explant with 21 years of implantation and failed McGhan textured explants with 5.5 and 3 years in vivo are presented for comparison.

A major reason for analyzing explants with the types of tools described in our protocol is to determine the effect(s) of implantation on shell properties. This is best accomplished by comparing explants to proper controls. Neither lot-matched controls nor controls that would yield shell property ranges were available for the saline explants listed in Table 7.6. Consequently, they were classified only by manufacturer and implantation duration and analyzed accordingly. The ultimate strength properties of tensile strength, elongation, and tear resistance are presented in Table 7.7 for the five as-received (nonextracted) shells. Table 7.7 also gives the average shell thickness determined from all the tensile and tear specimens. With no

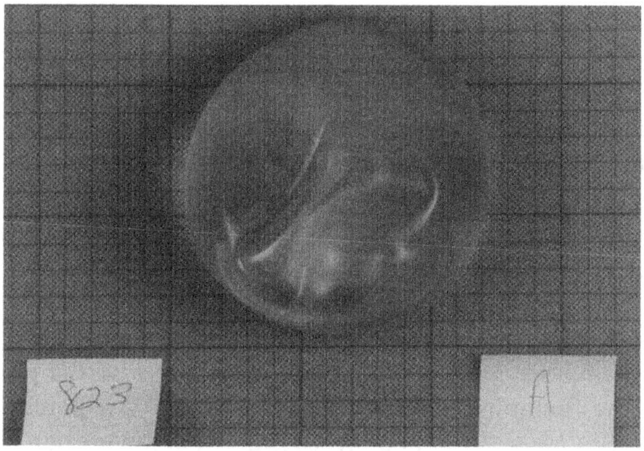

7.22 Intact Heyer-Schulte saline explant with 22 years of implantation. To our knowledge, the oldest US-made saline implant tested. Reprinted with permission from ref. 1. Copyright 2003 Begell House.

Table 7.7 Ultimate strength properties of five saline explant shells (reprinted with permission from ref. 1. Copyright 2003 Begell House)

Explant	Years in vivo	Tensile strength (psi)	Percentage elongation	Tear resistance (P/I)	Shell thickness (in)
Simaplast	23	866	299	74	0.023
Heyer-Schulte	22	371	387	33	0.018
Heyer-Schulte	21	284	421	25	0.018
McGhan	5.5	412	300	35	0.027
McGhan	3	642	420	52	0.023

psi = pounds force per square inch (1 psi = 6.895 kPa); P/I = pounds force per inch (1 P/I = 1.751 N/cm).

Table 7.8 Tensile strength and elongation of extracted saline explant shells (reprinted with permission from ref. 1. Copyright 2003 Begell House)

Explant	Years in vivo	Percentage extracted	Tensile strength (psi)	Elongation (%)
Simaplast	23	2.8	937	303
Heyer-Schulte	22	21.7	480	421
Heyer-Schulte	21	25.5	557	598
McGhan	5.5	2.7	449	373
McGhan	3	3.1	664	409

psi = pounds force per square inch (1 psi = 6.895 kPa).

controls available for these explants, any assessment of the effects of in vivo aging is limited because the values of the shell properties at implantation are unknown. We can, however, conclude that the shell thickness of the five explants are comparable. The tensile strength and tear resistance of the Simaplast explant are much higher than that of the other four explants, but its percentage elongation is the lowest. Elongation values for the Simaplast explant and the McGhan explant with 5.5 years in vivo are below the ASTM standard of 350% for unimplanted shells. Even so, the Simaplast implant remained intact for 23 years.

The properties of tensile strength and elongation for shells extracted with hexane prior to analysis are shown in Table 7.8, along with the percentage extracted. For the Simaplast and McGhan shells, the low percentages of material extracted (2.8%, 2.7% and 3.1%) indicate a higher percentage of monomer was incorporated into the elastomer. The large amount of material extracted from the Heyer-Schulte shells is comparable to the percent extracted from many silicone gel implant shells, which contain silicone molecules from the gel filler. As with silicone gel shells, property measurements of the unextracted saline shells are lower than those of the extracted shells. The failed Heyer-Schulte explant with 21 years of implantation had the greatest decrease in ultimate properties, with the tensile strength and elongation of unextracted specimens being about 50% and 30% lower than extracted specimens.

7.5.2 Effect of Betadine pocket irrigation

One of the few published studies on the mechanical properties of saline-filled breast implants investigated the effect of Betadine pocket irrigation on implant shell integrity.[18] The primary objective of this study was not an investigation of shell strength as a function of implantation time, but rather of the effect of implant exposure to Betadine pocket irrigation during implantation. Emphasis was placed on patch-shell delamination or disruption due to Betadine exposure. Shell strength properties were also measured and are reviewed here.

Because of concerns that exposure to povidone-iodine (Betadine) may lead to early breast implant failure, the US Food and Drug Administration (FDA) announced in 2000 that any contact between implants and Betadine is contraindicated. The evidence cited by the FDA primarily referred to Betadine added to saline implant filler solution and not to povidone-iodine used for pocket irrigation. After the FDA issued its directive against use of Betadine in breast implantation, one of the authors (V. L. Y.) began collecting saline-filled implants that had been exposed to Betadine pocket irrigation and later consecutively explanted. Standard, full-strength Betadine solution (povidone-iodine 10%) had been used. Because the same surgeon

Table 7.9 Mentor implants tested after pocket irrigation with Betadine and subsequent explantation (reprinted with permission from ref. 18. Copyright 2002 Sage Publications)

Implantation time (months)	Fill volume (cc)	Surface type	Explant status
0.2	525	Smooth	Intact
0.2	525	Smooth	Intact
1.0	775	Smooth	Intact
4.4	325	Smooth	Intact
16.0	300	Smooth	Intact
16.0	300	Smooth	Intact
20.0	350	Smooth	Intact
30.5	350	Smooth	Intact
30.5	350	Smooth	Intact
47.0	300	Smooth	Intact
47.0	300	Smooth	Intact
55.0	425	Textured	Deflated
55.0	425	Textured	Intact

had originally placed the implants, the precise durations of implantation were known, and Betadine pocket irrigation could be confirmed in the operative reports. It was also certain that no Betadine had been added to the implant filler solution. Within a few months, 13 explants manufactured by Mentor were identified and collected.

In our implant studies, we typically compare measurements from explanted implants to lot-matched controls or to the measured properties ranges (maximum to minimum) of controls for particular implant models. For the 13 Mentor explants tested in this study, we did not have either lot-matched controls or control range data. Thus, we could compare their mechanical properties only to ASTM requirements for breast implant shells.

Basic details about the 13 Mentor explants tested in this study are shown in Table 7.9, which gives implantation times, implant fill volume, shell surface type, and integrity status at a time of removal. The 13 devices were removed from eight patients who had undergone breast augmentation, of whom five underwent bilateral explantations and three underwent unilateral explantations. The mean duration of implantation was 24.8 months (range 0.2 to 55 months). All the explants were round, 11 had a smooth surface, and 12 were placed in the submuscular plane; one was a replacement implant inserted in a pre-existing subglandular pocket. All implants were filled with standard sterile sodium chloride U.S.P. solution for injection, implanted by the same surgeon who removed them, and placed in pockets that had been irrigated with standard, full strength Betadine solution (povidone-iodine 10%).

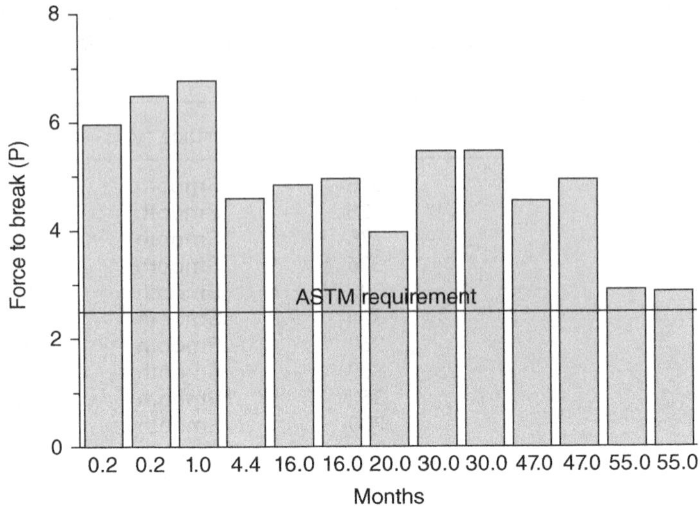

7.23 Force-to-break data plotted according to implantation time for the 13 Mentor explant shells subjected to Betadine pocket irrigation. P indicates how many pounds of force were applied to test specimens before the elastomer ruptured. Reprinted with permission from ref. 18. Copyright 2002 Sage Publications.

One of the implants with the longer time in vivo (55 months) began to deflate approximately a year before it was removed, but the patient delayed implant exchange. When explanted, this implant seemed to be leaking through the anterior diaphragm valve. The shell and posterior patch looked no different than the patient's contralateral textured implant. Specifically, the patch–shell interface was not disrupted, and there was no sign of shell or patch delamination. A detailed failure analysis of this explant was not performed, but we presume this one deflation resulted from a valve failure.

As stated earlier, we could not compare the mechanical properties measurements of the explants to lot-matched controls and therefore cannot comment on whether the shells exposed to Betadine pocket irrigation underwent any specific changes in their strength characteristics. Instead, we qualitatively assessed the mechanical properties of the explant shells, which are presented independent of control data.

Figure 7.23 presents force-to-break data, shown according to implantation time, for the 13 Mentor explant shells that were placed in pockets irrigated with Betadine. This bar graph, which represents the average of the tested specimens from each explant, shows how many pounds of force the elastomer withstood before the specimen ruptured. All explant shells exceeded ASTM requirements of 2.5 pounds for elastomer strength.

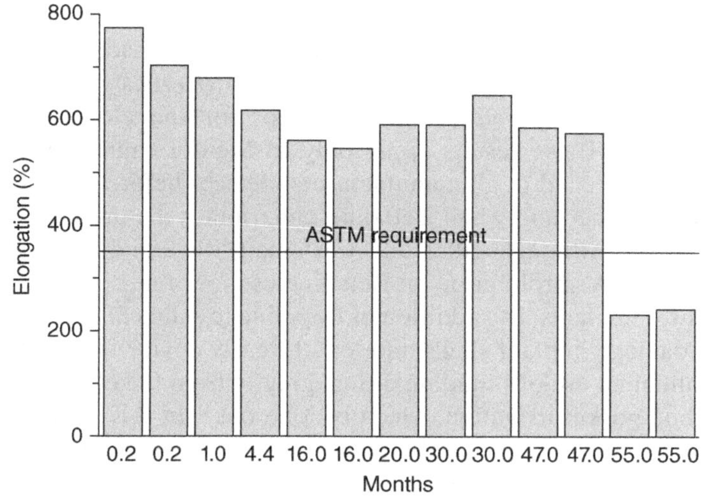

7.24 Percentage elongation before break of the 13 explant shells exposed to Betadine pocket irrigation shown according to implantation time. All smooth-surface shells exceed the ASTM requirement of 350%, but neither of the textured shells meet the minimum standard. Reprinted with permission from ref. 18. Copyright 2002 Sage Publications.

We also found that the shell thickness of a textured implant varies considerably. Furthermore, the thickness of the anterior surface is generally much thinner than the posterior surface. For both textured explant shells, the force-to-break at the thinner shell regions was less than 2.5 pounds, but the average for both the intact and deflated shells exceeded the ASTM specification.

Whereas force-to-break relates to the largest sustainable force the elastomer can tolerate, elongation refers to the longest endurable stretching deformation the specimen can withstand before rupturing. According to ASTM, the elastomer used in breast implant shells should be able to elongate 350% before the test specimen breaks. The average percentage (%) elongation for the 5 specimens tested from the 13 Mentor shells exposed to extraluminal Betadine is shown in Fig. 7.24. All tested smooth implant shells surpassed the ASTM requirement, but both textured shells were below the minimum requirement, with measurements of 233% and 245%.

We do not know why the mechanical properties of the two Mentor Siltex (textured) implants tested in this study were significantly lower than those of the 11 smooth-surfaced implants. However, we doubt that the difference is related to the use of Betadine pocket irrigation, because none of the explanted shells had delaminated or separated at the patch interface. A more plausible possibility is that the texturing process affects the mechanical properties of the shell. Our investigation found no evidence of patch or shell delamination. Furthermore, mechanical properties for the explants exceeded ASTM-required standards except for the elongation of the textured shells. These results apply only to Mentor saline implants, and more study is needed of all manufacturers' devices before researchers can determine whether and when Betadine undermines the integrity of breast implant shells. Although our study was small, we found no evidence to support the FDA's prohibition on Betadine use for breast pocket irrigation with Mentor implants. The addition of Betadine to saline filler solution does seem to damage implant shells and lead to early device failure. However, this intraluminal use of Betadine differs greatly from the common practice of Betadine pocket irrigation, which is done once. In this context, contact between an implant and extraluminal Betadine is transient and may not produce the same results as Betadine and saline solution in a sealed environment.

7.6 Breast implant rupture

7.6.1 Failure mechanisms

Breast implants can fail for a variety of reasons including: (1) inadvertent instrument damage during surgery, (2) open capsulotomy, (3) closed capsulotomy, (4) needle biopsy or hematoma aspiration, (5) shell wrinkling, (6) trauma, (7) mammography, (8) implantation surgery, (9) explantation surgery, (10) manufacturing defects, (11) cyclic fatigue, and (12) patch detachment. In addition, some published studies have indicated that implant failure can be explained on the basis of in vivo degradation of the shell mechanical properties with the exposure to a biological environment. For example, Marotta[13] concluded 'that a primary mechanism for rupture must be the progressive cyclic mechanical stress induced creation and enlargement of tears in weakened silicone fluid swollen silicone elastomeric shells.' This proposed failure mechanism is unsubstantiated. The shell extraction values measured by Marotta for Dow Corning explants were approximately 20%. Other studies have demonstrated that various types of silicone gel breast implants can remain intact in vivo with swelling of approximately 20% to 40%. A study by Wolf[19] demonstrated that the mechanical forces involved in the swelling process do not degrade the silicone shell, even when the elastomer is cycled through five swelling–extraction cycles with an aggressive swelling agent. The hypothesis that the material chemical bonds are not broken with swelling is also supported by the fair agreement of the ultimate properties of the extracted shells and the elastomeric dispersion used in the manufacture of Silastic I/Silastic 0 and Silastic II shells.[5,14]

7.6.2 Microscopy analysis of failed implants

There are several types of diagnostic techniques available for the analysis of ruptured implants. Visual inspection, physical examination, and photographic analysis provide an overall description of the implant shape and gross features of the shell failure region. These techniques allow categorization and documentation of the mode of failure, and are quite useful as a supplemental tool in the diagnosis of implant failure mechanisms. Microscopy techniques provide details of the ruptured shell region and can be used to determine the cause of breast implant failure. The use of optical microscopy and scanning electron microscopy (SEM) provide state-of-the-art techniques in the analysis of ruptured breast implants. Retrieval and analysis studies have used optical microscopy and scanning electron microscopy to describe the morphology of several types of breast implant failures. Several cases from published studies and a few new analyses are presented herein.

Optical microscopy is a common diagnostic technique used to analyze the failed regions of breast implant shells. The method is routinely applied in the analysis of retrieved failed devices. Many explants have been analyzed using the technique, and it is a reasonable approach to describe failed shell regions and to determine modes of shell failure. However, for many cases field emission SEM is needed to confirm or refute questionable failure sites and failure modes determined by optical microscopy. SEM can often be used to determine a failure mode by providing additional morphological features of a failure site. The SEM technique used to analyze failed explants has previously been described in the literature.[1,20,21] The FDA guidance document recommends the SEM technique for the characterization of the modes and causes of implant rupture.

Surgical instruments are used in both implantation and explantation procedures for breast implants. At the time of surgical implantation, an instrument can damage the shell or cut the shell, resulting in an immediate rupture, or it may cause minor damage to the shell that results in a rupture at a later time. If a shell surface has a slight cut or nick during the surgery, in vivo loading can cause the cut to propagate into a ruptured shell. Surgical instruments can also damage the shell at the time of explantation. Studies have been conducted on the physical characteristics of breast implants that have been intentionally damaged via a variety of surgical instruments. The studies were performed to provide information about device failure modes and the characterization of surgical instrument damage. The results collected from the studies may be used to provide information for failure analysis of explanted silicone gel devices. A few examples on artificially damaged shells are presented herein along with SEM analysis of failed explants.

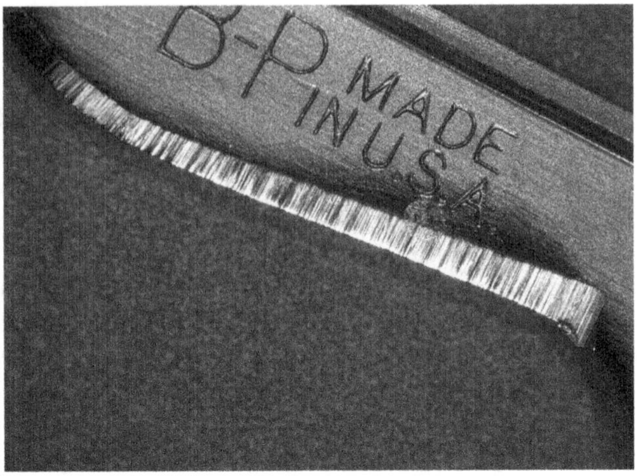

7.25 Optical micrograph of no. 15 scalpel. Reprinted with permission from ref. 21. Copyright 2007 Sage Publications.

A no. 15 surgical blade is the scalpel most commonly used in plastic surgery. With the proper lighting, parallel machining lines can be seen on the cutting surface of the surgical blade with the unaided eye. The lines appear only on the cutting surface of the blade and are created during the finish machining process to sharpen the blade. The lines can be called grind lines and are the result of the blade being sharpened by a grinding wheel during the last phase of the manufacturing process. The machined tracks, caused by the grains used in grinding wheels, are well known and documented in the manufacturing industry. The spacing between the grind lines will vary according to the grinding process. A detailed view of the grind lines is shown in Fig. 7.25, an optical micrograph of the scalpel.[21] The spacing between the grind lines was measured by use of a scale bar on a similar optical micrograph obtained with much greater magnification. The spacing between the grind lines varied from approximately 4.9 μm to 29.4 μm (0.20 to 1.2 thousandths of an inch). The most detailed description of the grind lines was obtained with scanning electron microscopy. On the basis of SEM analysis, the spacing between the grind lines varied from about 2 μm to 26 μm (0.1 to 1.0 thousandths of an inch).

A new cutting suture needle was also analyzed.[21] This was a typical needle used by plastic surgeons performing breast implantation surgery. Microscopy analysis revealed that the tip of the needle was formed by the intersection of three surfaces. The three surfaces did not have the same geometry, nor were they all planar. The geometrically simplest surface was the one along the inside curve of the needle. It was flat and fairly smooth. Each of the two outside surfaces was a cluster of three planes that intersected at low angles (producing a curved surface). The optical micrograph in Fig. 7.26

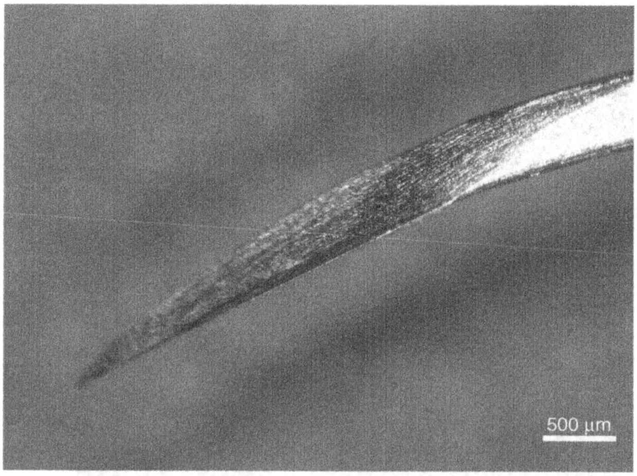

7.26 Optical micrograph of outside surface of cutting needle. Reprinted with permission from ref. 21. Copyright 2007 Sage Publications.

shows one of the outside surfaces. It shows that only fine-scale machining marks are on the tip of the needle surfaces. From SEM micrographs, the spacing of the grind lines on the needle tip varied from approximately 2.3 µm to 8.4 µm (0.092 to 0.33 thousandths of an inch), which is considerably less than the range of grind line spacing on the scalpels.

A shell damaged by a suture needle cut demonstrates various types of imprints. Figure 7.27 shows an SEM micrograph of the outside surface of a smooth shell that was intentionally cut with a suture needle. In this case the needle created a flap triangular in shape that protrudes from the puncture site and an additional cut that intersects the flap. A few striations are visible on the flap. Another needle cut produced the damage in Fig. 7.28. Multiple striations are visible in the micrograph. In a previous study,[21] no striations were detected by SEM in the surface of the shell after damage from a suture needle had occurred. This could have been due to the elastic property of the silicone shells analyzed or the resolution of the microscopy technique. Here the distance between striations from a suture needle range from about 2 µm to 6 µm on smooth shells.

An SEM analysis was conducted on a failed saline-filled explant manufactured by Ideal Implant Incorporated. Visual inspection revealed that the failure was due to a small pinhole on the anterior side. SEM micrographs obtained in the study for the failed region are presented in Figs 7.29 and 7.30. These results were obtained with the shell specimen folded at the cut. Both micrographs are of the outside surface of the shell. A millimeter or a micron scale is shown on the lower right hand side and the magnification is shown on the lower left hand side of each micrograph. Figure 7.29 shows

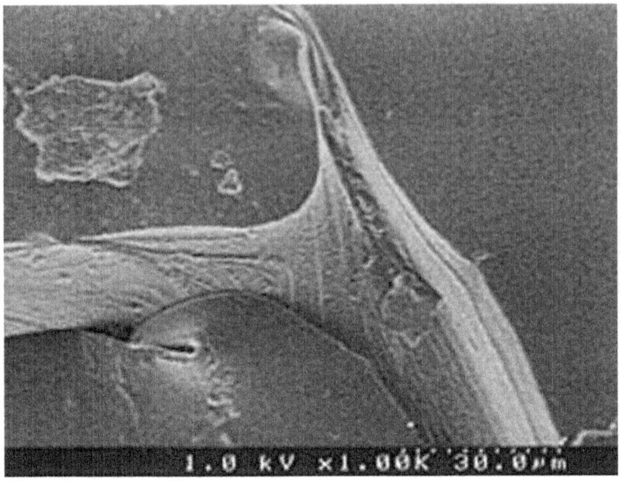

7.27 Smooth shell with suture needle cut initiated from the outside of shell. View is of initiation site. Striations are visible. Scale is 3.0 μm/division.

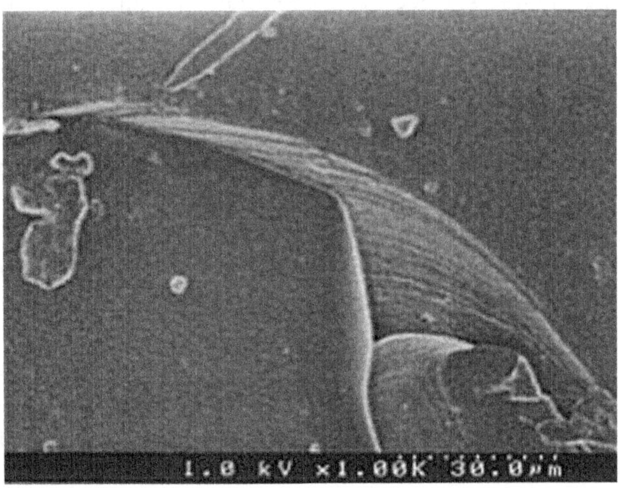

7.28 Smooth shell with suture needle cut initiated from the outside of shell. Again, striations are visible. Scale is 3.00 μm/division.

the entire pinhole which has a measured width of about 1.25 mm. The failed region consists of a flap that protrudes from the puncture site and an additional cut that intersects the pinhole. This configuration is typical of a failure caused by a suture needle cut. A higher magnification view of the failed region is presented in Fig. 7.30. The sharp edges of the cuts in the shell are indicative of failure by a surgical instrument. A few striations near the top

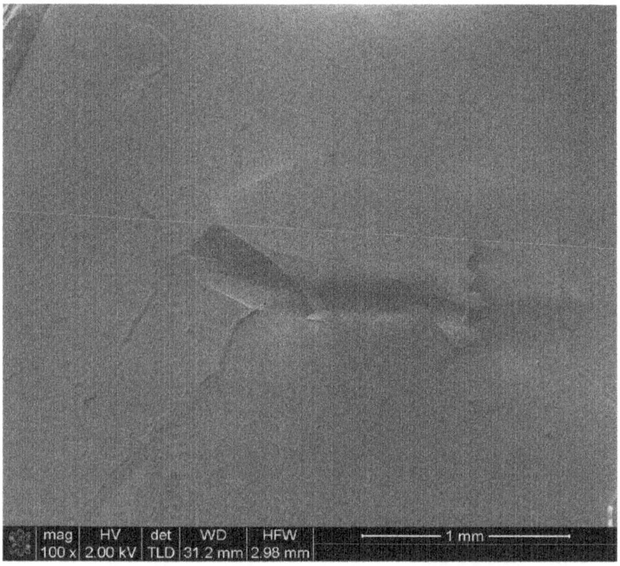

7.29 SEM micrograph, view of entire pinhole.

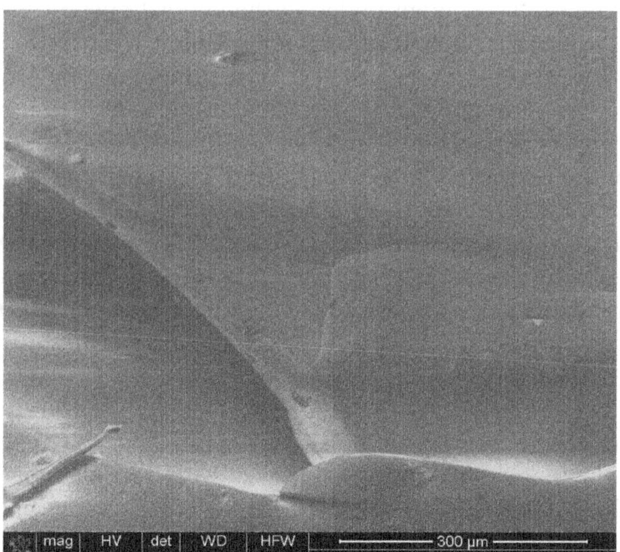

7.30 SEM micrograph, view of pinhole at higher magnification.

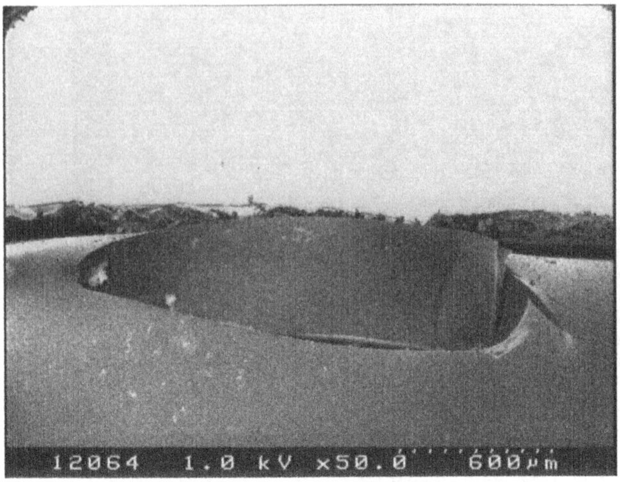

7.31 SEM micrograph, view of entire pinhole.

of the flap can also been seen. The spacing of the striations is about 7 μm to 12 μm.

An SEM analysis was also conducted on a second failed saline-filled explant manufactured by Ideal Implant Incorporated. Visual inspection revealed that the failure was due to a small pinhole (1 mm to 2 mm) on the anterior side about 0.5 inches from the outer perimeter. SEM micrographs obtained in the study are presented in Figs 7.31 to 7.33. These results were obtained with the shell specimen folded at the cut. All micrographs are of the outside surface of the shell. A micron scale is shown on the lower right hand side of each micrograph. Figure 7.31 shows the entire pinhole, which has a measured length of about 1.78 mm. The entire shell thickness is seen protruding up from the shell surface. Note the sharp edges of the pinhole on the right hand side. These sharp edges are indicative of a cut by a surgical instrument. Black tape that was used to hold the shell specimen to the SEM specimen holder can be seen at the upper edge of the specimen. A partial view of the shell thickness with striations is presented in Figs 7.32 and 7.33 at higher magnifications. The measured striation spacing ranges from about 3 μm to 6 μm. Therefore, the failure of this implant was caused by a nick from a suture needle.

A textured, silicone gel explant with 0.30 years in vivo ruptured because of a small tear on the anterior side. An SEM analysis[21] with views of the shell folded at the tear show a section of the cut with few striations in focus (Fig. 7.34), and another section of the cut edge with many striations in focus (Fig. 7.35). The striations are due to the grind lines on the edge of a scalpel.

A published study[22] has described the morphological features of the fatigue failure surfaces of saline-filled breast implants. Characterization of

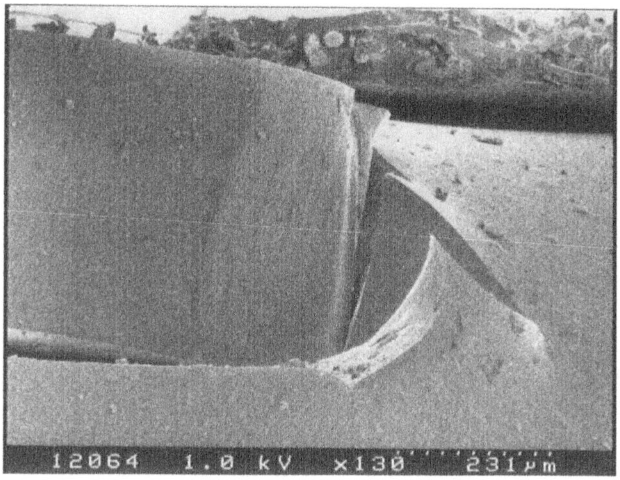

7.32 SEM micrograph, view of right side of cut at higher magnification.

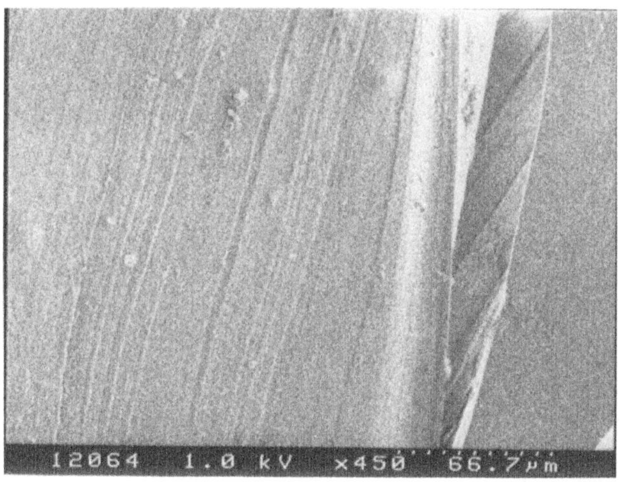

7.33 SEM micrograph, partial view of shell thickness with striations.

the morphological features of implant fatigue failure surfaces is useful in evaluating the modes of failure of retrieved failed explants. In the study, we describe the morphology of fatigue failure surfaces of smooth and textured saline-filled breast implants. The fatigue failure surfaces were created in a laboratory apparatus rather than in vivo, and the implants were unimplanted controls rather than explants. The current test methodology for fatigue testing uses flat plates that repeatedly compress the implant. The implant is loaded along a diameter from the center of the anterior to the

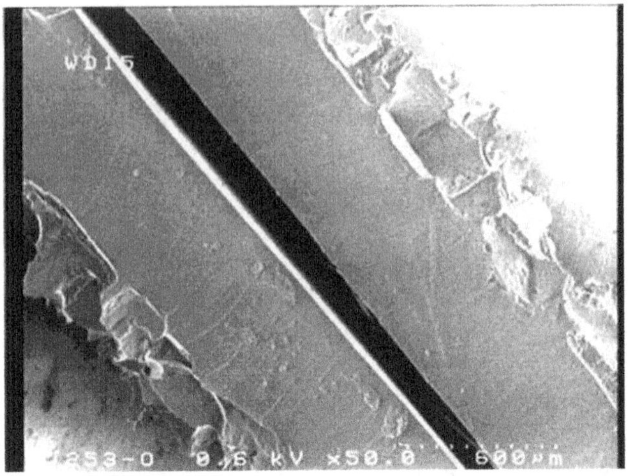

7.34 SEM micrograph of device, view of cut edges with few striations. Reprinted with permission from ref. 21. Copyright 2007 Sage Publications.

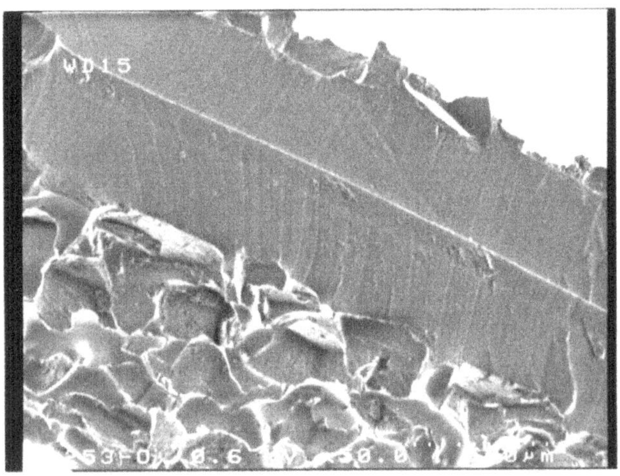

7.35 SEM micrograph of device, view of cut edges with many striations. Reprinted with permission from ref. 21. Copyright 2007 Sage Publications.

center of the posterior surface. Compressive loads in this direction create maximum tensile stress around the perimeter or equator of the implant, so the rate of fatigue damage accumulation is greater around the perimeter than at the top anterior pole or bottom posterior pole where the stress is less. This technique is not predictive of clinical failures, but rather provides information on the relative fatigue strength of breast implants during a standard test condition. One of the implants tested, implant C, was a smooth

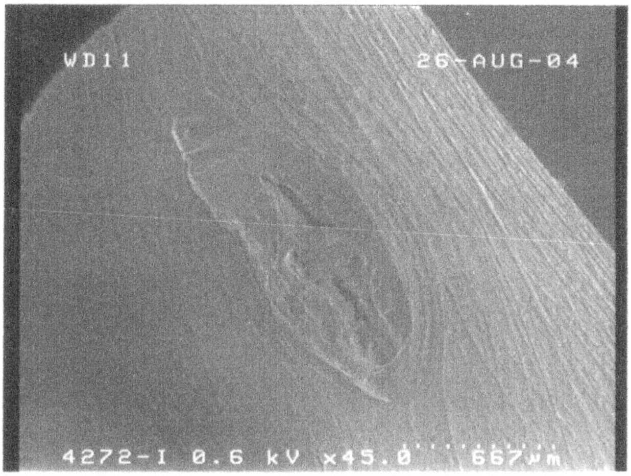

7.36 Shell C inside surface and pinhole (scale: 66.7 μm between adjacent dots). Reprinted with permission from ref. 22. Copyright 2006 Begell House.

shell that failed at 10801 cycles at a nominal cyclic load of 302 N. This implant was subjected to a relatively high cyclic load well above those experienced in vivo, and subsequently had a relatively short fatigue lifetime. The failure was due to a pinhole in the shell located on the perimeter of the implant. The oval shaped pinhole in Figs 7.36 and 7.37 has a maximum width of 1.5 mm on the inside surface and 0.50 mm on the outside surface of the shell. This hole size is representative of pinholes measured on failed explants. Surface extrusions and pits forming a band approximately 14 mm wide could be seen without magnification around the entire perimeter of the outside surface of the shell (Fig. 7.38).

A small pinhole can be induced in an implant shell by subjecting the shell to abrasion.[20] For example, the pinhole (1 mm to 2 mm wide) shown in Fig. 7.39 was generated by subjecting the control shell to cyclic abrasion in a linear reciprocating abrader. The top edge of a folded piece of shell was subjected to abrasion by a rod wrapped with another piece of shell. The rod cycled back and forth at 1.67 Hz. The entire abrading apparatus was submerged in a saline bath at room temperature. The shell surface immediately above the hole is rough, which is indicative of elastomeric abrasion. The rough regions are confined to the immediate vicinity of the failure site, whereas the rest of the shell surface remains smooth. Cracks and tears emanate from the failure site.

Damage similar to that shown in Fig. 7.39 has been observed on explants.[20] A section of a cleaned gel-filled shell, which was explanted after approximately 20 years in vivo, is shown in Fig. 7.40 (a). Flex fatigue due to a fold

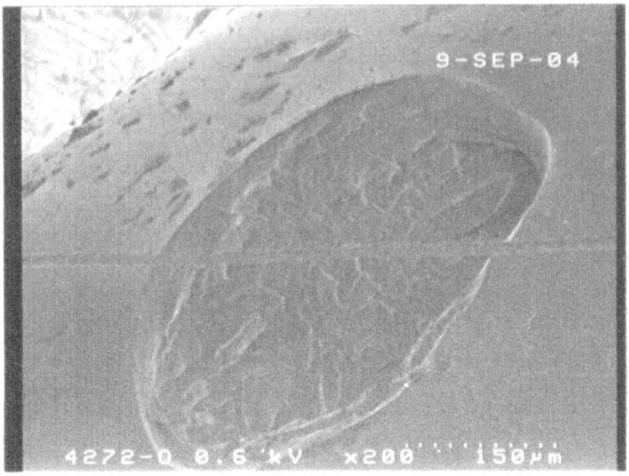

7.37 Shell C outside surface and pinhole (scale: 15.0 μm between adjacent dots). Reprinted with permission from ref. 22. Copyright 2006 Begell House.

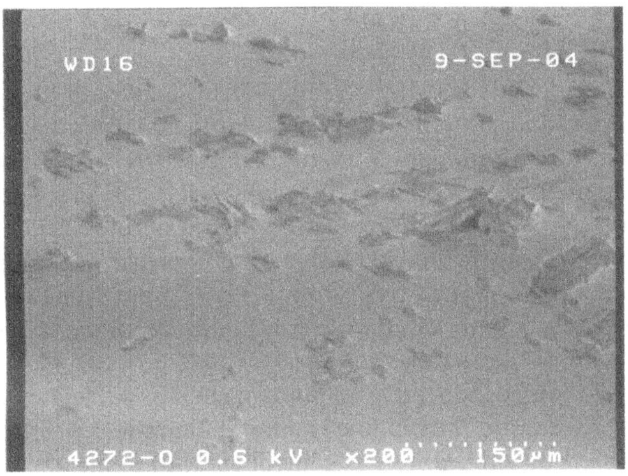

7.38 Shell C surface extrusions and pits typical of the surface texture around the perimeter (scale: 15.0 μm between adjacent dots). Reprinted with permission from ref. 22. Copyright 2006 Begell House.

in the shell created the feathered wear pattern. A micrograph of a similar gel-filled explant shell, which had remained in vivo for approximately 20 years, is shown in Fig. 7.40 (b). An advanced stage of wear in the fold created the material cracking pattern, which eventually formed the 1 mm hole in the shell. The flex fatigue lines shown in Fig. 7.40 (a) and (b), are spaced approximately 0.10 mm to 0.15 mm apart. Flex fatigue line spacing has been reported to vary from 60 μm to 350 μm.[23]

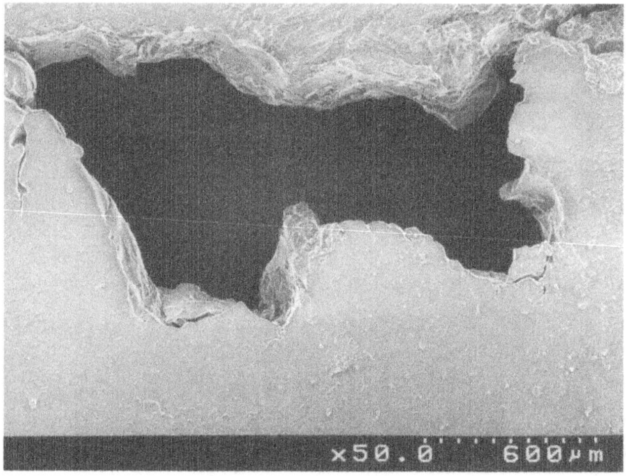

7.39 Pinhole artificially induced in an implant shell by subjecting the shell to abrasion (view normal to surface at 60.0 μm/division). Reprinted with permission from ref. 20. Copyright 2001 Wolters Kluwer Health.

The failure of a saline explant with 3 years in vivo occurred in a fold near the outer perimeter, where a small crack developed between two regions of wear.[1] The SEM micrograph of the inner shell surface for this saline explant (Fig. 7.41) shows that the failure site consists of a 0.06-mm hole with a crack propagating outward from the hole and extending a length of about 0.20 mm. (For comparative purposes, the width of the hole is about the size of a human hair.) An abrasion pattern around the small hole is also visible.

The last example is for a silicone gel implant that failed due to a small tear in a large crease on the posterior side.[23] The implantation time was unknown for this implant. SEM analysis revealed significant features on the inside surface of the shell. Figure 7.42 shows the inside surface of the shell near one end of the tear. Grooves due to mandrell machining lines are located in the upper portion of the SEM micrograph. The spacing of the grooves is approximately 14.5 μm. Much of the shell surface is smooth around the crease, which is indicative of a surface rubbing action. Hence, some shell abrasion did result due to the folding/rubbing phenomena. As shown in Fig. 7.42, a very small crack (0.15 mm) had also developed in the shell surface adjacent to the fold.

7.6.3 Fatigue and shell wrinkling

As discussed in this chapter, breast implants fail due to mechanisms that generate damage to the shell. Relating the mechanisms of damage growth

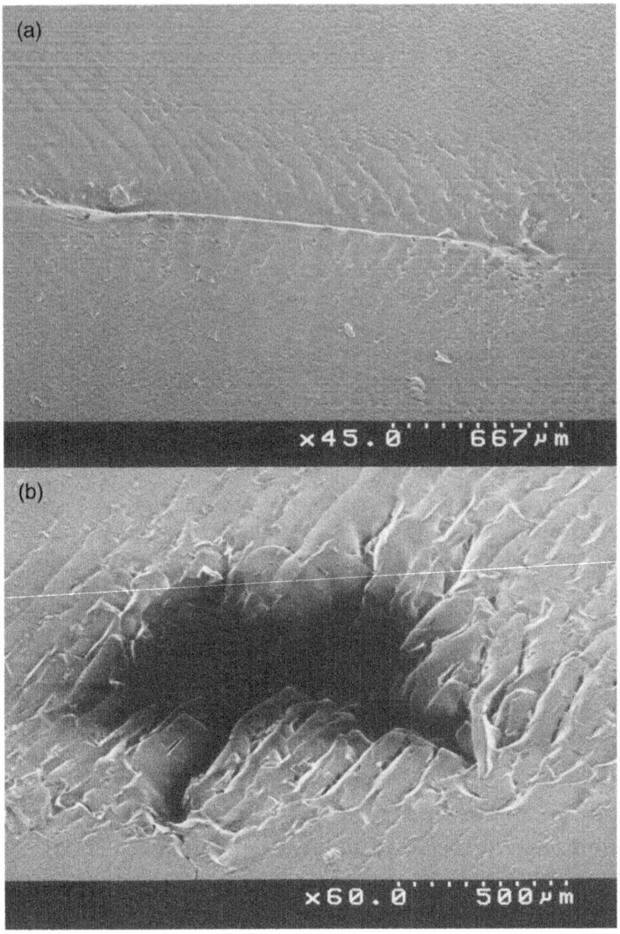

7.40 (a) Wear pattern around a crease in a gel-filled explant (view normal to surface at 66.7 μm division). (b) Hole produced by advanced stage of wear from flex fatigue (view normal to surface at 50.0 μm/division). Reprinted with permission from ref. 20. Copyright 2001 Wolters Kluwer Health.

and the modes of failure has been a focus of breast implant research during the past two decades. Daily activity body motion, such as walking and running, induces forces on implants. These in vivo forces are cyclic and repetitive. Over time the cumulative in vivo cyclic loading induces fatigue damage in the implant, which can result in failure of the implant. The rate of fatigue damage accumulation is greater at high stress than at low stress. At present, the FDA considers fatigue damage a potential cause of in vivo failure, since most materials have a finite fatigue life when repeatedly

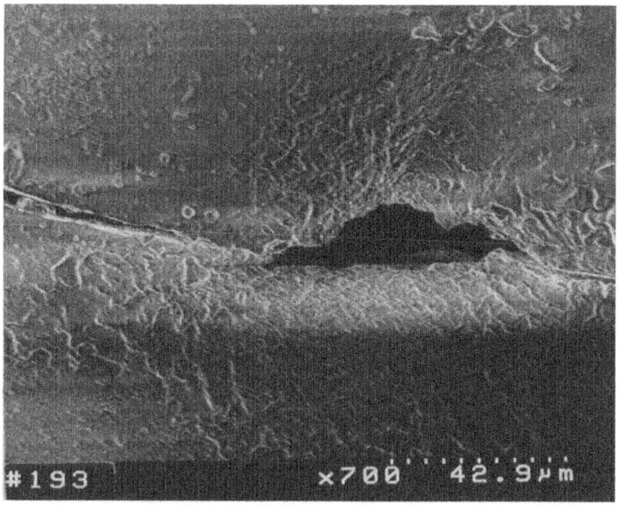

7.41 Textured McGhan saline explant with 3 years in vivo also failed in fold near outer perimeter, but abrasion evident around failure site. SEM micrograph of inner shell surface reveals 0.06 mm hold with crack propagating outward and extending about 0.2 mm. Reprinted with permission from ref. 1. Copyright 2003 Begell House.

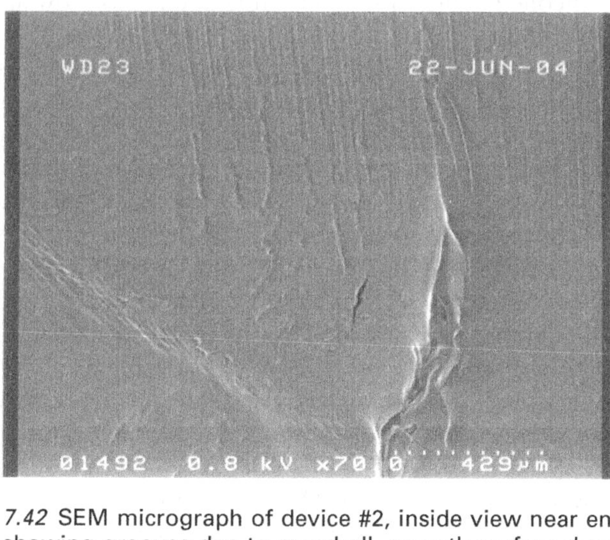

7.42 SEM micrograph of device #2, inside view near end of tear showing grooves due to mandrell, smooth surface due to rubbing, and small crack in shell. Reprinted with permission from ref. 21. Copyright 2007 Sage Publications.

stressed. Implants are designed so that induced cyclic load creates low cyclic stress. When the magnitude of this cyclic stress is small, the fatigue life is in excess of the expected implantation lifetime. Large cyclic stress will weaken the implant as fatigue damage accumulates and can result in failure during the implantation lifetime. In light of this fact, the FDA recommends fatigue rupture testing of breast implants for premarket approval (PMA) applications.

Very few studies of breast implant fatigue have been published. Inamed[24] reported fatigue testing of two types of silicone gel implants at an applied load of 30 pounds, and the implants withstood 6.5 million cycles without failure. Mentor[25] also fatigue tested two types of silicone gel implants with a net load of 20 pounds up to 10 million cycles without failure. Mentor also theoretically investigated cyclic loads by normal everyday activities like walking and jogging. These movements subject the shell of the implant to fatigue that occurs when it is repeatedly stressed. The Mentor study demonstrated that fatigue lifetime could be predicted solely in terms of the effects of local shell wrinkling and unwrinkling during walking, running, and jogging. The study did not consider the effect of abrasion/rubbing/wear associated with shell folding.

Only a few studies have been published that present data on the frequency of fold occurrences during implantation.[26–30] Folds have been observed in 15% to 67% of measurable gel or saline implant shells using methods such as palpation, mammography or observation at explantation. Although these studies demonstrate that shell folds have been observed in both saline and silicone gel breast implants, it is not known how applicable the published percentages are to all implanted breast implants. Data presented on the FDA website indicate that the percentage of patients with silicone gel breast implants that experience some form of wrinkling ranges from 1% to 8% after 4 years in vivo depending on the cohort. The extent of wrinkling is less severe in silicone gel breast implants due to the viscous property of the gel filler. Shell wrinkling is often transmitted to the overlying skin which produces an unattractive breast and patient dissatisfaction. In the extreme case, shell wrinkling can also produce a failure mechanism (fold flaw failure) resulting in implant rupture. Hence, shell wrinkling can affect aesthetic appearance and implant durability. In this section we present an analysis of shell wrinkling in saline-filled breast implants which should represent a worst case condition for all types of single lumen breast implants. Previous studies summarized by Young and Watson[31] have shown that fill volume plays a major role in saline implant deflation. Our present analysis demonstrates how fill volume, shell wrinkling, and implant shape are related. The analysis uses a combination of theoretical modeling and experimental contour mapping to describe the wrinkle geometry and implant shape when the device is subjected to gravity loading.

The theoretical analysis was conducted using a finite element computer program to predict how the shell behaves when exposed to a gravity load simulating a woman with implants in a standing position. The effect of the overlying skin and breast tissue was not included in the analysis. The experimental modeling was conducted on a saline shell whose posterior side was fixed to a flat vertical plate, and therefore exposed to gravity loading. Again, the overlying skin and breast tissue were not included in the experiment. The implant geometry was determined using 35 mm photography. Prior to the theoretical calculations, stress-strain properties were measured for a shell similar to the one used in the experiment for mapping the contour of the implant under gravity loading. The shell properties were then input into the finite element analysis. Figures 7.43 to 7.52 show the front view of a 240 cc saline implant with the posterior side fixed in the vertical direction such that the implant is exposed to a gravity load. Figures 7.43 to 7.47 give the experimental implant shape and wrinkle geometry obtained using 35 mm photography for the implant fill volumes of 200, 220, 240, 260, and 280 cc. Figures 7.48 to 7.52 give the theoretical implant shape and wrinkle geometry for the same fill volumes. The geometry pattern is due to the saline filler settling in the bottom portion of the implant. The empty upper portion collapses and wrinkles under gravity loading. The theoretically predicted implant geometries are similar to the experimentally measured implant shapes. Wrinkling occurs on the anterior side and the outer

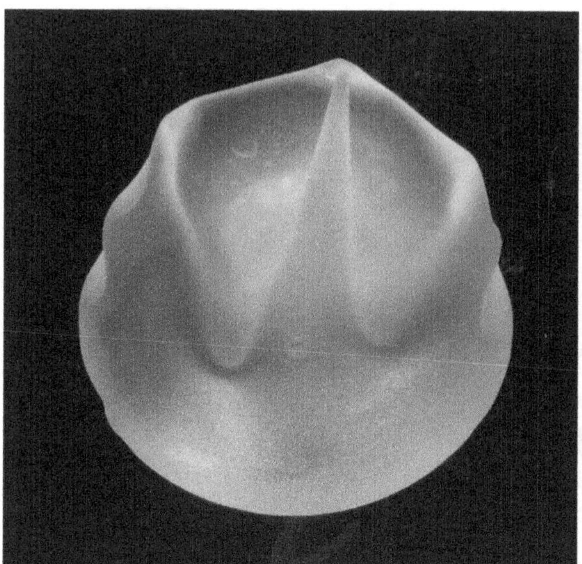

7.43 Actual implant shape for a fill volume of 200 cc.

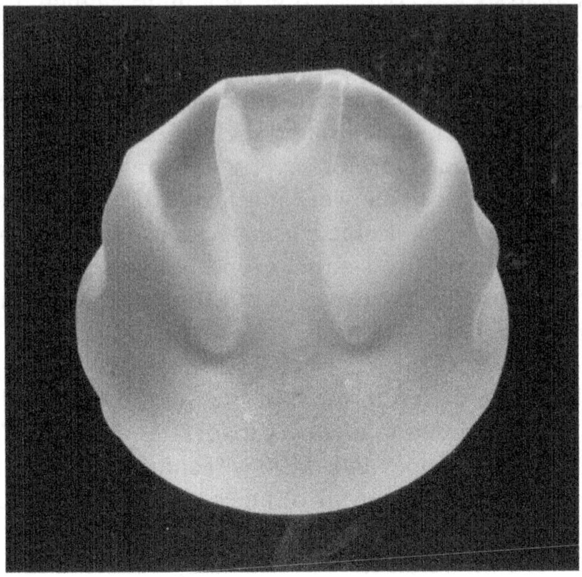

7.44 Actual implant shape for a fill volume of 220 cc.

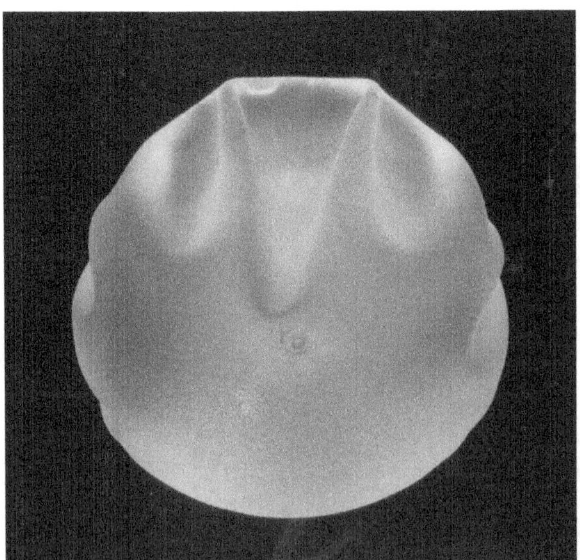

7.45 Actual implant shape for a fill volume of 240 cc.

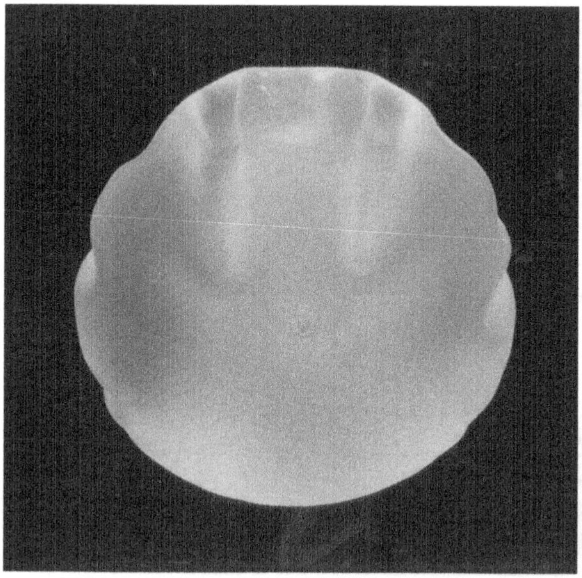

7.46 Actual implant shape for a fill volume of 260 cc.

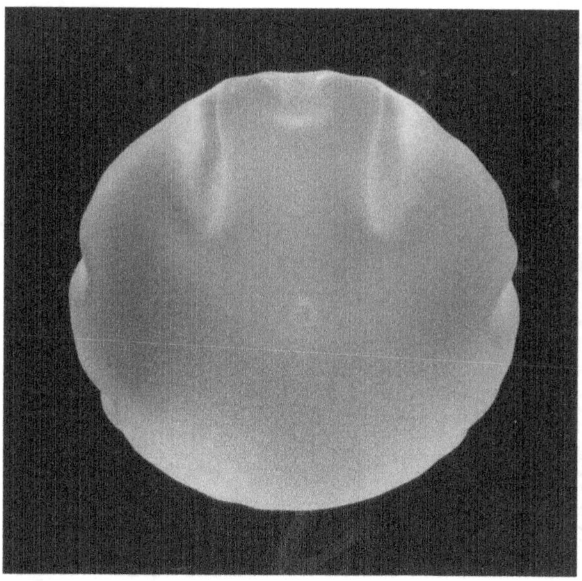

7.47 Actual implant shape for a fill volume of 280 cc.

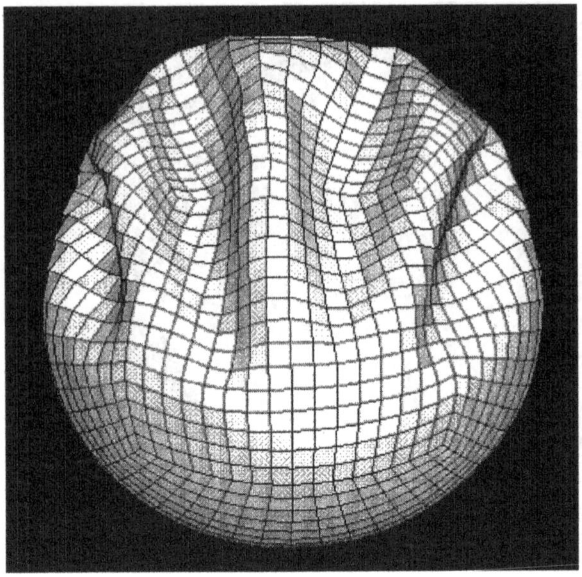

7.48 Predicted implant shape for a fill volume of 200 cc.

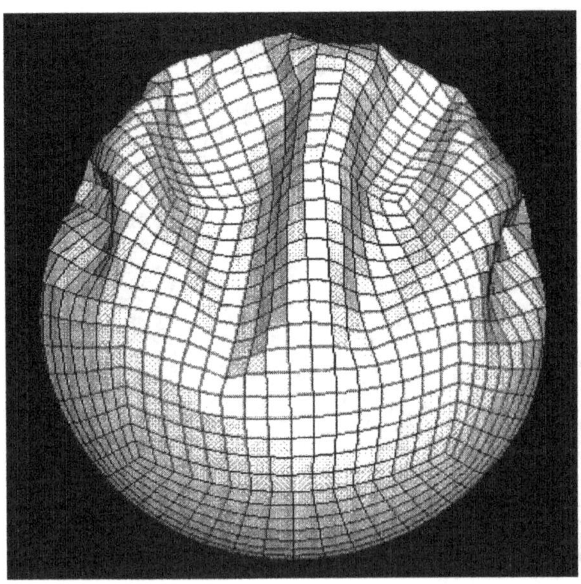

7.49 Predicted implant shape for a fill volume of 220 cc.

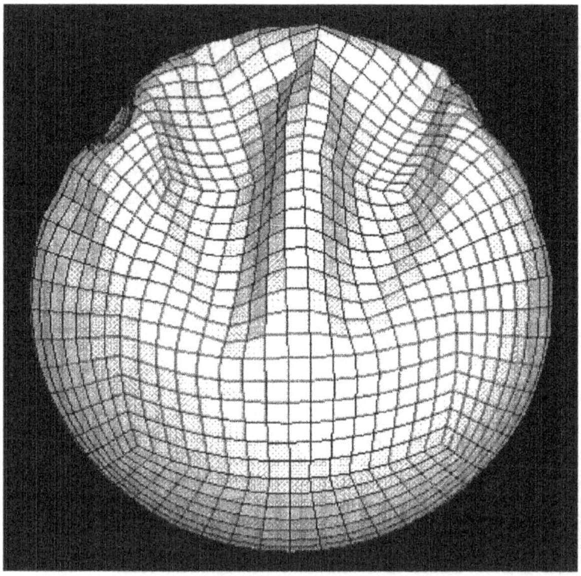

7.50 Predicted implant shape for a fill volume of 240 cc.

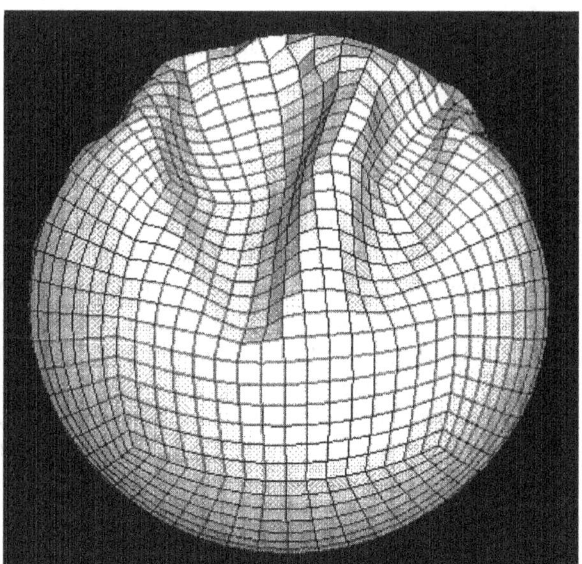

7.51 Predicted implant shape for a fill volume of 260 cc.

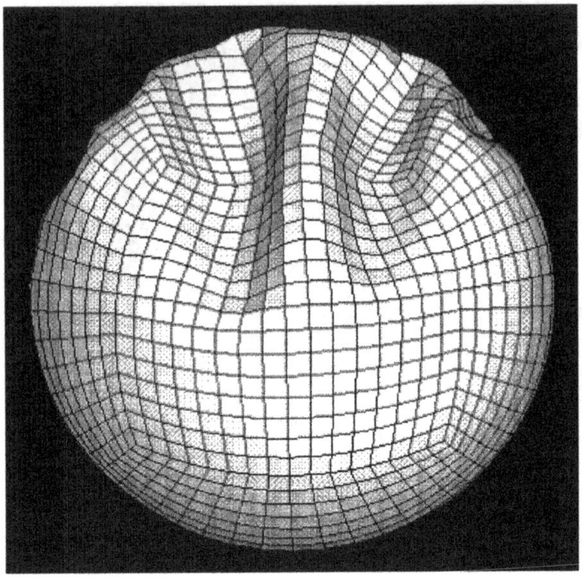

7.52 Predicted implant shape for a fill volume of 280 cc.

perimeter for the upper portion of the implant, but the degree of wrinkling significantly decreases with increasing fill volume. Improper device placement during implantation surgery and constraints imposed by the breast pocket could result in shell creases at other locations. Ideal Implant Incorporated (USA) has recently developed a new type of saline breast implant that significantly reduces wrinkling. Clinical trials are now being conducted on this device.

7.6.4 Implantation surgery

Breast implants are subjected to some degree of stress and deformation during the surgical procedure of insertion. Thus, implantation surgery itself could be a factor in affecting the durability of breast implants. The purpose of one of our studies[32] was to investigate whether the surgical procedure of insertion affects the mechanical properties of the silicone elastomer shell of gel-filled implants. We wanted to determine whether the procedure of inserting a breast implant might cause a decrease in the strength properties of the shell. Thirty-four Silastic® II gel-filled breast implants manufactured by Dow Corning were tested. All implants were from the same lot and had a volume of 300 cc. Twenty of 34 implants were tested without implantation to investigate variability within a lot and establish a baseline of control data for comparison with implanted implants. Fourteen of the 34 implants were implanted through an inframammary incision in the right breast of a cadaver. The effect of implantation surgery was investigated by comparing the mechanical properties of the anterior and posterior sides of the cadaver explants with those of the controls.

Statistical analysis of the data indicated that the mechanical properties of elongation and tear resistance were essentially unaffected by implantation surgery. However, the average tensile strength of the explants was reduced 4.9% to 6.2% (for shells extracted with hexane and unextracted shells, respectively) compared with the controls. Breaking energy averages for the explants were also reduced 7.8% to 5.9% (for extracted and unextracted shells, respectively) when compared with the controls and average moduli decreased by a similar magnitude. The surgical procedure of implanting a breast implant has a small but statistically significant effect on the average strength properties of the elastomer shell of the implant. It is unlikely that the small reductions are sufficient to be a factor in implant durability.

These reductions are quite small, though statistically significant, and refer to averages of the measurements obtained from hundreds of specimens taken from the 34 lot-matched implant shells. A summary of the stress-strain curves is shown in Fig. 7.53. The curves shown represent the averaged of the data; there were 20 control samples and 14 'explants', with six specimens (three from the anterior and three from the posterior side) from each shell for a total of 120 separate stress-strain curves from the controls and

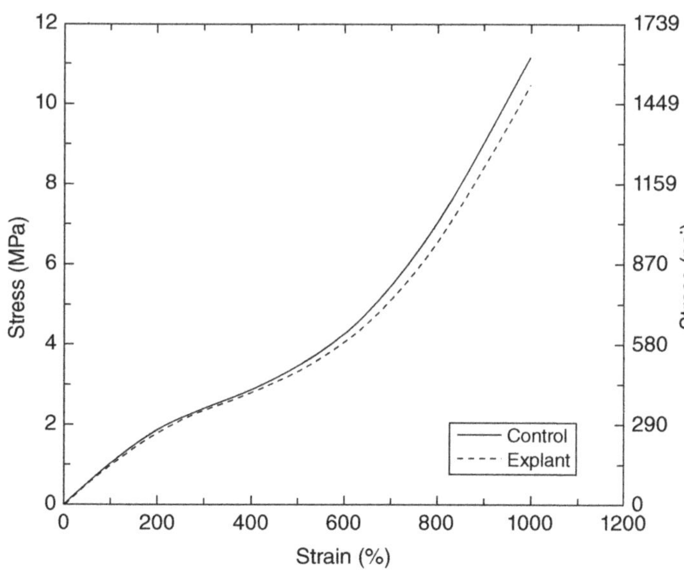

7.53 Averaged stress-strain curve for the controls (average of 20 samples) and explants (average of 14 samples). Reprinted with permission from ref. 33. Copyright 2000 Brill.

84 from the 'explants'. The results clearly indicate that the average mechanical properties of the shells after implantation are only slightly reduced when compared to their unimplanted controls. It should also be noted that we evaluated implants from one lot, one size and one manufacturer. Other factors not addressed in the study that could potentially affect strength properties of implants after implantation surgery include implant type, implant size, different manufacturers, the surgeon's technique, the location and size of the incision, and whether the implant inserted is a patient's first implant or a replacement.

Another study[33] is an extension of the previous investigation. In the follow-on study emphasis was placed on the effect of implantation on the shell region where the surgeon's fingers forced the implant through the breast incision. We addressed the question of whether the strength of the 'explant' shells had significant local weakening in those regions which were deformed by the surgeon's finger during the implantation process. Our results indicate that the implant shell can be locally damaged due to the implantation process. Tensile specimens were prepared from the clean shells with the specimen's gauge section cut across the regions where the surgeon's fingers forced the implant through the incision. A typical stress-strain curve in which the damaged region is compared to an undamaged adjacent site is shown in Fig. 7.54. Both curves illustrate the non-Hookeian behavior

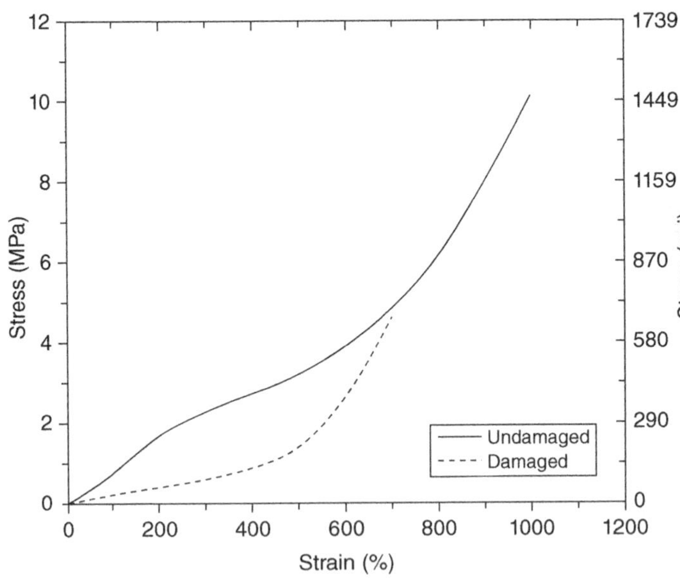

7.54 Stress-strain curve comparing a damaged region with an adjacent undamaged region. Reprinted with permission from ref. 33. Copyright 2000 Brill.

Table 7.10 Comparison of mechanical properties in damaged and undamaged regions of 'explants' (reprinted with permission from ref. 33. Copyright 2000 Brill)

Explant	Ultimate stress (MPa)	Elongation (%)
7-E control*	12.76 ± 0.54	1076 ± 16
7-E damaged	6.58	783
9-E control	12.66 ± 0.99	1045 ± 50
9-E damaged	11.40	910
10-E control	13.04 ± 1.93	1048 ± 44
10-E damaged	12.76	860
11-E control	13.13 ± 0.68	1063 ± 21
11-E damaged	8.28	854
12-E control	12.04 ± 0.43	1040 ± 97
12-E damaged	10.23	937
13-E control	12.06 ± 1.19	1009 ± 74
13-E damaged	12.39	969
14-E control	12.77 ± 0.61	1088 ± 66
14-E damaged	11.53	904
Undamaged (avg)	12.65 ± 0.39	1053 ± 26
Damaged (avg)	10.48 ± 2.30	888 ± 61

* All control values are the average of the analysis.

of elastomers, i.e. stress is not a linear function of strain. Furthermore, the overall shape of the two curves is quite different.

The stress and the elongation-to-failure of the damaged regions and the control regions are summarized in Table 7.10 for seven explants. The control values are the average of six measurements, three from specimens on the anterior and three from the posterior side of the implant in question; the standard deviation is also given. The values shown for the damaged regions are not averages since the number of the specimens tested depended upon the number of specimens which could be cut from the damaged region. The grand average for the undamaged sections of the explants are 12.65 MPa and 1053% for the ultimate stress and elongation, respectively. The strength range from the undamaged regions varies from 13.13 to 12.04 MPa or a spread of 9% (4% above and 5% below the average). Note that all values are the average of six determinations so that 42 separate stress-strain curves were evaluated. The elongation-to-failure ranges from 1088% to 1009%; the corresponding spread from the average is 3% (max) to 4% (min), a 7% spread. The values for the elongation-to-failure from the damaged region is, on the average, approximately 15% lower than that measured in the undamaged regions. As expected, the failure stress in the damaged regions exhibits a wide variation in values, ranging from 12.76 MPa to 6.38 MPa, a 50% variation in strength. It is interesting to note that several samples exhibit the same strength in the damaged regions as observed in the undamaged regions. The largest decrease in ultimate properties between the damaged and undamaged regions was observed in sample E-7. The maximum reduction is as much as 50% for strength and 30% for elongation. Obviously, not all shell regions that were in contact with the surgeon's fingers during the insertion were weakened. The strain required to significantly reduce mechanical properties remains to be determined. Local reduction in shell strength due to implantation surgery has not been reported in previous analyses of explants. However, some previously reported studies may have inadvertently included weakened shell regions in the determination of average shell strength properties.

The damaged regions may develop a slight irregularity or bulge in the shell surface contour. Whether or not this region has a greater tendency to develop wrinkles or rupture needs to be ascertained. Even though the implantation process has only a small weakening effect on the average strength properties of the implant shell, local damage can be imparted to the implant shell where the surgeon's fingers force the implant through the breast incision. The relationship between the local shell damage and implant failure needs to be addressed. Perhaps this shell-weakening mechanism was a cause of the high rate of failure for thin shell implants.

7.7 Rupture rates and reoperation rates

Breast implants are not lifetime devices and patients have to understand that they will be required to have secondary surgeries to remove and replace their implants. Mentor's and Inamed's core gel studies on reoperation rates are shown in Table 7.11; the main reasons for reoperation from Mentor are listed in Table 7.12, and for Inamed in Table 7.13. These results, available on the FDA website, are generally consistent with other reports in the literature, and on average one in five women undergoing primary breast augmentation can expect to need a second operation within 5 years. Numerous studies have reported rupture frequencies for a variety of manufacturers, styles, and generations of implants. Data from explantation studies are unreliable because they are inherently biased since suspected rupture

Table 7.11 Reoperation rates predicted in gel core studies (by patient)

	Mentor Kaplan-Meier risk Rate at 3 years (%)	Inamed Kaplan-Meier risk Rate at 4 years (%)
Augmentation	15	24
Reconstruction	27	41*
Revision	28	34

*High rate attributed to style 153.

Table 7.12 Main reoperation reasons for Mentor (silicone gel core study at 3 years, primary augmentation patients)

Reasons	Percentage (%)
Caps contracture	37
Patient request	15
Scarring	11
Hematoma/seroma	11
Need for biopsy	6
Asymmetry	5
Ptosis	4
Infection	3
Implant malposition	2
Delayed wound healing	2
Wrinkling	2

Table 7.13 Main reoperation reasons for Inamed (silicone gel core study at 4 years, primary augmentation patients)

Reasons	Percentage (%)
Caps contracture	29
Implant malposition	16
Ptosis	14
Need for biopsy	9
Hematoma/seroma	7
Scarring	6
Patient request	5
Suspected rupture	4
Asymmetry	4
Delayed wound healing	2

was the indication for surgery in many of the patients. Similarly, explantation studies cannot determine when failure occurred and therefore cannot determine a rate of failure. To establish a true rupture rate, a cohort of patients with known types of implants and implantation dates must be established. This cohort is then followed over time and studied at intervals with MRI to determine if their implants are intact. Although MRI is currently recognized as the most accurate method of evaluating silicone gel-filled implant integrity, it is inaccurate in approximately 10% of cases.[34,35,36]

Danish plastic surgeons have established a breast implant registry and some of the most reliable data on implant rupture comes from this source. Using the registry of patients, they conducted a study using MRI to determine the rupture rate for current generation silicone gel-filled breast implants. Women who had undergone primary breast augmentation were randomly chosen and given a baseline MRI followed by a second MRI 2 years later. They found a rupture rate of 5.3 per 100 implants per year. They also observed that failure was time dependent. Implant survival was 98% at 5 years and dropped to 84% by 10 years.[37–39] Hedén also reported on a European Union wide MRI study of Inamed third generation devices implanted between 1992 and 1994 with a mean implantation time of 10.9 years. The rupture prevalence rate at 11 years was 8%.[40]

Different generations of implants have significantly higher rupture rates in part because of variations in shell thickness and gel viscosity. This is illustrated in an MRI study on the Danish registry of patients. In this study, 94% of first generation implants were ruptured at 25 years, 52% of second generation devices were ruptured at 15 years, and 8% of third generation implants were ruptured at 5 years. There are variations in the definition of implant generations used in different references, which may be due in part to the implants being introduced at different times in certain countries. These varying definitions can cause differences in reported failure rates and add confusion to how long implants remain intact. For example, Peters (see Chapter 1) defines first and second generation implants as implants made from 1963 to 1972 and from 1972 to 1975, respectively. On the other hand, the Danish registry defines implants made from 1974 to 1978 as first generation implants and implants made from 1979 to 1987 as second generation implants. Present data suggests that the failure rate for current generation devices is in the range of 1% to 4% per year for the first 10 years. There is insufficient data to determine the failure rate beyond 10 years.

Inamed and Mentor both addressed the cause of implant failure as part of their premarket approval submission to the FDA and their results are available on the FDA website. Mentor found that the two most common causes of failure were sharp instrument damage and stress induced during implantation. Inamed reported failure analysis data and also found that evidence of surgical damage was the leading cause of failure. This means surgeons must be extremely cautious and meticulous when implanting these devices. The implants should not come in contact with sharp instruments, pickups, or electrocautery. Similarly, incisions must be of sufficient length to allow an atraumatic insertion and positioning of the implant. Using incisions which are too small can result in damage to the elastomeric shell, predisposing to early failure. A list of the breakdown of failure causes for each manufacturer is shown in Tables 7.14 and 7.15. Patients also need to be reminded to inform other specialists that they have implants when undergoing procedures such as breast biopsy, needle localization, mammography, and chest tube insertion.

Determining when failure occurs is much simpler with saline filled breast implants since imaging studies are unnecessary. The manufacturers' data indicate that the risk of deflation of saline filled devices rises over time.

Table 7.14 Failure causes up to 10 years: Mentor

Failure modes over time	Percentage of retrieved devices		
	0–5 yrs (*n* = 231)	6–10 yrs (*n* = 40)	>10 yrs (*n* = 3)
Instrument damage	48	13	67
Localized stress (*presumed cause*)	35	40	33
Shell/patch junction	8	10	0
Fold flaw	4	25	0
Shell/patch delamination	3	10	0
Patch internal	1	3	0

Table 7.15 Causes of rupture: Inamed

Failure modes over time	Percentage of retrieved devices		
	0–5 yrs (*n* = 148)	6–10 yrs (*n* = 27)	>10 yrs (*n* = 9)
Instrument damage	46	15	0
Style 153 post. opening	36	41	0
Sharp edge opening (cause unknown)	11	26	67
Manufacturing	3	15	11
Fold flaw	1	4	22
Surgical impact	3	0	0

Table 7.16 Saline deflation prevalence in non-prospective studies

	No. of implants	Follow-up time	Failure
Lavine 1993	2018	0.5–14 yr	4%
Mladick 1993	2863	17 yr (28 mo avg)	1% RTV 38% HTV
Rheingold 1994	326	0.3–14.5 yr	6%
Worseg 1995	167	2–20 yr (9 yr avg)	24%

Mentor reported failure rates in saline filled implants of 30% at 5 years and 39% at 7 years following augmentation. No comparable data is available for Inamed devices. Several authors[41–48] have reported failure rates for saline filled implants and the results are shown in Tables 7.16 and 7.17. Two studies[49,50] have also examined the effect of overfilling saline implants to their recommended maximum fill volume. These studies suggest that overfilling decreases failure rates (Table 7.18). Recognized causes of saline

Table 7.17 Saline deflation prevalence in non-prospective studies

	No. of implants	Follow-up time	Failure
Lantieri 1997	709	7 yr (avg)	7%
Rapaport 1997	289 033	6 mo	1%
Gutowski 1997	995	4–13 yr	5%
Raj 1999	345	7 yr	7%
Cunningham 2000	882	10 yr	4%

Table 7.18 Saline deflation: failure prevalence by fill volume

	Lantieri 1997 (n = 345)	Raj 1999 (n = 709)
Recommended value	4%	7%
Overfilled	4%	0
Underfilled	17%	16%

implant failure include injury at implantation, fold flow failure, valve failure, patch detachment, and manufacturing defects.

7.8 References

1. BRANDON HJ, YOUNG VL, WATSON ME, WOLF CJ, and JERINA KL (2003), Protocol for retrieval and analysis of breast implants, *J Long Term Eff Med Implants*, 13, 49–61.
2. FOOD AND DRUG ADMINISTRATION (2004), Draft Guidance for Industry and FDA Staff: Saline, Silicone Gel and Alternative Breast Implants, Jan 8, 2004, www.fda.gov/cdrh/ode/guidance/1239.html.
3. BRANDON HJ, JERINA KL, WOLF CJ, and YOUNG VL (2003), Biodurability of retrieved silicone gel breast implants, *Plast Reconstr Surg*, 111, 2295–2306.
4. MAROTTA JS, AMERY DP, WIDENHOUSE CW, MARTIN PJ, and GOLDBERG EP (1998), Degradation of physical properties of silicone gel breast implants and high rates of implant failures. *Proc Soc Biomater*, 374.
5. BRANDON HJ, JERINA KL, WOLF CJ, and YOUNG VL (1999), Ultimate strength properties of control and explanted Silastic I and Silastic 0 silicone gel breast implant shells, *Aesthetic Surg J*, 19, 381–387.
6. MAROTTA JS, WIDENHOUSE CW, MUTAZ BH, and GOLDBERG EP (1999), Silicone gel breast implant failure and frequency of additional surgeries: analysis of 35 studies reporting examination of more than 8000 explants, *J Biomed Mater Res*, 48, 354–364.
7. PHILLIPS JW, DE CAMARA DL, LOCKWOOD MD, and GREBNER CC (1996), Strength of silicone breast implants, *Plast Reconstr Surg*, 97, 1215–1225.
8. LOCKWOOD MD (1995), Strength, strain, energy, and toughness of silicone breast implant shells [Master's thesis]. University of Illinois; Urbana, Illinois.

9. MOREY SD and NORTH JA (1996), Final report on low bleed mammary implants: technical report to Dow Corning Wright from Battelle Columbus Division. Columbus, OH: Battelle.
10. POINTER SC JR (1992), The National Document Depository for Silicone Gel Breast Implant Products Liability Litigation. US Federal Court. Birmingham, Ala: US Federal Court. MDL 926.
11. BRANDON HJ, YOUNG VL, JERINA KL, and WOLF CJ (2001), Variability in the properties of silicone gel breast implants, *Plast Reconstr Surg*, 108, 647–655.
12. AMERICAN SOCIETY FOR TESTING AND MATERIALS (1986), Standard test method for rubber property-tear resistance. *Annual Book of ASTM Standards*, D412-87. West Conshohocken, PA: ASTM; 113–116.
13. MAROTTA JS, GOLDBERG EP, HABAL MB, *et al.* (2002), Silicone gel breast implant failure: Evaluation of properties of shells and gels for explanted prostheses and meta-analysis of literature rupture data, *Ann Plast Surg*, 49, 227–241.
14. BRANDON HJ, JERINA KL, WOLF CJ, and YOUNG VL (2000), Ultimate strength properties of control and explanted Silastic® II silicone gel breast implant shells, *Aesthetic Surg J*, 20, 122–132.
15. NECCHI S, MOLINA D, TURRI S, ROSSETTO F, RIETJENS M, and PENNATI G (2011), Failure of silicone gel breast implants: Is the mechanical weakening due to shell swelling a significant cause of prostheses rupture, *Journal of the Mechanical Behavior of Biomedical Materials*, 4, 2002–2008.
16. Silicone Gel Breast Implant Products Liability Litigation, Exhibits DCC285010031 to DCC285010257. Irondale, Ala.: National MDL926 Document Depository.
17. BRANDON HJ, JERINA KL, WOLF CJ, and YOUNG VL (2002), In vivo aging characteristics of silicone gel breast implants compared to lot-matched controls, *Plast Reconstr Surg*, 109, 1927–1933.
18. BRANDON HJ, YOUNG VL, JERINA KL, WOLF CJ, ADAMS WP, and MARLA ME (2002), Mechanical analysis of explanted saline-filled breast implants exposed to Betadine pocket irrigation, *Aesthetic Srgery*, 22, 438–445.
19. WOLF CJ, JERINA KL, BRANDON HJ, and YOUNG VL (2002), The effect of cyclic swelling (octamethylcyctetrasi-loxane) on the physical properties of silicone breast implant shells, *J Biomater Sci Polym, Ed.* 13, 27–41.
20. BRANDON HJ, YOUNG VL, JERINA KL, and WOLF CJ (2001), Scanning electron microscopy characterization of surgical instrument damage to breast implants, *Plast Reconstr Surg*, 108, 52–61.
21. BRANDON HJ, TAYLOR ML, POWELL TE, and WALKER PS (2007), Microscopy analysis of breast implant failure due to surgical instrument damage, *Aesth Surg J*, 27, 239–256.
22. BRANDON HJ, JERINA KL, SAVOY TL, and WOLF CJ (2006), Scanning electron microscope fractography of induced fatigue-damaged saline breast implants, *Journal of Long-Term Effects of Medical Implants*, 16, 71–82.
23. Brandon HJ, Taylor ML, Powell TE, and Walker PS (2006), Morphology of breast implant fold flaw failure, *Journal of Long-Term Effects of Medical Implants*, 16, 441–449.
24. INAMED CORPORATION (2006), PMA P020056 Silicone-Filled Breast Implants Briefing Document. pp. 13–14. Listed on FDA website. www.fda.gov.
25. MCMEEKING RM, ALLEN GM, and YANG P (2004), Parallel Plate Cyclic Fatigue Analysis of Gel-Filled Mammary Implants. PO30053, Attachment 11, Report M 028 listed on FDA website. www.fda.gov.

26. BONDURANT S, ERNSTER V, and HERDMAN R (2000), Safety of silicone breast implants. Committee on the Safety of Silicone Breast Implants. Washington (DC): Division of Health Promotion and Disease Prevention, Institute of Medicine, National Academy of Sciences.
27. FRANKEL SD, OCCHIPINTI K, KAUFMAN L, KRAMER D, CARLSON J, MINEYEV M, ESHIMA I, and FRIEDENTHAL R (1995), MRI findings in subjects with breast implants, *Plast Reconstr Surg*, 96, 852–857.
28. GANOTT JIA, KATHLEEN MH, ILKHANIPOUR ZS, and COSTA-GRECO MA (1992), Augmentation mammoplasty: Normal and abnormal findings with mammography and ultrasound, *Radiographics*, 12, 281–295.
29. GYLBERT LO, ASPLUND O, and JURELL G (1990), Capsular contracture after breast reconstruction with silicone-gel and saline-filled implants: A 6 year follow-up, *Plast Reconstr Surg*, 85, 373–377.
30. ROLLAND C, GUIDOIN R, MARCEAU D, and LEDOUX R (1989), Nondestructive investigations on ninety seven surgically excised mammary prostheses, *J Biomed Mater Res: Applied Biomaterials*, 23, 285–298.
31. YOUNG VL and WATSON ME (2001), Breast implant research: where we have been, where we are, where we need to go, *Clin Plast Surg*, 28, 451–483.
32. BRANDON HJ., YOUNG VL, JERINA KL, and WOLF CJ (1999), Effect of implantation surgery on the strength properties of Silastic II silicone gel breast implants, *Aesthetic Surg J*, 19, 197–204.
33. WOLF CJ, BRANDON HJ, YOUNG VL, and JERINA KL (2000), Effect of surgical insertion on the local shell properties of Silastic II silicone gel breast implants, *J Biomater Sci Polym Ed*, 11, 1007–1021.
34. *Plast Reconstr Surg* (2008) Nov, 122, 1591–1592; author reply 1592. Silicone breast implants and magnetic resonance imaging screening for rupture: do U.S. Food and Drug Administration recommendations reflect an evidence-based practice approach to patient care?
35. MCCARTHY CM, PUSIC AL, and KERRIGAN CL (2008), Silicone breast implants and magnetic resonance imaging screening for rupture: Do U.S. Food and Drug Administration recommendations reflect an evidence based practice approach to patient care, *Plast Reconstr Surg*, 121, 1127–1134.
36. HOLMICH LR, FRYZEK JP, KJOLLER K, BREITING VB, JORGENSEN A, KRAG C, and MCLAUGHLIN JK (2005), The diagnosis of silicone breast implant rupture: clinical findings compared with findings at magnetic resonance imaging, *Ann Plast Surg*, 54, 583–589.
37. HOLMICH LR, KJOLLER K, VEJBORG I, CONRAD C, SLETTING S, MCLAUGHLIN JK, FRYZEK J, BREITING V, JORGENSEN A, and OLSEN JH (2003), Prevalence of Silicone breast implant rupture among Danish women, *Plast Reconstr Surg*, 111, 2182–2189.
38. HENRIKSEN TF, HOLMICH LR, FRIIS S, MCLAUGHLIN JK, FRYZEK JP, PERNILLE HOYER A, KJOLLER K, and OLSEN JH (2006), The Danish Registry for plastic surgery of the breast: establishment of a nationwide registry for prospective follow-up, quality assessmentand investigation of breast surgery, *Plast Reconstr Surg*, 118, 303–308.
39. COLLIS N, LITHERLAND J, ENION D, and SHARPE DT (2007), Magnetic resonance imaging and explantation investigation of long-term silicone gel implant integrity, *Plast Reconstr Surg*, 120, 1401–1406.
40. HEDÉN P, NAVA MB, VAN TETERING JP, MAGALON G, FOURIE LE R, BRENNER RJ, LINDSEY LE, MURPHY DK, and WALKER PS (2006), Prevalence of rupture in Inamed silicone breast implants, *Plast Reconstr Surg*, 118, 303–308.

41. LAVINE DM (1993), Saline inflatable prostheses: 14 years' experience, *Aesthetic Plast Surg*, 17, 325–330.
42. MLADICK RA (1993), 'No-touch' submuscular saline breast augmentation technique, *Aesthetic Plast Surg*, 17, 183–192.
43. RHEINGOLD LM, YOO RP, and COURTISS EH (1994), Experience with 326 inflatable breast implants, *Plast Reconstr Surg*, 93, 118–122.
44. WORSEG A, KUZBARI R, TAIRYCH G, KORAK K, and HOLLE J (1995), Long term results of inflatable mammary implants, *Br J Plast Surg*, 48, 183–188.
45. LANTIERI LA, ROUDOT-THORAVAL F, COLLINS ED, RAULO Y, and BARUCH JP (1997), Influence of underfilling on breast implant deflation, *Plast Reconstr Surg*, 100, 1740–1744.
46. RAPAPORT DP, STADELMANN WK, and GREENWALD DP (1997), Incidence and natural history of saline-filled breast implant deflations: Comparison of blunt-tipped versus cutting and tapered needles, *Plast Reconstr Surg*, 100, 1028–1032.
47. GUTOWSKI KA, MESNA GT, and CUNNINGHAM BL (1997), Saline-filled breast implants: a Plastic Surgery Educational Foundation multicenter outcomes study, *Plast Reconstr Surg*, 100, 1019–1027.
48. CUNNINGHAM BL, LOKEH A, and GUTOWSKI KA (2000), Saline-filled breast implant safety and efficacy: a multicenter retrospective review, *Plast Reconstr Surg*, 105, 2143–2149.
49. AL-SABOUNCHI S, DE MEY AM, and EDER H (2006), Textured saline-filled breast implants for augmentation mammaplasty: does overfilling prevent deflation? A long-term follow-up, *Plast Reconstr Surg*, 118, 215–222.
50. RAJ J, and WOJTANOWSKI MH (1999), Spontaneous deflation in saline solution-filled breast implants, *Aesthetic Surg J*, 19, 24–26.

Index

acellular dermal products (ADM), 47–8
Adatosil 5000, 7
Akademikliniken method, 84
alcohol use, 143
Allergan, 71–2, 73, 101, 102
alternative filling materials, 44–5
amorphous silica, 66
anaplastic large-cell lymphoma, 138–40
atypical connective tissue disease, 126–7

Baker scale classification, 100–1
beeswax, 4
Betadine pocket irrigation, 182–6
  force-to-break data plotted according to implantation time, 184
  Mentor implants tested after subsequent explantation, 183
  percentage elongation before break of 13 explant shells, 185
Biocell, 72, 105–6
biocompatibility, 57–8
biomaterials
  breast implants, 16–23
  history in breast augmentation, 1–35
  inflatable implants, 27–33
  injectable materials, 1–10
  other texturing forms, 23–7
  sponges, 10–16
  Trilucent (LipoMatrix) implants, 33–5
breast augmentation, 69
  biomaterials history, 1–35
    implants, 16–23
    inflatable implants, 27–33
    injectable materials, 1–10
    other texturing forms, 23–7
    sponges, 10–16
    Trilucent (LipoMatrix) implants, 33–5
breast cancer, 137, 140–1
breast implants, 16–23
  alternative types, 44–7
    enhanced cohesive gel implants, 46
    filling materials, 44–5
    safety, 46–7
    textured surface implants, 45–6
  development, 40–8
  evolution, 41–4
    saline filled implants, 41–2
    silicone filled implants, 42–4
  future trends, 47–8
  history, 40–1
  implantation time effects on saline implants shell properties, 179–86
  lot-matched control study, 175–9
  polyurethane coated implants, 20–3
  polyurethane foam, 96–118
    capsular contracture prevention, 98–105
    disadvantages, 114—-16
    overview, 96–8
    safety, 110–12
    secondary procedure use, 112–14
    smooth and textured surface implants, 105–10

reoperation rates and rupture, 210–14
causes of rupture for Inamed, 213
failure causes up to 10 years for Mentor, 213
main reoperation reason for Inamed, 211
main reoperation reason for Mentor, 211
prediction in gel core studies, 210
saline deflation failure prevalence by fill volume, 214
saline deflation prevalence, 213, 214
retrieval and analysis on strength, durability and failure mechanisms, 154–214
rupture, 186–210
failure mechanisms, 186
fatigue and shell wrinkling, 197–8, 200–6
implantation surgery, 206–10
microscopy analysis of failed implants, 187–97
safety epidemiology, 121–44
cancer incidence, 136–41
connective tissue disease, 122–7
implant rupture, 129–34
local complications, 134–6
neurological disease, 129
offspring effects, 127–9
suicide occurrence, 141–3
silicone gel explants with longest implantation time, 155–60
silicone gel implants, 16–20
shell properties as function of implantation time, 160–75
silicones, 62–6
gel implants, 63–4
issues, 64–6
saline implants, 62
structural elements, 62

capsular contracture, 98–105, 134, 135
Baker classification, 100
electron microscopy of unused polyurethane foam, 103
histology of a capsule of a polyurethane foam covered implant, 104
histology of capsule of a smooth surfaced breast implant, 99
capsulectomy, 113
capsulorrhaphy, 113
cervical cancer, 137
cigarette smoking, 143
Cleopatra's Needle, 5–6
cohesive gel breast implants, 68–95
incision and surgical technique, 86–93
dual plane IV submuscular technique in body builders, 91
submammary scar, 87
overview, 68–70
breast asymmetry, preoperative marking and postoperative period, 70
preoperative planning, 84–6
problems and complications, 93–5
stable breast implants available form, 70–7
stable breast implants form selection, 77–84
Colorado, 89
condensation cure, 60
congenital malformations, 128
connective tissue disease, 122–7, 133–4
atypical, 126–7
established, 123–6
cosmetic breast implants
cancer incidence, 136–41
anaplastic large-cell lymphoma, 138–40
breast cancer detection, 140–1
suicide incidence, 141–3
cross-link density, 167–70
Silastic I implant shells as a function of time in vivo, 171
crystalline silica, 66
CTD screening questionnaire (CSQ), 123
cyclic siloxanes, 58

Dacron, 17
DCTG300, 71

dermatomyositis, 124
Direct Process, 55
double capsules, 94
Dow Corning 360, 5, 6
dual plane IV dissection, 90

enhanced cohesive gel implants, 46
epoxy resin, 4
Etheron sponge, 14

fatigue, 197–8, 200–6
  actual implant shape for fill volumes of 200–280 cc, 201–3
  predicted implant shape for fill volumes of 200–280 cc, 204–6
FDA Modernisation Act (1997), 7
fibromyalgia, 122, 125
Force FX, 89

gel bleed, 65
gel migration, 130, 131
gelatin, 61
glass balls, 4
goat's milk, 4
ground rubber, 4

haematoma, 135
hydrogel, 45

ILP-line, 84–6
implant asymmetry, 135
implant displacement, 135
implant malposition, 93–4, 115
implant rupture, 129–34
  connective tissue disease, 133–4
  incidence, 130
  prevalence, 130–3
implant vintage, 17–20
  first generation silicone gel implant, 17
  second generation silicone gel implant, 18
  third generation silicone gel implant, 19
implantation surgery, 206–10
  averaged stress-strain curve for the controls, 207
  mechanical properties of explants, 209
  stress-strain curve, 208
implantation time
  saline implants shell properties, 179–86
    Betadine pocket irrigation, 182–6
    ultimate strength, 179–82
  silicone gel explants, 155–60
    Cronin seamed explants with 32 years in vivo and a control, 159
    illustration, 156
    properties of control and explanted shells, 157
    properties of extracted control and explanted shells, 158
    Silastic II explant with 13 years of implantation and a lot-matched control, 160
  silicone gel implants shell properties, 160–75
    moduli and cross-link density, 167–70
    shell swelling effects, 170, 172–5
    ultimate strength of Silastic 0 and I implants, 160–3
    ultimate strength of Silastic II implants, 163–7
infection, 135
inflatable implants, 27–33
  Simaplast, 28–33
injectable materials, 1–10
  liquid silicone injections, 4–8
  other materials, 2, 4
  paraffin, 2
  polyacrylamide hydrogel (PAH), 8–10
intracapsular rupture, 129–30
Intrashiel, 19
Ivalon sponge, 11–13
ivory balls, 4

lanolin, 4
leachables, 64
light retractors, 89
LipoMatrix *see* Trilucent implants

liquid silicone, 41
injections, 4–8
mammography demonstrates multiple cystic masses, 8
local anaesthesia, 89
longer chain polymers, 58
lot-matched control study, 175–9
mean ratio of properties of the explant shell, 176
mean ratio of properties of the extracted explant shell, 177
outside surface of Silastic II, 179
outside surface of Silastic II explant with 10 years in vivo, 178
physical properties of explants, 176
lower ventral curvature (LVC), 84
lubrication, 92
lung cancer, 137

magnetic resonance imaging (MRI), 130, 131, 132, 133–4
mammography, 140–1
Micro Structured Implant (MSI), 45
microscopy analysis
failed implants, 187–97
optical micrograph of no. 15 scalpel, 188
optical micrograph of outside surface of cutting needle, 189
pinhole artificially induced in an implant shell, 197
SEM micrograph of device #2, inside view near end of tear, 199
SEM micrograph of device view of cut edges, 194
SEM micrograph of entire pinhole, 191, 192
SEM micrograph of right side of cut at higher magnification, 193
SEM micrograph partial view of shell thickness with striations, 193
shell C surfaces and pinhole, 195, 196
smooth shell with suture needle cut initiated outside of shell, 190
textured McGhan saline explant with 3 years in vivo, 199
wear pattern around a crease and hole produced by advanced wear stage, 198
mineral oil, 4
modulus, 167–70
values for Silastic I and II implant shells as a function of time in vivo, 168, 169–70
motor neuropathies, 129
multiple-lumen implants, 20
multiple sclerosis-like syndrome, 129
muscular rheumatism, 126

Nartelle, 71
nipple–inframammary fold distance, 84–5
no-touch technique, 92
NS-line, 84–6, 90

oesophageal disorders, 128
offspring effects, 127–9
optical microscopy, 187
organic polymers, 56–7
ox cartilage, 4

paraffin, 2
clinical status of a woman who had received paraffin injections, 4
warming chamber for liquefaction, 3
peanut oil, 4
peripheral neuropathies, 129
platinum, 65–6
polyacrylamide hydrogel (PAH), 8–10
clinical status of a Russian woman with injection into multiple sites, 11
MRI T1 weighted image of the breast, 9
removal through a bilateral inflammatory incisions, 10
polymyositis, 124
Polytech Silimed, 98
polyurethane coated implants, 20–3
contracted capsule from a silicone gel implant, 22

fragments of shed from an implant capsule, 22
Replicon implant, 23
silicone gel-filled implant, 21
polyurethane foam
breast implants, 96–118
capsular contracture prevention, 98–105
disadvantages, 114–16
overview, 96–8
history, 97–8
safety, 110–12
electron micrograph after enzymatic degradation, 111
secondary procedure use, 112–14
vs. smooth and textured surface implants, 105–10
histology of a capsule from a Biocell, 106
rash 2 weeks after implantation, 110
surface of explanted implant, 109
surface of unused implant, 108
surfaces of unused breast implants, 107
polyvinylpryrrolidone (PVP), 44
preoperative markings, 87, 88
preoperative planning, 84–6

radical cure, 59–60
radical crosslinking, 60
rash, 110, 116
Raynaud's syndrome, 133
rheumatoid arthritis, 122, 124, 125
Rochow–Müller Process *see* Direct Process
rubber, 4

sacs, 4
saline filled implants, 41–2
saline implants
implantation time effect on shell properties, 179–86
Betadine pocket irrigation, 182–6
ultimate strength, 179–82
scanning electron microscopy (SEM), 187
shell swelling, 170, 172–5
elongation-to-failure ratio, 173
percentage extracted as a function of time in vivo for Silastic I/0 and II implants, 174, 175
tensile strength ratio, 173
unextracted shell/extracted shell tensile stress ratio *vs.* percent extracted, 172
shell wrinkling, 197–8, 197–206, 200–6
actual implant shape for fill volumes of 200–280 cc, 201–3
predicted implant shape for fill volumes of 200–280 cc, 204–6
shellac, 4
Silastic 0 and Silastic I
ultimate strength, 160–3
elongation of shells as a function of time in vivo, 162
function of time in vivo, 161
status of explants at time of analysis, 161
tear strength of shells as a function of time in vivo, 163
Silastic II, 19–20, 159–60
ultimate strength, 163
average elongation-to-failure, 165
average tear resistance, 166
average tensile strength, 164
silica, 62
silicone elastomers, 59–61
silicone filled implants, 42–4
chemistry, 42–3
gel-filled, 43–4
silicone gel explants
longest implantation time, 155–60
Cronin seamed explants with 32 years in vivo and a control, 159
properties of control and explanted shells, 157
properties of extracted control and explanted shells, 158
Silastic II explant with 13 years of implantation and a lot-matched control, 160

silicone gel implants, 16–20, 41, 43–4, 63–4
  shell properties as function of implantation time, 160–75
    moduli and cross-link density, 167–70
    shell swelling effects, 170, 172–5
    ultimate strength of Silastic 0 and I implants, 160–3
    ultimate strength of Silastic II implants, 163–7
  structures, 63
silicone gels, 61
silicone oil, 6–7, 58–9
silicones, 52–66
  breast implants, 62–6
  main forms of siloxanes, 58–62
  overview, 52–6
    chemical composition, 53–4
    constituents, 54–5
    conversion of chlorosilanes, 56
    manufacturing, 56–7
    production, 54–6
    society, 52–3
    typical structure, 54
  properties, 56–8
    biocompatibility, 57–8
    difference between organic polymers, 56–7
    environment, 58
silicones D_4, 58
silicones D_5, 58
silk fabric, 4
siloxanes
  main forms, 58–62
    silicone elastomers, 59–61
    silicone formulation, 62
    silicone gels, 61
    silicone oils, 58–9
Siltex, 46, 72
Simaplast implants, 28–33
  Contemporary Mentor inflatable implant, 31
  Jenny inflatable saline-filled implant, 31
  second model with clear shell seamless filling tube, 29
  Varifil saline-filled implant, 32
Sjögren's syndrome, 122, 124
smooth silicone gel implants, 102, 105–10
Snoopy deformity, 113
soybean oil, 4
sponges, 4, 10–16
  case containing Pangman Ivalon double layered implant, 12
  double-layered Ivalon implant, 13
  polyethylene implants, 15
  SEM of capsule from the Ivalon implants, 14
stable breast implants
  available form, 70–7
    advantages, 73
    applications, 73, 75–7
    before and after breast augmentation, 71, 74, 76
    European patients confidence rate for implants, 73
    muscle tightening, relaxed side and site change after implant, 76
    patient with constricted lower pole tubular breast, 75
    side view before breast augmentation, 77
    textured implant surface, 72
  form selection, 77–84
    breast before augmentation, 82
    3D imaging with Canfield Vectra II camera and Precision Light software, 80
    existing breast width measured with a calliper, 81
    implant projection analysis using a calliper, 83
    implant sizers, 79
    postoperative nipple position prediction, 83
    synmastia complication, 81
State Food and Drug Administration (SFDA), 10
suicide, 141–3

Surgitek, 20
systemic lupus erythematosus (SLE), 122, 124
systemic sclerosis, 124

textured silicone gel implants, 102, 105–10
textured surface implants, 45–6
texturing, 23–7
  effect on capsular contracture, 24–5
  moratorium, 26–7
    fifth generation, contemporary, stable, Mentor cohesive gel implant, 27
  status of textured implants, 25–6
tilt test, 69
tissue–implant interface, 112, 113
2,4 toluenediamine, 107–8, 111–12
triglyceride, 45
Trilucent implants, 33–5
  radiolucent soybean oil-filled implants, 35
  silicone gel and saline-filled breast implants, 34
True Form, 71

ultimate strength
  properties, 179–82
    anterior surface of intact Simaplast saline implant, 180
    elongation of extracted saline explant shells, 181
    five saline explant shells, 181
    implantation time and status of five tested saline explants, 180
    intact Heyer-Schulte saline explant with 22 years of implantation, 181
  Silastic 0 and I implants, 160–3
    elongation of shells as a function of time in vivo, 162
    function of time in vivo, 161
    status of explants at time of analysis, 161
    tear strength of shells as a function of time in vivo, 163
  Silastic II implants, 163–7
    average elongation-to-failure, 165
    average tear resistance, 166
    average tensile strength, 164
unspecified rheumatism, 126

vegetable oils, 4
Velcro effect, 108
vulvar cancer, 137

World War II, 5

xenon head light, 89

CPSIA information can be obtained at www.ICGtesting.com
Printed in the USA
LVOW04*2020140914
404040LV00001B/14/P
9 781845 697990